THE HEALTHY SKIN DIET

Your complete guide to beautiful skin in just 8 weeks

ACHIEVE GORGEOUS, BLEMISH-FREE SKIN WHATEVER YOUR SKIN TYPE AND WHATEVER YOUR SKIN CONDITION

KAREN FISCHER

THE HEALTHY SKIN DIET

Your complete guide to beautiful skin in only 8 weeks

Karen Fischer

BHSc, Dip. Nut.

RODALE

Although every effort has been made to ensure that the contents of this book are accurate, and every precaution has been taken with the recommendations and advice given, neither the author nor the publisher can be held responsible for any loss or claim arising out of the use or misuse of the suggestions made. It is recommended that you consult with your own medical practitioner before embarking on any new health programme, particularly if you are elderly, pregnant, on medication or if you suffer from allergies or any other medical condition.

This edition published 2009 by Rodale
an imprint of Pan Macmillan Ltd
Pan Macmillan, 20 New Wharf Road, London N1 9RR
Basingstoke and Oxford
Associated companies throughout the world
www.panmacmillan.com

First published 2008 by Exisle Publishing limited
www.exislepublishing.com

ISBN 978-1-9057-4450-3

3 5 7 9 8 6 4 2

A CIP catalogue record for this book is available from the British Library.

Design by saso content & design pty ltd

Printed and bound by CPI Group (UK) Ltd, Croydon, CR0 4YY

This book is intended as a reference volume only, not as a medical manual. The information given here is designed to help you make informed decisions about your health. It is not intended as a substitute for any treatment that you may have been prescribed by your doctor. If you suspect you have a medical problem, we urge you to seek competent medical help.
Mention of specific companies, organizations or authorities in this book does not imply endorsement of the publisher, nor does mention of specific companies, organizations or authorities in the book imply that they endorse the book.
Addresses, websites and telephone numbers given in this book were correct at the time of going to press.

Visit www.panmacmillan.com to read more about all our books and to buy them. You will also find features, author interviews and news of any author events, and you can sign up for e-newsletters so that you're always first to hear about our new releases.

RODALE

We inspire and enable people to improve their lives and the world around them

To Mum and Dad, thanks for everything

' I trust Karen and her holistic, natural approach to beauty – this is an easy-to-follow program that will help you to have the beautiful skin you always wanted.'

Sophie Falkiner, television personality

'*The Healthy Skin Diet* is a fantastic book for those seeking healthy skin the natural way – Karen has so much experience treating sufferers of skin conditions, and her programmes, while really easy to follow, are so effective. *The Healthy Skin Diet* even caters for those with special dietary needs, like coeliac disease, which I suffer from. This book provides a natural, effective guide to getting beautiful skin from the inside, out.'

Holly Brisley, actor and television presenter

Contents

Part 1
Getting started

Introduction

You were *not* born to endlessly suffer from a terrible skin condition such as acne or psoriasis. You weren't meant to get wrinkles or cellulite prematurely either. You were born for a much better reason than to battle with your skin and feel terrible every time you glance in the mirror. Okay, so this might be an exaggeration in your case but I want you to not just hope, but *know* that you can improve your skin quality so you can enjoy having beautiful skin like the genetically blessed.

I know this is true because **the skin you have today will be totally renewed within two months**. Yep. Those wrinkles and that crop of whiteheads will be gone and new skin will be in its place in a matter of weeks, and it can either look exactly the same, worse or better, depending on the instructions and building materials you supply for it. In fact, the body you have today, all your cells and tissues, will be totally new within a year.

This is because your body turns over six *billion* cells each day and new ones are made to replace them. The pimple you have right now is not the one you had a month ago and it's certainly not the same blemish you had last year. You just haven't changed the underlying cause of your skin problems so they occur over and over again.

Whatever your skin condition may be, whether it is quite okay or out of control, you *can* improve your skin quality and have fantastic looking skin within eight weeks.

Want to know how?

The Healthy Skin Diet is designed to supply your body with the specific building materials to *make* gorgeous skin. Beautiful skin is created by a body that's functioning properly – by a body that is eliminating wastes efficiently, digesting food and transporting nutrients at lightning speeds around the body. It's not something exclusively reserved for the genetically blessed. You can have it too. The Healthy Skin Diet has eight basic guidelines that will take the guess work out of creating clear skin.

You don't even have to have bad skin to follow the Healthy Skin Diet, as this programme is fantastic for overall health and wellbeing. You can be in your nineties or starting school, and there is even information for parents with babies suffering from eczema.

I want to tell you a bit about my own health challenges. Please excuse me for talking about myself but I thought you might like to have a giggle about my 'ugly skin' days and believe me there were many of them. I also want to show you that you don't have to be blessed with the 'perfect' skin gene and you definitely don't have to settle for ho-hum skin.

I know what it's like to be so uncomfortable in your skin that you wish you were invisible. When I was at high school I had stick skinny legs, thin blonde hair and buck teeth (which braces eventually fixed), so I rarely smiled, and my teenage years saw the beginning of my skin worries with a regular crop of pimples decorating my oily forehead. I was not only shy, awkward and blemished, I was also unwell much of the time. I always seemed to have a runny nose or a headache and had dark circles under my eyes. Maybe I had 'poor genes' or maybe my health and skin problems occurred because of an epiphany I'd had in Year 2: 'I'm sick of eating sandwiches; I've been eating them all my life!'

I hated healthy food and I was a fussy eater so from that moment on I refused to eat homemade lunches and my parents didn't know what to do. On occasion a stranger in the street would rudely accuse my mother of not feeding me because I was so skinny and sickly. So in desperation, my mother gave me lunch money in the hope that I would buy healthy food of my own accord and put on some weight. But for the rest of my school years what did I buy? Meat pies, sausage rolls, hot chips, strawberry milk and cream buns (the ones with extra sugar and jam). I was not quite on the same page as my mum.

A vegetable never entered my radar when I was in the school playground. At home I did have some veggies with dinner thanks to Mum's persistence but I would only eat white bread, as the texture of the brown stuff just didn't feel right in my mouth and dairy was my addiction. I drank a litre of milk and ate two bowls of ice-cream nearly every day. We lived in Darwin, it was the 1970s and the health-food craze was decades away.

Inevitably my delectable childhood caught up with me as I became increasingly unwell. When I was a teenager, washing the dishes would make my hands peel until they were red, raw, painful and totally useless, and my face had never-ending red patches. I wasn't much of a help around the house either. Once I used a chemical-based furniture polish to clean the dining room table and I temporarily lost my vision – it was like I was looking through thick grey smoke – and then I vomited. Of course I suspected I was allergic to manual labour so I avoided it as much as possible.

In my twenties I joked 'I've been tired for ten years' but it was no laughing matter. I went to see various doctors about my constant lethargy and I rattled off a big list of symptoms. Then I would undergo various medical tests which would come back normal, so again I would be told there was nothing wrong with me. 'But I'm endlessly tired and so damned irritable,' I thought, 'and haven't you noticed my spotty forehead?'

I cut a fringe to cover my forehead so I had one less thing to worry about.

One doctor mentioned that I should eat healthy food but he didn't inspire me to investigate further. He had a good point though: my diet could have been a lot better. This doctor also said I would have more energy if I exercised. So putting on my baggy tracksuit (which practically covered me from head to toe), I went to the gym. But as usual, after one workout I got flu-like symptoms and felt too sick to exercise for the next week. Maybe it was all those toxins being mobilised in my body from years of eating fast food or maybe it was my lazy side winning the inner battle. Whatever the case, I would predictably lose motivation and go back to my sedentary lifestyle – listening to music in my bedroom as I scoffed strawberry milks.

However, my aversion to exercise sometimes worked in my favour. When I was 25 I had an audition for a TV presenting job and after I read the scripted dialogue, I had to talk for a minute about something I hated. Without a moment's hesitation I chose exercise as my topic. 'Exercise is for wacky people! You think about it ... To run on the spot on a noisy treadmill for an hour. Uh! Sounds absurd to me. I say pass me a tub of ice-cream and the remote control!'

To my surprise I got the job. This ended up being my first (and last) full-time job in television. The show was an afternoon cartoon programme, Channel Nine's *What's Up Doc?* (formerly *The Bugs Bunny Show*). We filmed every Monday and I was energetic all day. By Tuesday I was fatigued and the rest of the week I was miserable. I was still getting sick and it affected my work. It was no wonder, though: I would eat any junk food that was on set and the scriptwriter even dedicated a segment to my obsession with chocolate mousse. I think I ate seven tubs of the stuff that day.

During this time I got a debilitating flu and a couple of shooting days had to be rescheduled as I could barely speak. I went to see two doctors and both of them told me that antibiotics wouldn't work as I had a virus and they said I had to rest and drink plenty of water. I did and didn't get any better.

Eventually, after six weeks of complaining and moping around I decided to go into the local herbal dispensary to see a naturopath. The shop had always looked a bit too 'herbal' for me and I had never felt comfortable enough to go inside; but I was really sick of being sick and tired so I finally took the plunge. The naturopath looked into my eyes with an iridology torch and exclaimed 'You must be so tired!' We discussed my symptoms, my diet and lifestyle and then she told me about eating healthy food. She said, 'You are what you eat.' *Oh dear, I'm a walking chocolate mousse.* She made me a foul-tasting herbal mixture for my chronic flu and after two days of taking the herbs (and eating slightly more fruits and vegetables) I felt better. I was no longer a zombie extra in a low-budget movie.

After my battle with the never-ending flu, which would have been conquered quickly by a half-decent immune system, I decided to learn how to be healthy. I wanted to know what foods could make a difference to my energy levels and I wanted to find out how to look good without make-up on. I changed my diet very, very slowly (yes, I'm stubborn). I weaned myself off my dairy addiction, culled the chocolate mousse and made friends with wholegrains.

I also took up exercise (once again) but I started slowly and indulged in my body's natural aversion to movement for as long as I could. In my new-found yoga class I realised I had the flexibility of a brick and the 60-year-olds in the front row had better balance than me. At least the classes were 'beginner-friendly' so I could go at my own pace. Eventually I got better at exercising and choosing healthy food. It wasn't long before I began to feel better.

I was 27 and pregnant and I had more vitality than when I was a teenager. My complexion also cleared up and I no longer needed to kick-start my brain with a cup of coffee or four. That's when I realised I had been ripped off for all those years – some people get to enjoy health like this *all the time!*

During this period I completed my Health Science degree and a three-year Nutrition diploma. This introduced me to nutritional biochemistry, which is the study of how nutrients work in the body. This background knowledge has helped me to understand how different diets work and, more importantly, how some diets can be effective (with weight loss in particular) but also be unbelievably harmful to your health *and* skin.

However, I didn't become a nutritionist who specialised in skin health because of my own skin dramas. I did it because of my daughter. Two weeks after she was born she developed a severe case of eczema. Her face and the creases in her elbows and knees were red and painfully itchy. It also concerned us that eczema sufferers can develop asthma if the *underlying* cause of the inflammation is not treated.

My daughter's eczema persisted until she was seven months old when I put her on a 'friendly food' diet. However, this was a difficult diet that only offered temporary relief as her eczema would come back if the food programme wasn't followed strictly. I thought *there must be a better way ...*

After much research, I finally found an effective long-term solution to my daughter's inflamed skin. For years now she has been eczema-free and she's able to sleep with her fluffy toys without any irritation from dust mites (she had been diagnosed with dust mite allergy). She can now swim in any type of pool as the chlorine does not sting her skin and she can eat tomatoes, grapes and mangoes, and ALL of the other salicylate-rich foods she adores. She can also eat dairy products and go to kids' parties and scoff a few coloured lollies for the first time in her life without getting a flare-up!

My daughter and the other eczema sufferers I've treated over the years still have a genetic predisposition to eczema but they now have a simple health routine that they continue to follow which allows them to have a normal and rash-free life.

As fate would have it, my knowledge on skin health would be tested once again when my house was invaded by fleas (thanks to the gorgeous dog from next door).

After attempting to get rid of the mites without using harsh chemicals, I eventually flea-bombed the house with a pesticide bought from the supermarket. But after the chemical exposure, I got a small patch of psoriasis on my neck. Within a month the flaky patch had spread down my neck and all over my torso. My skin was scaly, dry and red. It looked so bad, I felt embarrassed when I went for a swim at the local pool. I began to avoid socialising as it continued to spread. I finally devised the Anti-psoriasis Programme. A month later my psoriasis had completely disappeared.

I feel very privileged to be able to pass on my knowledge on skin health to you, especially in a format that allows me to give you *all* the information you need to create gorgeous skin. And just so you know my skin health programme is really effective, I have also included scientific referencing at the end of the book so you can see for yourself that the Healthy Skin Diet has scientific merit.

Poor genes, enjoying too much of the good life or having an unhealthy, but delicious, childhood can leave you with bad skin. However, we all want to enjoy ourselves and not have to become Nancy-No-Fun in order to look good. I believe having fun and being kind to yourself is a really important part of healthy living and there are plenty of scientific studies to back me up! Therefore, the Healthy Skin Diet is designed so you can have *low* alcohol and coffee consumption. This enables you to hang out with your mates or have a couple of glasses of red with your partner over dinner if you wish.

As a health practitioner, it's my job to make being healthy accessible to you and I do this by not only giving you health information but also by setting activities for you, similar to the ones I've previously given my clients. The activities are your cue to take action and work towards gorgeous skin. I know you can do it!

This takes a bit of effort on your part because as you may already know, theory alone cannot make your skin beautiful. It's the process of *doing* that will get you the results you want. Your skin's health is in your hands. And no matter what kind of genes you were lumped with, I hope you now realise that when you follow the Healthy Skin Diet you can have gorgeous skin not unlike the genetically blessed. Of course you can simply read the book and get some fab skin-care tips. But I'm guessing you want more – gorgeous skin and vitality, and long-lasting results – or else you wouldn't be reading this book right now.

And I don't want to just sell you this book so it can gather dust on your bookshelf, either. I want you to follow the activities and complete the Healthy Skin Diet so you can then enjoy all the benefits of having beautiful skin. Just think: with clear, healthy skin you'd be able to focus on the rest of your life with confidence rather than worrying about skin-deep first impressions. I won't tell you not to stress about what other people may think of your skin. I will be honest and say yes, people can be unkind and leave you wishing you were invisible and yes, it's really wonderful when acquaintances remember your name or at least compliment you on your gorgeous complexion. And you can enjoy this too.

Be sure to let me know how you go!

Health and happiness,
Karen

FAQs

Q: 'My skin looks okay and my diet is already good. Can I find non-diet information in this book that I can use to look after my skin?'

A: *Yes, there are plenty of skin-care and lifestyle tips that you can follow to improve your skin's appearance even further.*

Q: 'I have a child with eczema. Is the programme suitable for her?'

A: *Yes! Since there are far too many children suffering with eczema, I've included food and supplement information specifically for bubs and children at the end of Chapter 15, 'Eczema/dermatitis' (see also 'Children's Clear Skin Programme'). The Healthy Skin Diet may be suitable for older children who eat the same food as their parents but for babies who are just starting on solids, there is a list of specific foods for them. I've had wonderful success at eliminating childhood eczema.*

Q: 'Can I follow the Healthy Skin Diet if I'm pregnant?'

A: *Yes you can, however you'll need to check with your health practitioner before taking any supplements. You should avoid vitamin A and liver detoxification supplements, as well as raw fish. You should also take a calcium supplement as this is a dairy-restricted diet.*

Q: 'I don't like taking supplements – do I need to take any while on the Healthy Skin Diet?'

A: *No, if you're just following the basic structured menu on the Healthy Skin Diet then you don't need to take any supplements.*

Q: 'I have rosacea, so is the Healthy Skin Diet suitable for me?'

A: *Yes! Part 3 has special programmes for severe skin ailments and Chapter 18 is dedicated to rosacea (redness of the skin and facial flushing). Acne, cellulite, eczema/dermatitis and psoriasis also have unique programmes: all you have to do is look up your skin condition in the index. This additional advice helps you to tailor the Healthy Skin Diet to your own specific needs.*

Q: 'Can I drink tea and coffee while on the Healthy Skin Diet?'

A: *During the **first three days** it's recommended that you avoid caffeine but after this time you can enjoy coffee and tea in moderation. If you have a **severe** skin rash it's recommended you avoid tea and coffee and substitute them with decaffeinated coffee or dandelion tea until your skin condition clears up.*

Q: **'Will the Healthy Skin Diet help me lose weight?'**

A: *Yes. Even though the Healthy Skin Diet is not specifically for weight loss, it will help balance your metabolism, improve fat digestion and increase elimination of wastes so you'll lose excess weight if you need to.*

Q: **'Can I still eat at restaurants while on the Healthy Skin Diet?'**

A: *Yes you can. Restaurant options are listed within the eight-week menu in Chapter 21. Once you have learnt the basic principles of the diet, you'll find it's relatively easy to spot a healthy meal when eating out. Of course, the specially designed recipes in the Healthy Skin Diet are likely to be superior for your skin so it's better to keep restaurant trips to a minimum.*

The Healthy Skin Diet is a unique eating and lifestyle plan because it's designed to integrate into your social, working and home routine so it can become a healthy *way of life* rather than a short-term diet that is hard to maintain for a long period of time.

Please note that I cannot mention brand names of beauty products in this book as product formulas can change; however, you can refer to www.healthbeforebeauty.com for an up-to-date review of suitable skin-care products.

Chapter 1

Who can benefit from the Healthy Skin Diet?

Everyone, including you, can gain all sorts of health benefits from being on the Healthy Skin Diet because it is a commonsense diet and lifestyle programme, designed to fit into your life. This means it's flexible so you have *no* excuses not to complete the eight-week programme.

Specific conditions which can be helped by the Healthy Skin Diet

- eczema/dermatitis/ contact dermatitis
- psoriasis
- rosacea
- dandruff
- acne
- cellulite
- hives
- premature ageing and wrinkles
- mood swings and irritability
- premenstrual syndrome (PMS)
- poor immunity to colds and flu
- hypoglycaemia (food related)
- poor digestion
- candida albicans (fungal infections)
- parasites in the bowel
- fatigue and sluggishness
- headaches
- body odour, bad breath
- abdominal bloating
- flatulence/wind
- food intolerances
- dull, sallow complexion
- inability to lose weight
- bags under the eyes
- dark circles under the eyes
- pigmentation

The Healthy Skin Diet is an **anti-inflammatory eating programme** that was originally designed for people with skin conditions such as **eczema**. The diet was also found to be effective in eliminating **acne, psoriasis** and **dandruff** and improving **mood swings**, **energy levels** and **rosacea**. And as the Healthy Skin Diet promotes production of anti-inflammatory prostaglandins, it's also ideal for people with **sinusitis, hay fever, asthma, arthritis** and **allergies**. However, please note that the

Healthy Skin Diet is NOT designed to prevent anaphylaxis allergic reactions so please continue to avoid your trigger foods.

The Healthy Skin Diet is suitable for people with **heart disease** and **high blood pressure** because the diet is low in red meat (two servings or less per week), it contains low GI (or low GL) meals and it's packed full of heart-protective antioxidants. Of course you should continue to take your prescribed medications and consult your doctor before taking supplements of any kind as they may interfere with your drug treatment.

The Healthy Skin Diet has many **low glycaemic load (GL)** recipes so it's fantastic for people with **blood-sugar problems** such as **type II diabetes** and **hypoglycaemia**.

If you have **poor digestion** with **bloating,** embarrassing **wind** and **constipation** then the Healthy Skin Diet has got you covered. There are recipes with natural digestives and the right types of fibre to enhance elimination of wastes. When you know the best foods to eat you won't get offensive **wind, BO** or **bad breath**! (Wouldn't that be nice?) **Parasites** and **candida albicans** can also cause really nasty bowel symptoms and skin problems; the Healthy Skin Diet is designed to significantly decrease harmful microbes within your bowels. Healthy bowels equals beautiful skin.

The Healthy Skin Diet is also designed to improve your **liver health** as it contains many foods that stimulate phase 1 and phase 2 liver detoxification (especially phase 2). I won't get all technical on you but phase 1 is where chemicals and hormones are made water soluble. This first phase can make a substance *more* toxic so you need phase 2 to finish the job and promote safe removal of these substances. Phase 2 also increases glutathione production which guards against **premature ageing**. You can feel lethargic and unwell if your phase 1 is high and your phase 2 is compromised, so the Healthy Skin Diet works to balance these reactions.

The Eight Guidelines for Healthy Skin detailed in Part 2 utilise the latest **anti-ageing** information so you can improve the texture and softness of your skin within the eight-week programme.

Fill out the following health quiz to check how the Healthy Skin Diet can help you. Answer each question by circling the number under 'often', 'rarely' or 'never' depending on what is most appropriate for you.

Health quiz

	Often	Rarely	Never
Do you suffer from dry skin and skin rashes?	5	3	0
Are you stressed, a worrywart or just too busy to look after yourself?	5	3	0
Do you suffer from acne or pimples?	5	3	0
Do you have asthma, arthritis or arthritic-like pain?	5	3	0
Do you have trouble losing weight?	5	3	0
Do you suffer from allergies and intolerances?	5	3	0
Do you have a dull complexion or signs of premature ageing?	5	3	0
Do you suffer from premenstrual syndrome (PMS)?	5	3	0
Do you get dandruff, bad breath or smelly body odour?	4	3	0
Do you have dark circles under your eyes?	4	2	0
Do you have cellulite?	4	2	0
Do you suffer from irritability, mood swings or depression?	4	2	0
Do you often wake feeling lethargic?	4	2	0
Do you suffer from constipation, wind, bloating or indigestion?	4	2	0
Have you taken antibiotics in the last six months?	3	1	0
Do you crave sugar or bread?	3	1	0
Do you need a coffee pick-me-up or something sweet in the afternoon?	3	1	0

Total score:

If your score was over 40 then you would get the most dramatic results from following the Healthy Skin Diet. You should also take a couple of the recommended supplements to speed up the process. If your score was between 20 and 39, you would greatly benefit from following the Healthy Skin Diet but supplements would be optional. If your score was below 20 and you don't have any specific undesirable skin conditions then you are probably quite healthy (or one of the lucky ones with fabulous genes). So you can use the Healthy Skin Diet as a food and lifestyle guide to help guard against premature ageing and preserve those wonderful genes. Enjoy!

Chapter 2

Your skin

What spirit is so empty and blind, that it cannot recognise the fact that the foot is more noble than the shoe, and skin more beautiful than the garment with which it is clothed?

– Michelangelo

Quite frankly, your skin is absolutely essential for your existence. Without it you'd die. It protects you from invading bacteria, it helps to regulate your body temperature and it keeps your insides from falling out. But you probably don't give a second thought to the role of your skin (why would you?). You're more likely to spend your day thinking about work, bills, fornication or worrying if you have food stuck between your teeth.

Your skin only grabs your attention once it lets you down. Your skin may start to wrinkle; it could become patchy with pigmentation; it might develop rashes and pimples or dimple all the way down your thighs. You wonder what you did to deserve a bum like yours and you think 'Are wrinkles and dimples a normal part of ageing?' You sit at the beach, practically covered from head to toe with zinc cream and tie-dyed sarongs, for fear of cellulite mockery and a nasty case of skin cancer. STOP! Don't be ridiculous. Your skin is simply telling you that something is amiss on the *inside* and it's hoping that you pay attention to its early warning signals.

Let's start at the beginning by getting the basic skin facts before we look at what your skin might be trying to tell you.

Quick skin facts:

- The skin is the largest organ of the body.

- Your skin is made up of three layers. The outside layer is the epidermis, the middle layer is the dermis and the inner layer is the subcutaneous layer.

- New skin cells form at the bottom of the epidermis and when they're ready they move towards the outer layer. This trip takes about four weeks. This is good news as it means that with the right building materials you can create better skin cells in four to eight weeks.[1]

Did you realise that in the minute or so you took to read this chapter, you've shed about 40,000 dead skin cells off the surface of your skin?[2] (It's enough to make you want to change the bed sheets pronto!)

Social skin

You may express yourself through words and actions but your body can also 'talk'. Yes, you've probably heard of body language, which involves your eyes and facial characteristics, but your body also 'speaks' through feelings of pain and energy output. Poor energy levels can mean just about anything, from nutritional deficiencies and poor posture to early warning of some disease states. So fatigue should *never* be masked by downing seven cups of coffee a day. Pain warns you when something is too hot for the skin; a headache could signal you're dehydrated; and back pain can indicate anything from poor posture to something as serious as cancer so it's essential that you learn to listen to the secret language of the body.

But what is your skin trying to tell you?

When trying to 'read' your skin it's like playing the game 'hotter and colder'. When you get further away from good health, your body will say 'colder' by making your skin look bad (your energy levels may also suffer, your breath could smell bad and so on). But as you get closer to good health, your skin will begin to look better and you will start to feel more alive. Your skin is saying 'You're getting warmer, keep going!' And when your skin looks awesome and you have no medical conditions, unexplainable fatigue or mysterious pains, then you're obviously on the right track. You're hot! So stick with it!

Let's get the facts

Your health is absolutely dependent on many different food and lifestyle factors. So when health experts only look at one bit of research or one body organ as *the* solution for optimal health it just seems a little crazy to me. It's the same with your skin – there isn't one solitary factor that can make you look gorgeous. This is why scientific studies can end up with inconclusive or negative results because they test a single theory or nutrient, such as vitamin E to cure eczema, and then they find that it doesn't work. Skin problems are rarely caused by a single nutrient deficiency. You can induce a solitary deficiency, such as vitamin B1, during a scientific experiment but in real life someone with poor nutrition or inadequate digestion will have a *whole range* of nutritional deficiencies and a single supplement won't fix their skin. A more holistic approach to health is necessary.

Poor skin health is more likely to arise from a *variety* of minor imbalances and the underlying cause of them needs to be addressed, not just masked with supplements or medical drugs.

Your skin is affected by the following factors:

- genetics
- diet (nutrition, hydration and pH or acid–alkaline balance)
- UV radiation from sunlight and the free radicals it causes
- liver health
- bowel and digestive health
- blood and lymph circulation
- stress
- sleep
- chemicals, cigarette smoke and drugs
- the weather (but we can't change that!).

Your skin's warning signals are trying to tell you that one, or several, of these factors are out of balance. How do you know which ones? The chapters in Part 2, 'Eight Guidelines for Healthy Skin', have questionnaires and all the information you need to work out what they may be. However let's consider your genetics first, as they are often blamed for those bad skin days ...

Genetics

According to the current research, it's estimated that the human body has between 24,000 and 25,000 genes. Your genes are what you inherited from your birth parents and they determine things like the colour of your skin, if you have freckles or not and how easily your skin tans when exposed to UV light.[3,4] Each gene in your body is a segment of DNA that can signal instructions to your cells.

Scientists, medical experts and nutritionists alike talk about how our genes play a role in our susceptibility to skin conditions and diseases. People talk about being blessed with 'good' genes – they rarely get sick and can drink truckloads of chocolate milk without getting a single spot. In the past I've cursed my 'bad' genes whenever my skin has broken out in a red, peeling rash. Our genes have a lot to answer for and there's no doubt that they can affect our skin; but are our genetics entirely to blame?

It's becoming clearer to researchers around the world that our genetically determined biology may not have had enough time to catch up with the radical dietary changes that have occurred in the Western world over the past ten decades. What does this mean for your health? Let's consider the diets of your ancestors. It's more than likely that your ancestors spent much of the day looking for food and making sure they had adequate shelter. Food processing and soft drinks were unheard of and artificial flavours and colours didn't exist. The traditional hunter–gatherers had diets that varied from region to region but taking these differences into account, scientists have worked out the basic universal characteristics of primitive diets.[5] It's estimated that our ancestors snacked on nuts, seeds, fruits, vegetables and wholegrains, and that they hunted for fish and chased after wild game then finished off the evening with a chocolate biccie and a cuppa (you know I'm joking).

Of course, your ancestral diet may have varied from this one, especially if you're of Inuit descent. You see, the primitive Inuits ate loads of seafood, so they consumed higher ratios of fat and omega-3 essential fatty acids. Grains weren't a staple part of their diet.

Whatever your ancestry may be, today you no longer have to search for nuts or sprint after a wild pig. You simply drive to the shops and select from rows and rows of fresh and packaged foods.

There's no argument that the modern Western diet varies greatly but it often consists of the following foods and drinks:

- farmed meats and processed meats such as ham, salami and sausages;
- dairy products, such as full-fat and low-fat milk, cheese and butter;
- white bread, pastries, cakes, biscuits, cereals, refined sugar and syrups;
- refined cooking oils and margarine;
- coffee, tea and alcohol;
- we also eat fruits, vegetables, fish, nuts, wholegrains and beans and pulses.[6]

As a general rule, the more processed foods you eat the less fresh and healthy food you end up consuming.

You've got to admit that packaged foods and pre-made meals are a godsend at the end of a busy day when you're too exhausted to prepare fresh food. Modern convenience has its place in our society, however this expediency may come at a heavy price and your skin could be the first thing to suffer.

In the *American Journal of Clinical Nutrition*, Loren Cordain and her colleagues say that our dietary changes began with the introduction of agriculture and animal farming about 10,000 years ago but that this may have occurred *too recently* for our human genetics to adapt.[7] Our biological make-up hasn't had time to become accustomed to the barrage of chemical preservatives and artificial sweeteners, not to mention heavily processed foods that are way too low in vitamins and minerals. Maybe many of us aren't victims of our genetic make-up after all – we're just confusing our poor little genes by eating foods that are unrecognisable to our bodies!

Many scientists now suspect that slow genetic adaptation to modern diets could be the reason diseases such as cancer, heart disease and acne are found in modern societies. Population studies show that acne is rare or non-existent in traditional cultures that eat unprocessed foods.[8,9,10]

According to Cordain and her colleagues, seven crucial nutritional changes occurred when food processing procedures were introduced:

1. The glycaemic load (GL) increased. Processed foods usually have a higher glycaemic index (GI) which elevates your blood glucose levels. This can damage blood vessels and lead to type II diabetes.

2. Fatty acid composition. Farmed animals don't get enough exercise so they are practically devoid of omega-3 and they've become higher in saturated fat.

3. The ratios of protein, carbohydrates and fat changed. More saturated fat and refined carbohydrates are being consumed.

4. We now have fewer micronutrients in our diet. Processed foods such as white bread and flour have had most of the vitamins and minerals removed.

5. Acid–alkaline balance has been altered. Western diets can cause low-grade metabolic acidosis that worsens with age. Having too much acid in the body can be detrimental to your health.

6. Sodium–potassium ratio has been altered. Higher intake of manufactured salt and lower fruit and vegetable consumption means there is less potassium in the modern Western diet. Researchers estimate there has been a 400 per cent increase in salt ingestion but we haven't increased our vegetable and fruit consumption at all; in fact, it has plummeted.

7. Fibre content has decreased. Refined sugars, vegetable oils, alcohol and dairy products are devoid of fibre, and refined grains contain much less fibre than wholegrains. The more nutrient-poor a flour product is, the whiter it looks.[11]

Today only a small number of primitive cultures continue to eat a natural diet that doesn't contain fast food, processed white flour and sugar. These cultures are fascinating to study as they give us glaring examples of how diets can affect skin health.

Another study, published in the *Archives of Dermatology*, detailed how acne can be affected by diet and made the following points:

- In modern societies where processed white flour, dairy and sugar-containing products are abundant more than 79 per cent of teenagers suffer from acne.

- And what's surprising is that more than 40 per cent of men and women over the age of 25 in Western cultures have acne.

- Inuits who eat a traditional diet are acne-free, whereas Inuits who make the transition to modern diets develop acne similar to that in Western societies.

- The native inhabitants of Okinawa, an isolated Japanese island in the South China Sea, eat traditional diets and don't have any signs of acne.[12]

The final word on genes

You can have a genetic predisposition to getting eczema, psoriasis, dark circles under the eyes and cellulite, but this doesn't mean you have to suffer with these conditions forever. A healthy diet and good lifestyle habits influence your genes every day. In fact, good nutrition can *switch off* a problematic gene! The gene for psoriasis can literally stop expressing itself and simply lie dormant within your body after you complete the Anti-psoriasis Programme.

If you suffer from acne, cellulite, dandruff, eczema/dermatitis, psoriasis or rosacea, then you'll be pleased to know that the Healthy Skin Diet has specialised programmes tailored for your condition (see Part 3). If you have a child with an undesirable skin condition then you can turn to the 'Children's Clear Skin Programme' in Chapter 16 and cradle cap is covered in Chapter 14. You can now skip to the corresponding chapter in Part 3, 'Specialised Programmes', before flipping back to the chapters in Part 2, 'Eight Guidelines for Healthy Skin'.

If you have another type of skin complaint or no specific skin problem (and

> **CAUTION**
>
> It's important not to self-diagnose your skin condition as there are many different types of skin abnormalities and some may be serious, requiring medical attention. If you haven't had a doctor diagnose your skin condition, then be a smart cookie and see a specialist before starting the Healthy Skin Diet so you can be sure to read the information that is right for you.

you just want to guard against premature ageing), then you can keep on reading the next section, Part 2, 'Eight Guidelines for Healthy Skin'. This outlines the principles of the Healthy Skin Diet and everything you need for beautiful skin.

Eight Guidelines for Healthy Skin

Healthy skin is not a mysterious phenomenon. There are eight basic guidelines that enable beautiful skin to exist. Some people can have luminous skin by only following four guidelines, maybe five. How many you need is unknown at present. To unlock the secret to beautiful skin, begin with all eight guidelines for healthy skin and see how good your skin looks after eight weeks.

These guidelines are based on anti-ageing research so they are very specific for decreasing the appearance of wrinkles and premature ageing. They can also eliminate undesirable skin conditions such as contact dermatitis, hives, acne, psoriasis, eczema/dermatitis, rosacea, dry skin and can reduce cellulite. Other skin conditions may also be improved when following these guidelines.

Some people are born with beautiful skin. For the rest of us, there are the Eight Guidelines for Healthy Skin because beautiful skin is also created. Expect to have it within eight weeks.

Chapter 3

Guideline No. 1: Think green and friendly

'Think green and friendly' is not a mantra for a hippy commune; it is an essential step for beautiful skin, involving 'friendly' gut flora and 'green' foods and drinks that have an alkalising effect on the body. Technically speaking, some parts of your body *should* be acidic, such as your stomach when it produces digestive acids and your outer layer of skin with its protective acid mantle. However in general, your body's tissues and blood should be slightly alkaline.

For years I ignored the concept of balancing the body's pH with alkalising foods. Now when I look back I feel so silly. This guideline is really simple and you quickly see *and* feel your health improving so you know it's working!

How is body acidity or alkalinity measured?

Your body has a natural acid and alkaline balance which is measured by the traditional pH scale (pH literally means 'potential of hydrogen'). For example, a pH of 1.0 is completely acid and a pH of 14 is all alkaline, and 7.0 is neutral. The pH of a substance is determined by how many hydrogen ions are in a substance. All acids in the body give off hydrogen ions as they dissolve in water.[1]

Now, for the body to remain *alive* and well the blood needs to be slightly alkaline – at a pH of 7.365 to be precise. If your blood pH becomes slightly acidic your blood would burn holes in your blood vessels. As you can imagine, you can't feel healthy if you have holes in your veins. In fact, if the blood pH was to vary by about one-tenth, your body's biomechanical function would fail and you'd die.[2] However the body, being the wise thing that it is, has many back-up plans to ensure the blood's pH balance is maintained:

1. The body uses its alkaline reserves such as alkaline minerals to keep the blood pH at the correct level. If you keep having an acid lifestyle, these stores run out and your body needs to go to back-up plan number 2 ...

2. Back-up plan number 2 involves quickly removing excess acids from your blood and storing them safely in your fat cells. Unfortunately, overweight people who have lots of acid stored in their fat usually have an incredibly difficult time losing weight because their body will do everything to avoid the influx of acid that would be released during weight-loss. An acidic body holds onto excess weight, making dieting extremely difficult.

3. After your body uses up its alkaline reserves and after it has stored acids in your fat, what happens next? Back-up plan number 3: your body takes alkaline minerals such as calcium from your bones. This is one of the reasons why people get osteoporosis and shrink as they get older. Their acid lifestyle is threatening to disrupt their blood pH and the body is protecting the blood by leeching calcium from their bones.[3] Unfortunately the modern Western diet is excessively acidic.

There are two ways you can find out how acidic you are. Firstly (and this is the more accurate way), your doctor can test your blood pH with a simple blood test. You need to ask for this test specifically as it is not a routine blood test. A healthy pH reading for your blood is between 7.35 and 7.45; as you can see it's a very narrow range.[4]

Secondly, you can test your saliva or urine pH with pH strips that you can purchase from your local pharmacy. These pH strips are made of litmus paper, which changes colour when acidic or alkaline substances come into contact with it. Dr Guerrero, a famous American doctor who studied traditional Chinese medicine and is the author of *In Balance for Life*, recommends testing the urine rather than saliva as the kidneys are one of the body's organs that eliminate acids. However the urine test is not as accurate as a blood test but it can reveal if you're acidic and you can do the test daily. This is useful because acid and base (alkalinity) levels fluctuate daily. When your body's pH is in balance, your urine pH will be between 7.0 and 7.5.[5]

What happens if your body is too acidic?

According to Dr Guerrero, acidosis can damage cells in your body. An acid-producing lifestyle can also reduce the amount and quality of collagen and elastin being produced so you can end up with premature ageing and wrinkles. Good quality collagen and elastin is essential for youthful-looking skin. Too many acids in the body can also cause demineralisation, which can lead to dry and cracked skin, fingernails that split easily and thin, brittle hair.[6]

According to Dr Guerrero, having an overly acidic system can also do damage to your red blood cells so they alter in shape, clump together and they can die prematurely. Your red blood cells should look like round, flat discs – a bit like red frisbees or a throat lozenge – floating freely through your blood plasma. They should also have a negative charge on the outside and a positive charge on the inside. When your red blood cells are negatively charged on the outside as they should be, they cannot clump together. They repel. Unfortunately, when acid strips some of your red blood cells of their negative charge they start *attracting* each other and they form clumps. Your red blood cells should not clump together unless you've cut yourself and the blood flow needs to be stopped from escaping. Otherwise your blood needs to flow without clotting.

Your skin is usually the first thing to suffer when red blood cell health is poor. Your red blood cells carry oxygen to your skin but when they are sticky and bulky they cannot give your outer layer a quick and efficient supply of oxygen. Your skin may also look dull and possibly even pasty or greyish from low oxygen supply.

You can also feel very lethargic if your blood is sluggish with damaged red blood cells that aren't supplying enough oxygen. No wonder people often wake up tired after eight hours' sleep and need a coffee pick-me-up!

Fill out the following questionnaire to see if your body is showing any signs of acidosis. Circle any symptoms you experience on a regular basis (three or more times a week):

Common symptoms of acidosis

fatigue, chronic fatigue syndrome

fatigue or weakness after eating meals

frequent colds and flu, low immunity

poor circulation, cold hands/feet

low blood pressure

burning sensation during urination

kidney stones

excessive urination

headaches

pallor, dull complexion

gastrointestinal problems: abdominal pains, cramps, acid reflux, diarrhoea, wind, ulcers

agitation, nervousness, anxiety, depression

lack of ambition, lack of joy

dental problems: bleeding or inflamed gums, cavities

cracked lips, loose teeth, tooth sensitivity

muscle cramps or spasms, tension in neck and shoulders

joint pain, arthritis-like pain

nail and hair problems: brittle hair, hair loss, split nails

allergies, runny nose, chronic bronchitis

vaginal discharge, candida albicans

skin problems: dry skin, eczema, acne, hives, itchy skin, red and patchy skin

osteoporosis, brittle bones

insomnia, restless sleep.[7]

If you have circled four or more symptoms then you may have too much acid in your body. Cross-check this by doing a pH urine test for five days in a row (to get a more accurate average). Do the urine test first thing in the morning, on rising.

What causes excess acidity in the body?

acid-forming foods, poor diet

stress (covered in Chapter 10)

coffee and other products
   containing caffeine

alcohol

smoking

chemicals

dehydration/not enough water

parasites (worms)

candida albicans

drugs, including prescriptive
   medications

constipation/poor bowel health.

Acid-forming foods

There are many types of acid-producing foods and the most common ones come from animal produce. Now these foods don't seem acidic before you pop them in your mouth – they contain some acids but they also *form* acids once they're digested. Acid-forming foods are okay in moderation but when your body is continually trying to counteract an acidic state, acid can become poison to your system.

When you have an acidic system, your body will eventually tire of shunting calcium away from your bones and storing acid in your fat. And if you're a thin person, with limited fat cells, then you're in a worse predicament than an over-weight person.[8] Where is your acid being stored? As you can imagine, skinny people can get sick very, very quickly. This means that Skinny-Minnies need to be *extra* healthy to feel great and have beautiful skin.

You can probably guess most of the common acid-forming foods as they're also the usual 'offending' foods that already have bad reputations, such as sugar, white flour products, foods high in saturated fats and damaged (trans) fats, meat, dairy, soft drinks, chips and alcohol. But what you may find surprising is that when you chomp on a piece of fruit, it creates acid during digestion. This is because *most* fruits have an extremely high sugar content. Yes, these are natural sugars but they promote acidity and they provide a quick and easy meal for thriving microbes.

Acid-forming foods – the worst offenders

vinegar
liquor/spirits/whiskey
pork
beef
processed fruit juice
yellow cheeses
kefir
yogurt sweetened with fruit, sugar
   or artifical sweetener
carp
processed meats/ham/luncheon meat
crayfish
herring
salmon
lobster
mackerel
black tea
artificial sweeteners
sugar
cocoa/chocolate
coffee
milk
soft drinks
tap water

wine
hydrogenated fats
margarine
peanut and walnut oils
commercially made tomato sauce
pickles and mustard
processed table salt
chickpeas
peanuts
hazelnuts
pecans
pistachios
sunflower seeds
walnuts
blackcurrants
kiwi fruit
mandarins, nectarines
oranges
pineapple
millet
white rice
white flour products
white/yeast breads
soyabeans[9]

Acid-forming foods – the milder ones

beer	cashews
wholegrains, whole wheat	coconut
amaranth	pine nuts
brown rice	sesame seeds
oats	apples
barley	fresh apricots
quinoa	blueberries
spelt	cherries
soft cheeses	figs
eggs (whole)	grapes
plain organic yogurt	mangoes
chicken	melon, watermelon
flounder	pears
lamb	plums
oysters	pomegranates
trout	strawberries
sole	most dried fruits
kidney beans	carbonated mineral water
lentils	(heated) cold-pressed oils
haricot beans	organic mustard[10]
peas	

READER QUESTION

Q 'I've heard that acid-forming foods are bad for me. Do I have to totally avoid them to be healthy?'

A *No! The foods and liquids that exert the strongest acid-producing effect can be enjoyed in moderation. However, during the Healthy Skin Diet these substances will be strictly limited to no more than three servings per day. Two servings is two glasses of alcohol or one coffee and salmon or chickpeas for dinner. Keep your animal protein servings small – about the size of the palm of your hand – especially if you're eating meat*.*

* Pork is not included in the eight-week programme as it is the most acidic meat.

When eating at restaurants, you usually can't control the serving size of your meats so choose less acidic protein such as chicken, trout, lamb, kidney beans or lentils.

Acid-forming fruits are also fine in moderation – two servings per day or less. After all, fruit supplies plenty of cancer-protective phytochemicals, vitamins and minerals but it can also supply too many simple sugars that parasites thrive on. Two servings per day is equivalent to two apples, or a small handful of blueberries and half a mango.

READER QUESTION

Q 'My dad has alkalosis; what is it?'

A Alkalosis is basically the opposite of acidosis as it's an overly alkaline condition in the body. Alkalosis is rare; however it is most commonly caused by **alkalising** drugs such as ulcer and anti-heartburn medications. Alkalosis can also be caused from chronic vomiting or diarrhoea and it can also occur from hyperventilation (as breathing is one of the ways in which the body expels acids and breathing in a rapid, anxious manner can result in alkalosis). Symptoms of alkalosis include over-stimulation of the nervous system resulting in tetany, muscle spasms/cramps and extreme nervousness.[11]

Coffee and other products containing caffeine

READER QUESTION

Q 'I know I have to hydrate my body but do coffee and tea with milk count as fluids and are they okay for my skin?'

A No, coffee and black tea with milk can't be counted as hydrating fluids because caffeine has a dehydrating effect on the body; however, caffeine may not be harm-ful to the skin in small doses.

NEVER have more than two cups of coffee or tea per day because caffeine trig-gers the stress response in the body, releasing cortisol, and you don't want to over-stimulate this hormone as it contributes to premature ageing. Caffeine also causes the adrenal glands to work overtime so it can cause puffy eyes and dark circles under the eyes.

If you have **eczema, rosacea, acne, cellulite** or **psoriasis** then I recommend you avoid caffeine or switch to **decaf coffee** as it is less likely to exacerbate your condition. Look for water-decaffeinated coffee as opposed to decaf that has been produced with chemicals. Another alternative I recommend to everyone is to have dandelion tea once a day as it helps the liver safely eliminate skin-ageing chemi-cals. Here are some guidelines for tea and coffee drinking:

- One to two cups of coffee or tea is permitted while you're on the Healthy Skin Diet.

- Instant coffee and decaf coffee are decaffeinated with chemicals so choose water-decaffeinated coffee or have (weak) freshly brewed bean coffee.

- Avoid soft drinks containing caffeine (cola and energy drinks).

- You can drink green tea twice a day as it has liver detoxifying and antioxidant benefits (remember that green tea also contains caffeine).

- Drink dandelion tea/coffee – it is a great coffee alternative. It's caffeine-free and tastes great. Look for the Soya Dandé recipe in the back of the book.

- Suddenly abstaining from caffeine can result in withdrawal symptoms such as headaches, so wean yourself off caffeine slowly.

Activity

If you drink more than two cups of coffee or tea per day, begin to reduce this amount today. If you normally drink six cups, cut down to five cups today and then only have four cups tomorrow. You aim is to reduce your intake to two weak coffees per day (do this over the period of a week).

Please note for the first three days of the Healthy Skin Diet, during the Three Day Alkalising Cleanse, caffeine-containing drinks and foods are not permitted.

Alcohol

READER QUESTION

Q   'Can I still drink alcohol while on the Healthy Skin Diet? I've heard I should be drinking red wine; is it good for me?'

A   *Yes you can occasionally drink alcohol while on the eight-week programme although you need to limit consumption as alcohol is very dehydrating and acidic so it may slow down your progress to beautiful skin.*

Scientists may say that red wine is packed full of antioxidants but they don't mention that red wine also contains sulphite preservatives that can cause allergic reactions such as anaphylaxis (in very sensitive people). If you love your wine, have the preservative-free kind during the eight-week programme. If you want a dose of heart-protective antioxidants eat red grapes, blueberries and raspberries and drink green tea.

- *One glass of red wine can cause red flushing and rashes in sensitive individuals with rosacea.*
- *Drinking excessive amounts of alcohol can lead to skin disease.* [12]

If you have a severe skin condition, the best thing you can do for your skin is abstain from alcohol, at least until your complexion clears. However this can be hard to do, especially if your job is very social. So I've devised some options so you don't have to completely ditch your social life while on the Healthy Skin Diet:

- *Keep alcohol intake low.*
- *When socialising have no more than two standard alcoholic drinks.*
- *Have at least four alcohol-free days per week.*
- *Make a rule to never drink alone or at home.*

*If you have **eczema, psoriasis** or **rosacea** it's best to ditch the alcohol altogether; however, if you want to have the occasional drop, your best choices would be '**low chemical' alcohol** which doesn't contain salicylates, amines or MSG, such as: vodka, gin and whisky. Have them with mineral or soda water (**not** tonic water, cola or lime cordials).*

Smoking

READER QUESTION

Q **'Can I smoke while on the Healthy Skin Diet?'**

A *No. You probably already know that cigarette smoking can alter your physical appearance dramatically and not for the better: smokers with a history of heavy smoking are five times more likely to have wrinkles than non-smokers.[13] And smoking decreases vitamin C levels in the body and it affects the body's ability to form healthy collagen in the skin.[14,15]*

Activity

Enrol in a quit smoking programme today, or better still decide to 'choose health' instead of focusing on 'not smoking'. Focus on what you want rather than what you're trying to avoid. When you have a craving for a cigarette, take five slow, deep breaths and 'drink in' the fresh air. Imagine yourself looking fit and healthy, with beautiful skin. Gradually decrease how many ciggies you have and don't be too hard on yourself if you occasionally fail. Even if you only have a few less than usual, you are on your way to being healthier.

Chemicals

Synthetic chemicals are also acid-producing. You are bombarded with small (and not-so-small) doses of chemicals every day and these increase acid in the body – when you walk beside a busy road, when you drink chlorinated tap water and when you put on your favourite perfume or moisturiser.

But even though your environment is laced with thousands of synthetic chemicals there is no need to ditch your life and become a chemical-phobic hermit. And it is not essential to eat strictly organic food, and you don't even have to give up wearing make-up or polyester high-waisted trousers (unless they're out of fashion, which is nearly always). You just need to *reduce* your chemical load so you can decrease the amount of acids you are ingesting or inhaling.

Chemicals can be found in:

oven cleaner	pesticides, fly spray
window and kitchen cleaners	furniture polish
bleach	nail polish, beauty products
processed and packaged foods	make-up
fried foods	carpets
preserved foods and drinks	paints
perfumes	plaster

Decrease your chemical exposure by following these three key steps:

1. **Open windows daily to ventilate your home and car.** Chemicals are emitted from carpets and furnishings, and if you use chemical cleaning products the chemicals can accumulate in enclosed spaces, so open your windows and let in the fresh air.

2. **Soak fruits and vegetables in water and vinegar.** If you cannot afford organic food, you can minimise chemical load by washing your fruits and vegetables in a bowl of water containing two tablespoons of vinegar. Soak vegetables in the water solution for five minutes and scrub hardy vegetables (you can't scrub leafy greens as they will bruise). Vinegar helps to remove pesticides and it also kills bacteria. In the old days, before refrigerators were common, vinegar was used to wash mouldy meat to kill the bacteria and this often prevented food poisoning. Apple cider vinegar is the best choice as it's alkalising. White vinegar is the budget option.

3. **Check food labels.** Avoid preservatives, artificial colour, flavours and flavour enhancers. Look for products with natural preservatives such as vinegar (although vinegar is acid-producing, it is the healthier option). Follow the guidelines below:

   Avoid chemical preservatives. When buying bread, look on the labels for 'preservative free', there are plenty around. Avoid preservative 282, calcium propionate. Avoid preserved dried fruits, preserved wines and flavoured drinks.

   Avoid artificial sweeteners. Avoid aspartame and saccharine as they can cause adverse reactions. Favour natural sweeteners such as honey, dark brown sugar and agave nectar. Agave nectar is a natural liquid derived from the cactus of the same name. It has a naturally low GI and is useful for baking and cooking.

   Avoid yellow, blue and red food colouring. You don't need fake-coloured foods! There are natural alternatives everywhere – just check the labels.

   Avoid flavour enhancers 621 and 635 by saying no to chicken salt, chips and potato crisps, and Thai and Chinese takeaway that still uses MSG (all you have to do is ask 'Does your food contain MSG or any other flavour enhancers?').

   Avoid fried food and you will automatically avoid BHA. At the fish and chip shop order grilled fish, if available, or simply avoid eating the batter, and if you must have chips, also grab a big green salad for a dose of alkalinity.

   You can make your own cleaning products with ingredients such as vinegar and baking soda or check out biodegradable brands from your local health food shop – or see the cleaning product recipes at the back of this book.

Drugs, including prescriptive medications

Drugs, especially antibiotics and other pharmaceutical medications, are acid-forming once digested. So if you're the type who pops a pill every time you have a minor sniffle or ache then you may want to reconsider as you could be making your health more fragile in the long term. Often a headache or runny nose can be alleviated by drinking plenty of water and having a decent nap. However, if you have a serious medical condition requiring prescriptive drugs then you may *harm* your health by suddenly abstaining from your medications so you shouldn't take the risk. In this case, keep taking your medications as prescribed and eat the nutritious food on the Healthy Skin Diet to help prevent acid accumulation.

Constipation and poor bowel health

Being constipated on a regular basis can also increase acidity in the body. Ideally you should do a poo every day, even twice a day. But many people experience irregular bowel movements where they don't do 'number twos' for days. Although not ideal, it's okay if you only have one bowel movement every second day. However, if you're only going once every three days, or worse – once a week – then toxins from your poo are being reabsorbed by your body and as you can imagine this can lead to skin problems such as acne and rashes, and health problems such as arthritis, aching limbs and fatigue. If you have constipation or any other bowel complaints then it's essential that you improve your bowel health immediately. Positive solutions for constipation include:

- Overheating can cause dehydration. In winter use blankets rather than a duvet as they allow excess heat to escape as you sleep and they 'breathe' better than duvets.

- Drink eight to ten glasses of water each day plus 2–4 teaspoons of chlorophyll in water as chlorophyll promotes bowel movements (see Green Water recipe on page 304).

- For every glass of alcohol you drink, follow it with one glass of natural mineral water.

- Add 1–2 tablespoons of flaxseed oil to your meals.

- Take laxative herbs such as dandelion root tea (see the recipe for Soya Dandé on page 305).

- Foods that promote bowel movements include green leafy vegetables, papaya/pawpaw, coconut, cabbage, prunes, peas, black sesame seed, sweet potato, asparagus, figs, oat bran, wheat bran and rice bran.

- Have a high fibre diet. Eat brown rice, wholegrains and lots of vegetables.

- Make sure you don't have parasites and do the Three Day Alkalising Cleanse.

What is your gastrointestinal tract like?

Do the following questionnaire to see if you have poor bowel health.

Bowel health questionnaire

Circle any symptoms you experience on a regular basis (three or more times a week or enough to disrupt your life):

foul-smelling wind or stools

excessive wind

excessive burping

bloating

food allergies, food sensitivities

abdominal discomfort/pain

fatigue after eating

premature ageing

constipation and/or diarrhoea

nausea

reflux

headaches

constant hunger

irregular bowel movements

skin blemishes or rashes

undigested food particles in your stools (other than seeds and corn, which are normal)

'pellet' poos

pale, hard-to-flush stools

irritable bowel syndrome

unexplained back/shoulder/ abdominal pain*

blood in stools*

* You should tell your doctor if you experience pain or notice blood in your stools.

If you've circled three or more symptoms then pay particular attention to the advice in this chapter.

Dehydration/not enough water

READER QUESTION

Q 'I'm not used to drinking water as it makes me go to the toilet too often. How can I drink more water without the side effects?'

A *If you don't usually drink water then it is important to **gradually** increase water intake over the period of a week as you need to drink enough hydrating fluids to prevent dehydration. Dehydration is associated with increased acids in the body, constipation, dry skin, acne, blood pressure problems, headaches, moodiness and lethargy. Dehydration also quickly increases the appearance of wrinkles.* [16]

A good indicator is to increase water consumption as your urine output increases. Your body needs time to adapt to the extra water so increase intake little by little so your body benefits without feeling waterlogged. If you are still going to the toilet too frequently then add liquid chlorophyll and a pinch of good quality sea salt to your bottle of water. You may also want to check for chromium deficiency and supplement if necessary (see Chapter 5, 'Guideline No. 3', for questionnaire, dosage and cautions).

Water prescription

Work out how much water your body requires using the following equation: your body weight in kilograms (kg) x 0.033 = how many litres of water to drink.

For example, if you weigh 75kg: 75 x 0.033 = 2.47, so you would need approximately 2.5 litres of water per day for optimal health.

(If using pounds, divide your body weight by 2, so body weight in pounds ÷ 2 = ounces of water to drink each day.)[17]

How to make water consumption more enjoyable

- Buy a water filter that attaches to your kitchen sink or buy a water filter jug.

- Serve your water chilled with ice and a splash of real lime or lemon juice (as they're alkalising).

- Drink natural mineral water.

- Drink other hydrating beverages such as herbal teas and fresh vegetable juices (keep fruit to a limit as it's mostly acid forming).

- Drink one to two glasses of water in between meals to leave your digestive tract well lubricated for digestion. This also prevents excessive thirst during meals (a sure sign you are not drinking enough water in between meals).

- Drinking too many liquids during meal time can dilute digestive juices and prevent proper digestion.

Activity
Drink a glass of water right now.

Parasites

Q **'I've heard probiotic supplements contain friendly gut flora. What is this?'**

A *'Friendly' gut flora doesn't look anything like pretty little flowers in the gut lining. Gut flora are microscopic bacteria, such as acidophilus, that are* **beneficial** *to health. They work by adhering to your gut wall and 'policing' the bad bacteria and other microbes so they can't multiply.* *

Parasites and candida albicans thrive when good intestinal flora is absent.

An acidic lifestyle can create a desirable breeding ground for worms and candida albicans. Microbes love an acidic environment. That is why this guideline is so important for health. You can't avoid picking up germs from unclean surfaces, contaminated people and the great outdoors. Have you ever walked barefoot in public toilets or change rooms? Do your pets lick your face or sleep in your bed? Have you ever forgotten to wash your hands before eating lunch or just couldn't be bothered? Like most people you probably have, but these harmless habits can unfortunately lead to little wriggly health problems **if** *you also have an overly acidic body.*

The World Health Organization (WHO) states that parasitic infections, if left untreated, weaken your body's defence system (immunity) because of blood loss, anaemia, malnutrition and tissue and organ damage.[18] Luckily we have great health care facilities in the Western world so parasite treatments are readily available to us. Non-specific symptoms include fatigue, nausea, abdominal pains and loss of appetite. Sometimes worms can be spotted in the faeces.[19]

Vitamin A deficiency can also occur as worms need this vitamin to survive.[20] Vitamin A deficiency symptoms include rough and dry skin, frequent infections, bumpy skin and poor sense of smell.

How do you know if you have a worm problem? Take a look at the following questionnaire.

---

* Not many strains of bacteria adhere well but they can still have a beneficial effect.

Parasite questionnaire

Circle any symptoms you experience three or more times per week:

general weakness

facial pallor

anaemia

vitamin A deficiency

withered yellow look

huge appetite (may cause weight gain) or loss of appetite (and weight loss)

nausea

muscle wasting, unexplained thinness

bluish specks in the whites of eyes

white coin-sized splotches on the face

anal itching (especially at night)

itchy ears

poor sleep

excessive nose picking

grinding teeth during sleep

cravings for sweets or dried foods

cravings for raw rice or dirt (usually kids)

cravings for charcoal or burned foods

abdominal pain

digestive complaints: diarrhoea, wind, bloating, belching, constipation, irritable bowel syndrome, mucus in stools

gluten intolerance

low blood sugar (hypoglycaemia)

high blood sugar

allergies

skin rashes

acne

depression

moodiness

hyperactivity (in children)

If you have more than five of these symptoms then you could have a parasite problem.

READER QUESTION

Q 'I think I have worms. What should I do?'

A *If you suspect you have parasites then you have a number of options. You may want to speak to your doctor and get a stool test done to confirm what sort of worms you have so you can get the specific drug treatment. However keep in mind that even with medical treatment, if your microbe problem is caused by an acidic lifestyle then your parasite problem can quickly come back to haunt you. A multi-faceted approach is by far the most helpful option. The first step is to make the microbe's environment (your body) so undesirable that they will stop multiplying* and start dying. You can do this when you alkalise your body using the information in this chapter.

There are also various anti-parasitic herbs that may be useful, but the most important supplement to take is a probiotic so you have plenty of the good guys to take over as the undesirables die. You can take anti-parasitic herbs for ten days if you have a severe infestation or you can simply follow the Healthy Skin Diet for eight weeks with the simple addition of a probiotic supplement and garlic.

Anti-parasitic herbs and seeds include:

Black walnut extract

Black walnut's chief compound is called juglone and studies have found it to have a strong anti-parasitic, anti-fungal and laxative effect, which is really handy as it not only kills pesky worms but also helps to flush them out.[21,22] The adult dosage is 1000mg, three times per day with water (taken before meals). Short-term use only.

> **CAUTION**
>
> Do *not* use black walnut during childhood, pregnancy or when breastfeeding as there is a lack of reliable information regarding its safety during these periods.

Clove oil

Clove oil contains the constituent eugenol, which can destroy parasite eggs, candida albicans and bacteria such as staphylococcus and E coli.[23]

> **CAUTION**
>
> Don't use clove oil supplements if you're pregnant or breastfeeding.

Pumpkin seeds

Cucurbita, a major compound in pumpkin seeds, is anti-parasitic, making pumpkin seeds useful for eradicating tapeworm. Pumpkin seeds are a safe treatment for worm-infested children as long as they're old enough to chew the seeds.[24,25,26] Eat a handful of pumpkin seeds daily.

Other extracts that are fantastic for treating worms and candida include thyme oil, grapeseed extract, the herb pau d'arco and garlic oil.

Anti-parasitic foods

I've already mentioned pumpkin seeds but there are plenty of other food sources that help to control microbes. Foods, herbs and spices that exhibit a *strong* anti-microbial effect include raw garlic, raw onion, cinnamon, cloves, radishes and mustard. Herbs and spices that have a *moderate* anti-microbial effect include allspice, basil, bay leaf, caraway, cumin, coriander, nutmeg, oregano, sage, rosemary and thyme. Other foods and herbs include avocado, coconut, sauerkraut, seaweed, raw honey, extra-virgin olive oil, black pepper, red pepper (capsicum) and ginger.[27,28,29,30] Foods that promote good bowel flora include miso (Japanese fermented soya paste that can be used as a soup base) and chlorophyll-rich foods such as dark leafy green vegetables and alfalfa greens.[31]

Tips for avoiding future worm infestations

- Avoid sugary foods – cakes, sweets, pastries, doughnuts, white flour desserts, dairy desserts, sugar in coffee/tea, dried fruits and chocolate that contains sugar (these foods create a breeding ground for parasites in the body).

- Have plenty of alkaline-forming foods such as leafy green vegetables, almonds, lemon and avocado.

- Take a probiotic supplement.

- Filter your drinking water with a filter jug or tap fitting.

- Wash hands thoroughly before eating meals.

- Wash all fruits, vegetables and meats with apple cider vinegar and water before use. Soak them for five minutes as this will remove any pesticide residues and kill microbes.

- When travelling to foreign countries, only drink bottled water and eat thoroughly cooked foods (avoid uncooked salads, iced teas, ice etc.).

- Avoid consuming raw fish/sashimi (good quality wasabi is a green paste made from horseradish and it's a natural anti-parasitic so consume it whenever you eat raw fish).

- Eat garlic every day. Have one small clove of garlic with every meal.

- Avoid constipation.

- Chew food thoroughly so your food can be digested properly. Parasites thrive in poorly digested foods.

- Drink Green Water daily (see the recipe on page 304).

Candida albicans (thrush, fungal or yeast infection)

Candida albicans can be present in the vagina in women and the digestive tract of both sexes. It may also be present externally on the skin and as a toenail fungal infection or tinea. Women are eight times more likely to suffer from a yeast infection than men, which may be due to higher antibiotic use, higher oestrogen hormones in the body and birth-control use.[32]

Answer the questions in the following questionnaire to see if you have any signs of candida albicans.

Candida questionnaire

Write 'yes' or 'no' beside any lifestyle factors or symptoms you relate to. For questions such as 'Do you crave alcohol' only write 'yes' if you crave it regularly (three or more times per week):

Have you taken antibiotics for more than a month in the last six months?

Have you taken the birth-control pill for more than two years?

Have you taken any cortisone-type drugs for more than two weeks?

Do perfumes, insecticides and chemicals make you feel unwell?**

Do you have athlete's foot?

Do you frequently crave sugar and bread?

Do you frequently crave alcohol?

Does cigarette smoke really bother you?

Do you have unexplained fatigue?

Do you often feel drained or spaced out?

Do you frequently suffer from constipation or diarrhoea?

Do you have bloating, wind or belching?

Do you have vaginal itching, burning or creamy discharge?**

Do you have a loss of sex drive?

Do you have PMS or period cramps?

Do you have frequent mood swings?

Do you have frequent attacks of anxiety or crying?

Are you shaking or irritable when hungry?

Do you have an inability to concentrate?

Do you have frequent headaches?

Do you have food sensitivities and intolerances?

Do you have rectal or nasal itching?**
Do you have excessive body odour not relieved by deodorant use?
Do you have bad breath?[33,34]

If you answered yes to more than five symptoms then you may have candida albicans. If you said yes to any of the symptoms marked by ** then you are highly likely to have candida albicans. If you suspect you have candida albicans you should take a probiotic supplement and consume alkalising foods and drinks. Your candida albicans should magically disappear; if it doesn't improve within a week, see your doctor as it may be a different condition.

Case study

A 30-year-old woman suffered from skin rashes and vaginal itching (her doctor diagnosed candida albicans). She reported insatiable cravings for sweet foods and frequent colds and flu, which were occasionally treated with antibiotics. Green Water, probiotics and garlic were recommended to improve her gut flora and she did the Three Day Alkalising Cleanse. She replaced sugary foods and white bread and rice with good quality vegetables, protein, brown rice and wholegrains. She also had to do some light exercise and relax at the end of the day (to restore her immune system). Her vaginal itching stopped two days later and after three weeks her skin rash began to clear and her cravings stopped. Six weeks later her skin rash was completely gone.

What types of probiotics are suitable for treating candida albicans?

In the *Journal of the Australian Traditional-Medicine Society*, naturopath Jason Hawrelak noted the benefits you get from probiotic supplements are *strain-specific*: they do not all work in the same manner.[35] For example, the probiotic supplement that is good for treating irritable bowel syndrome *won't* be beneficial for eczema. See Chapter 15, 'Eczema/dermatitis', for probiotic strains specific for this condition. Probiotics can be used therapeutically for treating digestive problems, poor immunity, eczema and candida albicans but you need to know the *specific* strain that has been scientifically proven to suit your needs.

Probiotics for candida albicans:

- L. acidophilus LA5
- L. rhamnosus GG
- L. acidophilus strain NAS
- L acidophilus NCFM.[36]

Probiotics for digestive complaints:

- L. rhamnosus GG
- L. johnsonii La1, L. plantarum 299v
- L. paracasei Shirota
- propionibacterium freudenreichii HA-101 and HA-102
- Eat sauerkraut.[37]

Probiotics for compromised immune system:

- L. acidophilus LA5
- L. rhamnosus GG.[38]

To remove confusion Hawrelak also listed where to find the specific strains of good bacteria. However, product companies can change their supplement formulas so I have listed the specific brands on my website so this information can be updated when necessary.

Dosage: Take the dose as recommended by the manufacturers. For adults, the general rule is one capsule two to three times per day on an empty stomach (in between meals or at least 15 minutes before meals). Probiotics should be ingested with room-temperature water or almond/rice/soya drink. Avoid having probiotics with excessively cold or hot drinks as they may damage the beneficial bacteria. For children's dosage see 'Children's Clear Skin Programme'.

How do you 'think green'?

Green drinks such as those containing chlorophyll (see page 53) and wheat grass are the best way to create a good acid–alkaline balance in your body. Drink them every day for the best results. Being vegetarian may also help, but only if your food choices are healthy ones. Some vegetarians eat a lot of dairy, processed white breads and sugar-rich desserts so they too can end up with an acid problem.

Foods that are mildly alkalising

asparagus

cauliflower

garlic

onions, shallots

radishes

endives

turnips

egg yolk

whey (fresh)

brazil nuts

avocado

bananas, dried bananas

grapefruit

tomatoes (uncooked)

dates

raisins

almond milk

herbal teas

natural mineral water
   (non-carbonated)

spring or filtered water

butter, buttermilk (uncooked)

cold-pressed extra-virgin olive oil
   (unheated)

herbs

sea salt/Celtic salt (unrefined)

spices[39]

Foods that are strongly alkalising

most vegetables:

   dark leafy greens

   artichoke

   beets, beet greens

   broccoli

   carrots

   cucumber

   dandelion greens

   green beans

   cabbage (white, red)

   lettuce (not iceberg)

   potatoes

   sweet potatoes

spinach

squash

sweet peppers

yams

courgette

almonds

lemons

limes

freshly made vegetable juice

apple cider vinegar

green drinks:

   chlorophyll

   wheat grass[40]

The lists above contain some surprises as the notorious *acidic* fruit tomato is actually alkalising to the blood. And isn't lemon usually acidic? Yes, but only before consumption; once it has been digested, lemons and limes have an alkalising effect that is beneficial for your blood. I guess you can't always judge a fruit by its bite!

The alkalising fruits are lemons, limes, grapefruit, avocado, apricots, banana and tomato.

When referring to the acid and alkaline lists in this chapter you may notice that butter is a better choice than margarine as butter is slightly alkalising (but only when it's unheated). Apple cider vinegar is super alkalising so it's a great addition to salads. However, you can see from the acidic list on page 34 that *all* other types of vinegar are highly acidic and should be avoided or limited.

During the *first three days* of the Healthy Skin Diet you'll have approximately 95 per cent alkaline-forming foods and drinks, and 5 per cent acid-forming substances. This is to give your body a major cleanse to decrease acidity. This cleansing programme is fantastic for your bowels, your skin and your whole body.

READER QUESTION

Q   'If alkalising foods are so good for me, would I be even healthier if I ate 100 per cent alkalising foods and avoided all the acidic ones?'

A   *No! You shouldn't eat an all-alkalising, all-cleansing diet every day for months because this is not good for you. An alkalising cleanse is beneficial for short periods but one week should be your maximum. People who eat salads and vegetables with no protein such as beans or fish can end up feeling unwell and may get sallow-looking skin that has poor tone. In fact many overweight people who have lost the extra kilos by eating nothing but salads end up with very saggy skin. This is often (but not always) caused by protein deficiency.*

All of the recipes in the Healthy Skin Diet have a healthy ratio of alkalising and acid-forming foods. This balance, where there is approximately 50 per cent alkalising and 50 per cent acid-forming foods within one meal, allows you to enjoy many of your favourite foods such as meat, breads and the occasional sweet treat.

READER QUESTION

Q   'I hate vegetables so how can I create a good acid and alkaline balance in my body without eating them?'

A   *To be honest, I don't know if you can be healthy without consuming vegetables. Scientists have concluded without doubt that eating lots of vegetables decreases your risk of diseases such as cancer, heart disease and strokes.*

*A diet **low** in vegetables increases your risk of getting severe skin conditions such as acne.[41,42,43] And studies show that a **high** intake of fruits and vegetables lessens the damaging effects of sun exposure and protects against premature skin wrinkling.[44,45,46]*

*Scientists, nutritionists and other health experts may argue about what a healthy diet is (and is not) but when reviewing the scientific literature they all agree that **a diet rich in vegetables has the strongest and most consistent association with disease prevention**. Can you believe it? All of the health experts agree on something!*

What is chlorophyll?

Chlorophyll is the name of the green pigment found in plants. It is formed as the plant's leaves capture sunlight in a process called photosynthesis. Chlorophyll is structurally very similar to our own blood. The only difference is that chlorophyll has the mineral magnesium at the centre of its structure and we have iron. Magnesium and iron are both essential for our health and can be obtained by eating leafy greens such as spinach and parsley.

A chlorophyll drink made from a liquid chlorophyll supplement can give you an extra dose of vegetables daily. It can help to neutralise acids in the body so your blood is less likely to clump together and become sluggish and inefficient. Chlorophyll drinks taken in the morning can also stimulate a bowel movement so they're a great way to prevent constipation and toxic build-up.

What types of green drinks are the best?

There are many types of green drinks and supplements available from health food shops, however most of them taste unpleasant (such as wheat grass) or they don't have the correct alkalising effect (such as spirulina, which is acid producing). Barley grass is suitable, however plain liquid chlorophyll not only tastes pleasant it's also cheap and effective (see the Green Water drink on page 304 in the recipe section).

What to look for when choosing a liquid chlorophyll supplement

Liquid chlorophyll is available from health food shops, online and from places where health products are sold. Look for the following:

- Choose a liquid chlorophyll that is *preservative free* as preservatives are acid-forming and can irritate the skin (especially if you have eczema).

- Choose a supplement that is low strength* – look on the ingredient panel for a chlorophyll concentration of around 200mg per 100ml.

- Other suitable ingredients in a chlorophyll supplement are spearmint oil, alfalfa extract and vegetable oil. Lactic acid or ascorbic acid may be present in small quantities.

  * I prefer to use and only recommend low-strength chlorophyll because it is not only very effective at treating skin conditions, it also has a more pleasant colour and taste than higher-strength chlorophyll. High-strength liquid chlorophyll supplements (with 2000mg per 100ml) usually appear black and as a result of the dense colour it may stain your teeth after regular use. If you wish to use high-strength chlorophyll then reduce the dosage and clean your teeth afterwards.

Let's get practical

Alkalising and energising recipes in the Healthy Skin Diet include Green Water; ACV Drink; Flaxseed Lemon Drink; Almond Milk; Anti-ageing Broth; Skin Firming Drink; Spicy Green Papaya Salad; Sweet Raspberry, Avocado and Watercress Salad; Roasted Corn and Cauliflower Soup; Therapeutic Veggie Soup; Tasty Antioxidant Salad; Tabbouli; Rich Mineral Salad; Roasted Sweet Potato Salad; B-rich Avocado Salsa; Avocado Dip with Dipping Sticks and Avocado Beauty Snack (see recipes chapter).

For breakfast you could have the Flaxseed Lemon Drink plus a handful of almond and brazil nuts; or if you want to have a 'standard' Western breakfast you could try the Designer Muesli or Gluten-free Muesli with homemade Almond Milk.

Key points to remember

- Drink Green Water every day.
- Limit/avoid caffeine as it is acid-forming in the body.
- Avoid alcohol if possible, or when socialising have no more than two standard alcoholic drinks. Have at least four alcohol-free days per week.
- Avoid smoking and passive smoking.
- Eat two servings of fruit and at least five servings of vegetables per day.
- Drink eight to ten glasses of filtered water per day (this includes having Green Water twice a day).
- Take a suitable probiotic supplement daily.
- Eat anti-parasitic food daily, such as garlic, onion, ginger and herbs and spices.
- Eat dark leafy green vegetables every day; they are like gold! They increase your energy stores and create strong, healthy red blood cells. Have two handfuls of leafy greens per day.

Chapter 4

Guideline No. 2:
Eat moisturising foods

Imagine you've spent a lot of money on a brand new sports car. Now, you wouldn't go and fill it with the wrong type of petrol, would you? If your car's manufacturer said it needed premium unleaded for enhanced performance and mileage you'd buy the good stuff so it ran as well as it should. So too with your body: eating the *wrong types of fats* can decrease your performance and leave you looking not so hot. On the other hand, eating the *right types of fats* can make your skin look fantastic. You see, certain fats are moisturising to your skin. They moisturise you from the inside out and they're more effective than even the most luxurious skin cream.

That's the good news but the not-so-good news is that Westerners like to eat the type of fats that decrease performance and mileage – the ones that can cause inflammation, dry skin, premature ageing and enhanced feelings of pain. They also increase your risk of heart disease, asthma, eczema and acne.

In this guideline you will learn about fats that are The Good, The Bad and The Beautiful, for gorgeous, healthy skin and vitality.

Prostaglandins

You need fats in your diet to make powerful hormone-like chemicals called prostaglandins. Prostaglandins are made by your body and they affect your hormones, your heart, your blood vessels, your cells and your skin's appearance.

The human body has over 30 different types of prostaglandins and they're grouped into three families called series 1, 2 and 3 prostaglandins. **Which series a prostaglandin falls into depends on what type of fat it's originally made from –** omega-3, omega-6 or saturated fats.[1] Each prostaglandin has a highly specific function but they're short-lived so you need to keep supplying the 'building materials' – the fats and synergistic nutrients – required to make them.

Okay, so you still may be thinking 'Prosta what?' Prostaglandins can be a bit difficult to visualise, but just imagine your prostaglandin biochemical pathways as three parallel streets, like the ones on a road map. Imagine that Street 1 and Street 3 are the 'good' streets that lead to two smooth, clear lakes set in tropical surroundings and Street 2, the 'bad' street stuck right in the middle, leads to the illegal rubbish tip.

Now you also have 'inner traffic' that travels along these three streets. Imagine your inner traffic looks like yellow dump trucks bringing fats to add to either the clear lakes or the rubbish tip. If a dump truck is full of fat, which street do you want it to go down? Do you want the truck to dump out fats that may harm your health at the end of Street 2 or do you want it to go down Street 1 or 3 and dump out fats that will keep the lake looking lovely and smooth? I'm guessing you said Streets 1 and 3 and by now you may have pieced together that the 'rubbish tip' down Street 2 is rough, like skin inflammation and the smooth lake at the end of Streets 1 and 3 represents skin that is healthy and smooth.

Prostaglandins are still relevant to you even if you've never suffered from a skin rash because prostaglandins can help to prevent acne, heart disease, arthritis, asthma, hay fever and sinusitis.

Let's work our way up from series 1 to series 3 prostaglandins ...

The Good

The first group of prostaglandins is series 1, which is made from a polyunsaturated fat called linoleic acid, but you may know it by its common name 'omega-6'. Omega-6 is an **essential fatty acid** but it isn't as famous as its cousin 'omega-3'. Maybe this is because our Western diets are usually overflowing with omega-6 as we get it from cooking oils, seeds, nuts, margarines and some veggies so there's no big buzz about omega-6's goodness because we're not usually deficient in it. Omega-3 and omega-6 are **essential fatty acids** (EFAs) and they are named so because they are *essential* for our health – our body cannot manufacture them and deficiency symptoms can occur when our diet is lacking. Series 1 prostaglandins (Street 1) have been found to improve circulation, lower blood pressure and decrease inflammatory responses such as eczema, PMS and arthritis-like pain – but only if the pathway (or 'street') is unblocked.

Omega-6 food sources include the oils of corn, sesame, safflower, sunflower seeds, rapeseed (canola), soyabean, walnuts, pumpkin seeds, borage oil*, evening primrose oil*, blackcurrant seed*, flaxseed (linseed) and green leafy vegetables.[2] (Those marked with an asterisk contain GLA, which your body can more easily convert to silky smooth Street 1 or series 1 prostaglandins.)

Is your Street 1 blocked and causing dry and damaged skin?

As you know, Street 1 leads to the smooth, clear lake (and gorgeous, clear skin) but this doesn't always occur. Smooth Street 1 can be blocked by various dietary and

How fats can make good and bad prostaglandins

STREET 1 'The Good'	STREET 2 'The Bad'	STREET 3 'The Beautiful'
OMEGA-6 Vegetable cooking oils, margarine, nuts and seeds, rapeseed (canola) and soya oils	**Saturated fats** Dairy, meat, fried foods (trans fats), tropical seafood, eggs, high meat/protein diet	**Omega-3** Flaxseeds, flaxseed oil, walnuts, omega-3 eggs, fish, leafy greens
Delta-6-desaturase* NEEDS... biotin, B6, zinc and magnesium		**Enzyme reation delta-6-desaturase**
GLA Also supplied in borage oil, blackcurrant seed and evening primrose oil	**Arachidonic acid(AA)** (blocked by EPA & DHA)	**EPA and DHA** Salmon, trout, sardines, herring, tuna oil, mackerel
DGLA	**DETOUR** (if blockage then omega-6 slowly converts to AA...)	
Prostaglandin Series 1 Inhibits inflammation, and high blood pressure, promotes heart health, healthy skin and prevents release of AA from cell membranes.	**Prostaglandin Series 2** Promotes inflammation, salt retention, heart disease, pain and fever, increases allergic reactions, asthma, arthritis, eczema, dermatitis, psoriasis, hay fever, dandruff and sinusitis.	**Prostaglandin Series 3** Inhibits inflammation, decreases blood pressure, reduces pain and depression, prevents heart disease, promotes beautiful skin and prevents release of AA.

*Delta-6-desaturase is a slow enzyme conversion which may be blocked by too much meat and dairy/saturated fat (AA), high stress, high GI (high insulin), alcohol and trans fats, and d-6-d dysfunction can be genetic or occur as you age.
AA (Arachidonic acid), DGLA (dihomogamma-linolenic acid), EPA (eicosapentaenoic acid), DHA (docosahexaenoic acid), GLA (gamma-linolenic acid).[3, 4]

lifestyle factors and then a traffic diversion is set up like a roadworks detour that redirects your healthy omega-6 fats into the inflammation-making rubbish tip down the end of Street 2. It's very important to work out if your Street 1 is blocked as all your omega-6 polyunsaturated fats may be diverting to inflammation-making Street 2 right now.

Fill out the following questionnaire to see if you have any omega-6 blockage or deficiency signs.

Omega-6 questionnaire

Circle any of the following symptoms you experience on a regular basis (three or more times per week):

eczema-like skin eruptions

loss of hair

premature ageing

behavioural disturbances, hyperactivity

kidney or liver degeneration*

excessive water loss through the skin (dry skin), combined with excess thirst*

frequent infections such as colds/flu/thrush

poor wound healing

sterility (in males)*

miscarriages*

arthritic-like pain*

period pain, PMS, breast pain during periods

breast/ovarian cysts*

heart and circulation problems*

growth retardation in childhood*

If you've circled three or more symptoms then read 'Can you repair a Street 1 roadblock?' below.

If you have severe dry skin, premature ageing and wrinkles, adult eczema or premenstrual syndrome (PMS) then an evening primrose oil (EPO) supplement may help. EPO should be used in conjunction with omega-3 foods or supplements. See dosages and cautions. If you (or your child) have any conditions that are marked above with an asterisk* you should speak to your doctor as these symptoms can also be caused by other factors.

Can you repair a Street 1 roadblock?

There are two enzymatic reactions that need to occur in order for your omega-6 oils to be converted to GLA and then into substances that make smooth, lovely skin. These reactions are called delta-6-desaturase and delta-5-desaturase (see diagram on previous page). However, one or both of these enzymatic reactions may be genetically faulty or temporarily blocked by the following:

- chronic stress or anxiety

- high insulin responses (from high GI foods)

- the presence of trans fats (found in fried foods, biscuits, dairy, pastries, cakes, chips, margarines and products containing 'shortening' or 'hydrogenated vegetable oil).

Your genetics play a part in your body's response to omega-6 fats but even with genetic blockage you can 'fix' the problem with dietary modifications. Through client feedback I have also found that drinking Green Water daily can prevent omega-6 blockage signs from occurring; this may be due to liquid chlorophyll's high magnesium content or its alkalising effect.

There are also six enthusiastic 'roadworkers' who can fix delta-5 and -6 and remove the roadblocks and they can help you to have good quality skin.

The six key nutrients that unblock Street 1 are: vitamin B6; biotin; zinc; magnesium; vitamin B3; vitamin C.

> Evening primrose oil (EPO) supplementation increases skin hydration, smoothness and resilience, especially when used in conjunction with omega-3 and the six key nutrients.[5]

READER QUESTION

Q 'I've tried evening primrose oil and it didn't work. I took two capsules a day, like the manufacturer suggested, and my skin was still extremely dry. What am I doing wrong?'

A *The dosage was too low. If you have severe dry skin that is ageing fast and crying out for moisture then try evening primrose oil in **therapeutic** doses. I've never seen anything work so quickly and so dramatically at reversing dry skin and some signs of ageing. However, it can cause spots (as EPO also increases arachidonic acid in the body) – to prevent this from happening always use EPO in conjunction with omega-3 (see 'The Beautiful' for more on omega-3).*

Evening primrose oil supplementation is good for adults with severe dry skin, premature ageing and wrinkles, eczema and premenstrual syndrome (although EPO is not essential in the Anti-eczema Programme in Chapter 15).

Dosage: *Adults should take 5000–6000mg (5–6g) EPO per day, in divided doses (this equates to approximately 500–600mg of GLA at the end of the day). Check the information panel on your supplement to see how many grams are in each capsule. If each capsule contains 1000mg of evening primrose oil then you'll need to*

take two capsules with breakfast, two with lunch and two with dinner. Have EPO
supplements with liquid, and for best results have EPO with a protein-containing
meal. See the caution box below.

CAUTION

EPO can make symptoms worse in a select few people. This reaction usually means
they have an omega-3 deficiency which prevents series 3 prostaglandins from
being made in the body. EPO actually *increases* AA in the body but this does not
occur if you have omega-3/EPA at the same time (for the relationship between
omega-3 and EPA see page 63, 'The benefits of omega-3'). Always have a daily
dose of omega-3 from foods such as ground flaxseeds, flaxseed oil or oily fish such
as salmon, sardines, trout, herring and mackerel as the EPA made from these
foods has been shown to help EPO relieve inflammation. Avoid taking EPO if you
are on phenothiazine drug therapy for schizophrenia. EPO can make drugs, such
as chlorpromazine and trifluoperperazine, less effective. If you're on any
medications see your doctor before using EPO.

The Bad!

You've met The Good but have you heard about The Bad? You may have these
troublemakers living in your street...

The thugs that may be vandalising your body right now are called leukotrienes
and thromboxanes. These substances can cause skin inflammation, constrict blood
vessels, trigger asthma attacks and increase feelings of pain so they're nasty fellas.

Leukotrienes are implicated in asthma attacks, atopic eczema/dermatitis,
psoriasis, arthritis and heart disease (atherosclerotic plaques).[6,7,8,9,10,11]
Thromboxanes are wanted for questioning for excessive constriction of blood
vessels and blood platelet aggregation, which can lead to cardiovascular
disease and pre-eclampsia during pregnancy.[12,13]

Where do leukotrienes and thromboxanes come from?

Leukotrienes and thromboxanes are made from arachidonic acid (AA), which
comes from saturated fats.[14] I call these fats 'The Bad,' but they're not all strictly bad.
Saturated fats are all right when eaten in moderation and if they are 'policed' with

foods that prevent the 'bad prostaglandins' from being made (see 'How do you stop "The Bad" from damaging your health?'). Your body can also make AA from omega-6 (polyunsaturated cooking oils, margarine, nuts and seeds).

AA comes from animal produce – food with eyes – including: beef (including liver and all offal, steak etc.); egg, especially the yolk; chicken; turkey; lamb; veal; tropical seafood; and dairy products including milk, cream, cheese and ice-cream. It is therefore best to limit these. And due to poor quality or extra high saturated fat content you need to avoid chicken and turkey skin, pork, cheap mince, hamburger mince patties (unless you make your own lean patties), fatty beef, wagyu; many desserts; and deep fried foods and margarine as they contain damaged trans fats that behave like saturated fats in the body.

Case study

A 25-year-old woman came to me because she was concerned about her infertility, irregular periods, fatigue and spots around the chin area. Her periods consisted of occasional spotting and no menses for about ten weeks. Her diet for the past 17 weeks had consisted of an egg white omelette or a protein shake for breakfast, fish or chicken with salad for lunch and red meat and vegetables for dinner, occasional fruit, protein bars and coffee. She later confessed to being on a high protein, low carb diet. She was taken off this low carb diet and put on the Healthy Skin Diet. After a week her energy levels improved and six weeks later her periods returned to normal and her spots cleared.

How do you stop 'The Bad' from damaging your health?

Certain foods can help to protect your health from the damaging effects of 'bad' fats and these include: onion, garlic, ginger, turmeric, flavonoids from high fruit and vegetable intake, vitamin E, selenium, carotenes (from brightly coloured fruit and veg such as carrots), and EPA from salmon, trout, sardines, herring and mackerel (and fish oil supplements).[15,16,17,18,19,20,21]

Scientists have found that therapeutic amounts of EPA can inhibit the substances that cause inflammation and blood vessel constriction so it might be worthwhile whipping up a salmon stir-fry tonight.[22] Make sure you include plenty of red onion, garlic, ginger and greens, or you could make a delicious trout or chickpea curry with turmeric, onion, garlic, ginger and carrots. It's also important to reduce saturated fat intake so you will need to temporarily avoid dairy products and reduce meat intake.

Calcium

READER QUESTION

Q 'If I need to avoid dairy products then how do I get my calcium and how much is enough?'

A *The Healthy Skin Diet is a **dairy-free programme** as dairy can cause inflammation in sensitive individuals. The fastest way to clear up acne, eczema, cellulite and age-related skin conditions is to remove milk and other dairy products from the diet. You can get calcium from other food sources (see 'Non-dairy calcium sources' below), however calcium supplementation may also be necessary if you are pregnant, breastfeeding, over the age of 40 or a child.*

- *Children with skin complaints should have 500mg of calcium daily for the duration of the Healthy Skin Diet.*

- *Adults with skin problems should have 800mg of calcium per day for the duration of the Healthy Skin Diet. Pregnant and breastfeeding women may need 1000mg of calcium daily.*

Note that calcium competes with skin-repairing nutrients such as zinc and copper, and too much calcium can cause iron deficiency so do not have calcium intake in excess of 1000mg per day until your skin condition improves. After your child's skin condition clears up they can have 800–1000mg of calcium per day.

Non-dairy calcium sources (Calcium amount is shown in brackets)

240ml (8 fl oz) fortified soya milk^ (300mg)

255g pink salmon* (543mg)

37g tin sardines w/bones (111mg)

255g rainbow trout* (219mg)

185g (7oz) refried beans (155mg)

150g (5½ oz) chickpeas/garbanzo (210mg)

145g (5oz) soya flour (180mg)

115g (4oz) soyabeans (edamame), cooked (90mg)

225g (8oz) yellow beans* (110mg)

2 tablespoons ground flaxseeds (80mg)

85g baked snapper (34mg)

220g (8oz) cooked kale (150mg)

170g (6oz) haricot beans (130mg)

150g (5½ oz) cooked broccoli (90mg)

3 teaspoons tahini (192mg)

150g (5½ oz) canned kidney beans (138mg)

2 tablespoons carob powder (56mg)[23]

^ fortified with calcium (look for soya milk that is organic and made from 'whole' soyabean, not soya isolate

* cooked (note tinned salmon with bones has a higher calcium content)

And The Beautiful

I've briefly mentioned omega-3 so let's find out where it comes from and why it's so beautiful.

Omega-3 is abundant in cold-water fish such as sardines, trout, salmon, mackerel and herring. Flaxseed oil and ground flaxseeds contain around 50 per cent omega-3 and lesser amounts are found in fresh walnuts and green leafy vegetables.

The benefits of omega-3

Omega-3 is beneficial in a number of ways. It converts to eicosapentaenoic acid (better known as EPA), which decreases inflammation and improves skin moisture.[24] Omega-3 also helps to normalise blood pressure and is beneficial for cardiovascular health, and it can reduce your risk of certain cancers.[25,26,27]

Fill out the following questionnaire to see if you have any signs of omega-3 deficiency.

Omega-3 questionnaire

Circle any of the following symptoms you experience three or more times per week:

weakness

growth impairment in childhood*   behavioural changes, hyperactivity

poor vision*, need to wear glasses   tingling sensations in arms/legs*

learning difficulties   dry skin[28,29]

poor coordination*

If you have circled three or more symptoms then you may have a deficiency in omega-3; however, please keep in mind that these symptoms can also be caused by other factors. If you or your child has any condition marked with an * you should let your doctor know.

You can also check to see if you have any conditions that may be helped by adding omega-3 foods to your diet. According to researchers, omega-3 can be beneficial in treating the following: high blood pressure*; high triglycerides, sticky platelets*; fluid retention*; mental deterioration*; slow metabolism*; retina/eye problems – inflammation/ischemia; risk of premature birth/low birth weight; Crohn's disease; asthma (however, current evidence is inconsistent); risk of stroke* (risk may decrease by 43 per cent); risk of death by heart disease* (risk may decrease by up to 38 per cent if fish is eaten weekly).[30,31,32,33,34] If you suspect you need to increase your omega-3 intake, eat oily fish two to three times a week and use freshly ground flaxseeds or fish oil supplements on the days you don't eat fish. Have approximately 2000mg of EPA/DHA per day for a therapeutic effect. Deficiency symptoms may take up to 12 weeks to reverse. As with the questionnaire, if you have any of the symptoms or diseases marked by an *, please see your doctor.

Omega-3 food sources

There are high amounts in flaxseeds and flaxseed oil, and lesser amounts in soyabeans (edamame), wheatgerm, walnuts, blackcurrant seed oil, brown and red algae and dark leafy green vegetables. (Omega-3 amount is shown in brackets.)

2 tablespoons flaxseeds (3500mg)

60g (2oz) walnuts (2200mg)

113g salmon (2000mg)

113g scallops* (1100mg)

113g halibut, baked (620mg)

2 omega-3 fortified eggs (1114mg)

115g (4oz) soyabeans (edamame)*
(700mg)

113g tofu (360mg)

150g (5½oz) squash (340mg)

150g (5½oz) cauliflower (210mg)

2 teaspoons cloves, ground (200mg)

2 teaspoons mustard seeds (200mg)

150g (5½oz) broccoli, steamed
(200mg)

75g (2½oz) kale (180mg)

75g (2½oz) cabbage* (170mg)

* An asterisk indicates the food is cooked. Note that omega-3 amount shown in brackets equates to less EPA/DHA content than the therapeutic amount.

Good food sources of EPA and DHA (omega-3 in its converted form)

100g Atlantic salmon
(1090–1830mg)*

100g fresh tuna (240–1280mg)*

100g herring (1710–1810mg)*

100g sardines (980–1700mg)*

100g rainbow trout (840–980mg)*

100g mackerel (340–1570mg)*

100g canned tuna in water, drained
(260–730mg)*

1 tablespoon flaxseed oil (850mg)

1 tablespoon flaxseeds, ground or
whole (220mg)

2 slices soya-flaxseed bread (180mg)

supplements/capsule (300–500mg)

* The range varies according to the region fish is sourced from, quality of storage, if fish skin was left intact and cooking method.

According to Udo Erasmus, author of *Fats that Heal, Fats that Kill,* in order to get the most health benefits from eating fish, choose fresh fish, avoid frying, and eat the fish skin as the skin contains much of the beneficial oils. The top tip is to steam fish whole so the oils are not destroyed by oxygen, light and high temperature. Erasmus says that after you've eaten oily, deep sea fish, it takes two to three weeks for the EPA and DHA to be useable in the body.[35]

Avoid the following omega-3 (EPA and DHA) sources

- White bread with added omega-3 – liquid 'invisible' omega-3 goes rancid when it's baked. It's best to choose grainy bread where you can see whole flaxseeds.

- Omega-3 margarines (which contain damaged trans fats) – you are better off having natural butter, fresh avocado or extra-virgin olive oil and leaving your omega-3 intake to more natural sources.

- Pre-ground flaxseeds and LSA (a mixture of ground flaxseeds, sunflower seeds and almonds) that is not refrigerated (they may be rancid even if shopkeepers store it in the fridge).

- Packaged walnuts (if they taste bitter or unpleasant do not eat them, ESPECIALLY if you are pregnant as the nuts may be rancid). Walnuts should taste mild and be pleasant to eat.

READER QUESTION

Q 'How do I take an omega-3 (EPA/DHA) supplement?'

A *You need to take any oil or omega-3 supplement with food, especially good quality protein because this is how lipids occur in nature. Good quality protein includes free-range eggs, antibiotic-free chicken, oily fish, seafood, lean meat, beans and lentils. Protein with your oil supplements guarantees better absorption. If you get negative digestive symptoms after taking fish oil then improve your digestion (as suggested in the previous chapter) and resume taking the fish oil two weeks later.*

How much omega-3 do adults need?

To avoid deficiency, your EPA + DHA dosage should be 600mg per day. However, if you're an adult with **acne, dandruff, dry skin, cellulite, eczema, psoriasis, rosacea or wrinkles and premature ageing**, take the following therapeutic dosage: 2000mg EPA/DHA per day* in divided doses – for example, have two capsules with breakfast, two with lunch and two with dinner (see notes and caution box below). On the days you eat fresh omega-3 rich fish you can skip taking an omega-3 supplement. Also, have 1 to 2 tablespoons of flaxseed oil per day (50 per cent is omega-3).

* Between 2000 and 4000mg EPA/DHA is needed for a therapeutic effect (adult dosage). You want a therapeutic effect so take the equivalent of 2000mg of EPA/DHA per day. For children's information see 'Children's Clear Skin Programme'.

CAUTION

Fish oil and flaxseed oil naturally thin the blood so avoid supplemental omega-3 if you are a haemophiliac, undergoing surgery or taking blood-thinning medications such as aspirin. If diarrhoea occurs from flaxseed oil then reduce the dosage.

Storage tips: Flaxseed oil goes rancid very easily. Only buy refrigerated flaxseed oil and choose one that's packaged in dark glass (not plastic). To keep it fresh always refrigerate the oil and use within five weeks. Flaxseed oil can be stored in the freezer to keep it fresh for longer. Heat damages flaxseed oil so never heat it or add to hot food. Whole flaxseeds are more heat resistant.

NOTE: 2000mg equals approximately six capsules per day. To check capsule amount see labelling: if a product says 180mg of DHA and 120mg of EPA per capsule then there is a total of 300mg of EPA/DHA in each capsule. 300mg x 6 capsules equals 1800mg of EPA/DHA so you need to also get omega-3 from food sources (such as dark leafy greens, flaxseed oil and ground flaxseeds).

READER QUESTION

Q   'Is olive oil good for me?'

A   Yes. Your humble bottle of olive oil is rich in omega-9 fats, but omega-9 isn't **essential** like omega-3 and -6 so you won't keel over if you don't have it. However this fragrant oil has many health benefits, especially the cold pressed 'extra-virgin' variety. Extra-virgin olive oil contains a phenolic antioxidant called hydroxytyrosol and this little compound is wonderful at protecting your DNA against deadly mutations. Extra-virgin olive oil also contains an unusually high amount of squalene, which has antioxidant properties that can reduce your risk of cancer.[36,37,38]

Did you know that when you barbecue or brown (or burn) meats, the charcoaled portion is full of cancer-promoting substances and scientists are now calling barbecued meats 'carcinogenic'? This sounds bad, however, scientists tested fried hamburger patties and discovered that cooking meat with extra-virgin olive oil **reduces** the amount of cancer-promoting compounds.[39] So extra-virgin olive oil can make your barbecued meats a little bit healthier! Keep in mind that extra-virgin olive oil can be damaged if it's cooked on high heat and you'll know it's forming trans fats if your oiled pan starts to smoke.

Don't skimp on quality by buying plain 'olive oil' as it won't protect your barbecued meats in quite the same way as extra-virgin olive oil. This is because most processed oils, during the refining process, have lost all the health goodies such as phenols and vitamin E.

Let's get practical

To get more omega-3 in your diet, eat deep sea/oily fish at least twice a week – and I don't mean a piddly little can of tuna either, I mean the fresh stuff that's packed full of EPA and DHA, so you may need to visit your local fish shop. Also, eat omega-3 fortified eggs that are free range or organic (rather than battery/caged chicken eggs), and have ground flaxseeds and flaxseed oil on a regular basis.

Omega-3 rich recipes in the recipe section of this book include Marinated Whole Steamed Trout; Salmon Steaks with Peas and Mash; Rainbow Trout with Honey Roasted Vegetables; Creamy Tuna and Mushroom Mornay; Smoked Salmon and Eggs; and Smoked Salmon and Avocado on Toast.

If you don't eat fish or you want to have some fish-free days you can add 2 tablespoons of flaxseeds to your breakfast cereal or use flaxseed oil in one of the skin drinks such as the Skin Firming Drink, Berry Beauty Smoothie, Flaxseed Lemon Drink and Pear Flaxseed Drink for Sensitive Skin. Flaxseed oil is a fantastic addition to homemade salad dressings. To get the most out of your high omega-3 diet, reduce the amount of saturated fats you eat.

When cooking meat, use a bit of extra-virgin olive oil to grease the hot plate or pan and after cooking use a paper towel to blot away excess oil and fat from the meat. One cooking-savvy scientist also suggests that we add 'rosemary extract' into our bottle of extra-virgin olive oil to help retain its anti-cancer properties during storage.[40]

Key points to remember

- The right fats can literally moisturise your skin from the inside out.
- The Good and The Beautiful are GLA (evening primrose oil), EPA, DHA (fish) and omega-3 (flaxseeds).
- Limit sugary, processed foods, saturated fats, dairy and stress as they are 'The Bad' (not so good for gorgeous, hydrated-looking skin).
- Have red meat less than twice a week and protein servings should be no bigger than the size of the palm of your hand (thickness-wise too).
- Avoid dairy products for the duration of the Healthy Skin Diet.
- Have 1 to 2 tablespoons of ground flaxseeds per day or 1 to 2 tablespoons of flaxseed oil (flaxseed oil contains more omega-3 than the ground seeds).
- Eat deep sea fish two to three times per week (trout and sardines are the best choices as they promote less acid production than the other omega-3 rich fish).
- Adults have approximately 2000mg of EPA/DHA per day for a therapeutic effect.
- Use extra-virgin olive oil when cooking.

Guideline No. 3: Eat less!

I must confess I have not followed this principle until recently. In fact, I did the complete opposite. I previously ate three whopping big main meals a day and had lots of snacks in between. My partner used to say 'You never stop eating!' And I used to suggest that clients eat lots of small meals throughout the day. This principle was designed to speed up their metabolism so they could eat lots of food and burn it off quicker. The well-worn theory being: if you *never* give your body the chance to be hungry, it will store less fat as there's no need for it to save fat if your body never experiences a hint of famine.

It's true; this method *does* speed up your metabolism; however, this popular nutritionist's theory is flawed. The problem with eating lots of meals to speed up your metabolism is that it also seems to speed up the ageing process. Scientists are *not* discovering 'eat more and live longer' or 'snack all day and look younger'. No wonder my skin was ageing rapidly; I was eating enough for two people!

On the other hand, there are hundreds of scientific studies that have produced the same results over and over again: eat less and live longer; eat less and delay the onset of ageing; eat less and reduce your risk of cancer.[1,2,3,4] One explanation is that eating less increases the production of anti-ageing hormones, such as melatonin.

Melatonin

Melatonin is a night-time hormone that is largely released during sleep. It's secreted by the pineal gland in the brain, and according to scientists melatonin exerts an antioxidant effect that helps to protect against DNA damage. This is important because your DNA gives instructions to your skin cells and damaged DNA can lead to age-related skin damage. Melatonin also stimulates production of an anti-ageing substance called glutathione peroxidase. There is also evidence that melatonin helps to strengthen the immune system and decrease feelings of stress.[5,6,7,8]

Children naturally have high levels of melatonin. However (and this is the bad news), as you age your body's ability to produce melatonin plummets. In fact, many scientists believe that a decline in night-time levels of melatonin not only occurs with age but also *contributes* to the physical symptoms of ageing such as wrinkles and changes in pigmentation.[9,10,11,12]

When your body doesn't produce enough melatonin the following can occur:

- the onset of ageing
- difficulty falling asleep at night
- waking up after eight hours' sleep feeling drowsy
- irregular periods
- early menopause.

Lower melatonin levels may also shorten your lifespan. Eek! Luckily scientists have discovered a way to influence how much melatonin is released as you get older. That's right, released from *your* body not from a pharmaceutically patented drug. So you can have good melatonin secretions at any age.

A study published in the *Journal of Clinical Endocrinology & Metabolism* showed how melatonin levels can be manipulated by diet. Scientists did a 12-year study on rhesus monkeys because these mammals have a dramatic drop in melatonin secretions as they age, just like humans. Forty-four monkeys were put on a calorie-restricted diet and they ate 30 per cent less food than the control group of 50 monkeys. The monkeys were categorised by age as either 'old' or 'adult'. This long-term study and many others like it found that the animals eating smaller portions of food were the ones who ended up with fantastic melatonin levels. In fact, the *old* monkeys eating less produced remarkably more melatonin than the *young* monkeys who ate bigger meals.[13]

Monkey and rat studies have found that **sensible calorie restriction** not only improves melatonin production in ageing animals, but also: reduces body fat (but we knew that already); lowers blood glucose levels; and best of all, delays and greatly reduces age-related problems and the risk of cancer.[14,15,16,17,18,19,20] And it's not just animal experiments that are showing dramatic results. Longer life and smoother skin in calorie-restricted humans has also been documented (read 'The village of long life' on page 85).

However don't get all excited and put yourself on a three-month calorie-restricted diet and then expect awesome melatonin levels and long life. You see, scientists have also noted that eating 30 per cent less food for *short periods of time* such as two to three months (the duration of most diets) does *not* improve your melatonin levels and it may only have a minor anti-cancer effect or none at all. They've found that you have to eat sensible amounts of food as *a way of life* to get a lowered risk of cancer or a significant melatonin boost and long-term anti-ageing rewards.

READER QUESTION

Q 'How do I eat 30 per cent less food all the time? Do I need to count calories for-ever?'

A *No! But if you already know how to calorie count, and you want to, then go ahead. However you should not count calories for more than a month (or at all!) as I believe it's a slow and arduous way to prepare food. In fact, it may put you off having a healthy lifestyle because it takes the fun out of mealtimes.*

For the easiest ways to reduce calorie intake, follow these two tips:

1. Use a standard sized dinner plate and fill half the plate with salad or cooked vegetables. The other half of your plate is for a small serving of protein (about the size and thickness as the palm of your hand) as well as a small serving of whole-grain carbohydrates. Don't overstuff this side of your plate!

- If you're an active male you will need to consume slightly more calories, but never eat more than what can comfortably fit on a standard sized dinner plate.

- *Avoid* going back for second servings.

- And if you want to lose weight, skip dessert.

2. If you're having a heavier meal such as pasta and meat then serve up a plate of food (dinner plate sized) and remove 30 per cent or approximately one-third of your meal (this isn't exactly 30 per cent but it's easy to calculate). You can add a side salad if you need more food to satisfy your hunger but don't have any more bolognese.

- Have approximately three dinner plates of food per day (minus the 30 per cent, or with 50 per cent of the plate consisting of vegetables).

- Make sure there are lots of greens on your plate as they're the most anti-ageing of all the veggies and they ensure your body is less acidic and more alkaline.

CAUTION

If you already eat like a sparrow then DO NOT cut your meals by a further 30 per cent. If you suffer from anorexia or bulimia, or only eat one small meal a day then you are doing yourself no favours: you will accelerate wrinkles and you could also get very sick. *Please don't mistake calorie restriction with starvation.* Starvation or *severe* calorie restriction harms your appearance and your health.

Q 'I'm overweight and I look disgusting. I know I should eat less – I've tried but I just don't have the willpower to exercise and say no to desserts. How do I stop sabotaging my weight loss routine?'

A *If you have poor willpower and sabotage your health routine then it's a sign you have programmemed yourself to fail. You can undo this with positive self-talk and self-confidence-building exercises (but they must be done daily and with enthusiasm). You also need to get an attitude of 'I've had enough, I deserve more!' Then you'll be ready to pursue your health goals.*

   *If you're an overeater also remember that food is **not** love. It's just fuel to give your body energy to live. Nothing more, nothing less. I know food can be a great comforter but it's better to comfort yourself with reassuring words. Positive, comforting words said by yourself will not give you any negative side effects – you can't gain weight from self praise. If you overeat then read Chapter 20, 'How to be beautiful', to find out how to prevent self-sabotage and poor willpower.*

   Now, you know to eat 30 per cent less food, but what types of foods should you be eating?

- good quality carbohydrates
- good quality protein
- more anti-ageing foods.

Eat good quality carbohydrates

Q 'What are carbs and are they bad for me? I keep reading conflicting information.'

A *Some carbohydrates are good for you and others (processed white flour products) are giving carbs a bad name, as they're not so good for you. Carbohydrates are basically food components such as sugars, starches and certain kinds of fibre. Carbohydrates can make food taste sweet. They are the natural sugar in fruit and the refined sugars added to junk food items such as soft drinks and cakes. Carbohydrates are also the starchy parts of potatoes, bread, pasta, rice and cereals. Vegetables, beans and pulses also contain carbs and dairy products contain milk sugar (lactose), which is a carbohydrate.[21]*

   Good quality wholegrains are essential for your health and vitality. Did you know that carbohydrate is the only source of fuel your brain can use? Your brain needs glucose that has been broken down from the carbohydrate portion of your food.

Without a slow and continual supply of glucose, your intellectual ability suffers, you can't concentrate as effectively, and your body goes into survival mode.[22] Your body then starts the arduous task of converting fats and protein into brain fuel. This makes you feel tired. If you have a good quality carbohydrate meal, your brain function returns to normal. Carbs can be your friend if you eat them in moderation and pick the ones that are good for you.

*This is probably familiar to you, but I want you to get to know the two types of carbs a bit better. These aren't the **official** names for the two categories, these are nicknames used to make it easier to remember carbohydrates' potential effects on your body. The first group is the 'Hit and Run' carbs and the second is the 'Commitment' carbs.*

Now the Hit and Run carb is here for a good time, not a long time. Take Mr Doughnut for instance – he wants to give your taste buds a moment of pleasure you'll never forget. He'll happily supply your brain with a hit of energy that will make you feel great in an instant, then he'll quickly get 'cold feet' and leave you to cope with an energy crash all by yourself. So you reach out for Mr Cake this time and hope that he'll be the one to make you feel satisfied; but yet another moment of pleasure comes and goes and now the energy he gave you is nowhere to be found (it's probably hiding on your thighs).

*There is yet another problem with the Hit and Run carbs: although they supply you with a glucose hit, many of them are very low in nutrients so your body can't utilise their glucose gift properly. So Mr Doughnut and Mr Cake both end up making **you** pay for all the nutrient 'extras' with your own vital body stores of vitamins and minerals. They steal your chromium (if you have any) and this mineral helps the glucose transfer into your cells. This produces a burst of energy but your chromium stores are getting more and more depleted and the energy is short lived. Yes, the Hit and Run carb is a lot like a con artist who offers you a moment of pleasure, then robs you blind while you're sleeping.*

The Hit and Run carbs

The Hit and Run carbs include:

doughnuts	white bread, Turkish bread
cakes, buns	wholemeal bread
biscuits	muffins, English muffins
pretzels, water biscuits	scones, crumpets, bagels
sauces	most white rice, especially jasmine rice
pastries, waffles	

rice/corn cakes, rice crackers (even the wholegrain ones)

potato, especially mashed

packet mix pancakes

chips, crisps

corn pasta, corn cakes

most breakfast cereals, including many corn and bran flake cereals

some breakfast bars

lollies, sweets, ice lollies

coffee

sports drinks[23]

As you can see, this is not a complete list. There are too many processed and packaged foods to name them all, however this will give you a good idea what to look out for.

The Hit and Run carbs are the food and drink products that have a high glycaemic index *and* don't supply enough nutrition for their utilisation in the body.
The Hit and Run carbs aren't good for the skin because they 'steal' many of the best nutrients that are needed for skin health.
Eating Hit and Run carbs can lead to skin complaints such as spots, rashes and signs of premature ageing.[24,25,26]

What do high GI and low GI mean?

The glycaemic index or 'GI' is a measure of how foods, specifically the carbohydrate content of food, affect our blood glucose levels (commonly called blood sugar). The fantastic research on the GI and 'glycaemic load' of foods has been really beneficial to the advancement of our health. Low GI foods fall in the range of 0–55, medium GI is 56–69, and high GI foods are above 70[27].

The Hit and Run carbs list is largely derived from the GI research available in the book *The New Glucose Revolution*. However, the Hit and Run list doesn't include some of the healthier high GI foods such as amaranth (97), dates (103), millet (71), parsnip (97), pumpkin (75), tapioca (70), watermelon (72), brown rice (66–80) because they supply an acceptable amount of goodness. (Yes, many of them bring along their own vitamins and minerals so they offer more than just glucose.)

READER QUESTION

Q 'Why are high GI foods so bad for me?'

A   High GI foods can be bad for you if you eat them every day or in excessive amounts. High GI foods give your pancreas a lot of work to do and, like all overworked organs (and people!), it can eventually malfunction. Over time your pancreas may begin to make mistakes in measuring how much insulin it needs to release.

This is not so disastrous at first ... your silly old pancreas starts dumping out too much insulin – or too many 'orders' – causing your blood sugar levels to drop so low that your brain is suddenly left without fuel. So you're left feeling lethargic. You may also feel confused, irritable and have weakened muscles. These are all signs of hypoglycaemia and in extreme cases where blood sugar levels drop dangerously low, loss of consciousness can result (hopefully you'll have a good quality grainy snack before this happens).

If your pancreas is healthy it'll respond to the changes in blood sugar levels by promptly releasing insulin into your bloodstream. If your pancreas is tired from making too many insulin 'orders' (from you eating Hit and Run carbs for too many years) then it may begin to make mistakes and you can end up with blood sugar disorders such as hypoglycaemia and type II diabetes.

Case study

A 27-year-old woman came to me suffering from recurring muscle weakness, mental fogginess, insatiable thirst not relieved by water, spots on her forehead, lethargy soon after eating (to the point of needing to lie down) and frequent colds and flu. I advised her to see a doctor for a glucose tolerance test, which showed she had hypoglycaemia (her blood sugar level dropped dramatically within 30 minutes of the glucose test). The woman was prescribed a chromium supplement that contained B vitamins and magnesium, and she was put on the Healthy Skin Diet. One week after commencing the new regime, her lethargy after meals ceased and thirst decreased, and she had clear skin by the fifth week.

Have no more than one Hit and Run snack/item per day. This means having only one coffee per day or two weak ones and ditch the white bread for 'nice guy' grainy bread.
Commit to choosing your carbs wisely!

The Commitment carbs

Enjoy the Commitment carbs, which include:

- most fruits, especially cherries, berries and apples
- avocado
- most vegetables
- wholegrains
- rolled oats
- basmati rice
- almonds
- brazil nuts (and other nuts)
- seeds, flaxseeds, pumpkin seeds etc.
- wheat pasta
- tomato-based pasta sauces
- hummus dip
- carob
- sushi
- beans
- honey, especially yellow box, stringy bark and red gum
- agave nectar (a natural sweetener)
- soya milk
- lentils, chickpeas[28]

You've met the Hit and Run carbs so now I'd like to introduce you to the Commitment carbs. Mr Commitment carb has a lot to offer: he's a strong, good looking and dependable guy with a healthy nutrient account. And he likes to take it slow. A Commitment carb such as Mr Wholegrain Bread takes his time because he can't be digested quickly and as a result he offers slow-release glucose for sustained energy. Your brain will just adore him!

You may recognise the Commitment carb as he often has a tough exterior – he's not all white and fluffy with no substance like Mr Hit and Run. The Commitment carb regularly comes with his own edible packaging and he may be naturally sweet and delicious. He's your fruits and vegetables, he's your grainy breads and some of the more natural low GI products available at your local supermarket.

> Commitment carbs keep your brain stimulated and supply slow-release fuel so you feel good for longer.
> Most high-protein foods such as meat, seafood and eggs have a GI rating of 0 as they contain little or no carbohydrate.[29]

Wholegrain carbohydrates supply *slow-release* glucose, for greater mental clarity and sustained energy. Wholegrains are also Commitment carbs because they supply their own carbohydrate-processing nutrients such as the B-group vitamins and chromium (so they're less likely to rob your supplies). However, be warned: product advertising regarding 'wholegrains' can be misleading. A cereal or bread product may claim to contain healthy wholegrains but **if you can't *see* the grainy bits then it's not wholegrain – it's wholemeal.**

More about chromium

READER QUESTION

Q 'I've heard chromium is good for me. Should I take a chromium supplement?'

A *Maybe ... This little mineral is so important for your health and wellbeing because it's the key to getting glucose into your cells. If you have chromium deficiency signs then you should take this supplement immediately as it is difficult to reverse these deficiency signs with diet alone.*

A nutritional deficiency in chromium may contribute to fatigue associated with low blood sugar as well as the opposite: high blood sugar and type II diabetes.

Chromium questionnaire

Circle any symptoms you experience on a regular basis (at least three times per week):

dizziness and irritability after several hours without food

acne/spots

anxiety

the need for frequent meals

cravings for sweets and carbohydrates

excessive hunger

excessive thirst

weakness in legs

fatigue

excessive sweating

ADD, ADHD

depression

If you have three or more deficiency symptoms then take a chromium supplement for the duration of the Healthy Skin Diet (eight weeks) and if symptoms persist, see your doctor because many of these symptoms relate to type II diabetes.

How much chromium do you need?

Adults require 120–200mcg (micrograms) of chromium per day according to the US Food and Drug Administration (no recommended dietary intake [RDI] has been set in the UK). You should get this from a variety of sources including supplementation and food intake.

Adults who are showing chromium deficiency signs should supplement their diet with 60 to 200mcg of chromium per day, especially when consuming carbohydrates. It is recommended that you take chromium with protein to help with its absorption. Those in the 12- to 15-year-old bracket who are showing chromium deficiency signs should take 30 to 50mcg of chromium per day.

Use chromium picolinate as it is easier for the body to absorb. I've found that not all chromium supplements have measurable benefits, however I have consistently seen positive results from a chromium supplement that contains a combination of chromium picolinate, chromic chloride, vitamins B1, B2, B3 (nicotinamide), B5, B6, B12, vitamin C, vitamin D3, folic acid, magnesium, manganese and zinc.

> **CAUTION**
>
> Do not take more than 250mcg of chromium per day as exceedingly high doses may inhibit insulin production.
> If you have insulin-dependent diabetes, seek advice from your doctor before supplementing with chromium as it alters blood sugar levels, which could be dangerous if combined with insulin drug therapy (insulin would need to be reduced if you were taking chromium but do this *only* with your doctor's supervision as this could be dangerous).

Good sources of chromium include (amount of chromium in brackets):

- 1 tablespoon brewers yeast (up to 60mcg)
- 28g wheat bran/germ (32.5mcg)
- 150g (5oz) broccoli (22mcg)
- 100g organic liver (42mcg)
- 65g (2oz) raw onion (12.4mcg)
- 120g (4oz) romaine lettuce (15.6mcg)
- 100g turkey meat (10.4mcg)
- 175g (6oz) raw tomato (9mcg)
- 240ml (8fl oz) grape juice (7.5mcg)
- 140g (5oz) cooked peas (6mcg)
- 1 teaspoon dried garlic (3mcg)
- 1 wholemeal English muffin (4mcg)[30]

Case study

A 70-year-old woman presented to me with elevated blood glucose levels (a reading of 6.3, which is bordering on high). She had been told by her doctor that she needed regular monitoring with blood tests every four months to see if these high readings were a precursor to type II diabetes. However I recommended she take a chromium supplement, which she took two or three times per day with food, for four months. Her diet stayed basically the same (as she ate vegetables and grainy bread already), but minus cakes and biscuits at morning tea and she stopped putting sugar in her coffee. Her doctor retested her blood sugar level four months later and her reading had reduced to 5.8 and was now within the normal range. Her doctor was amazed. Her twin sister also had slightly elevated blood glucose and she took the same chromium supplement; three months later the twin's blood glucose levels had also dropped 0.5. The twin sister had not changed her diet in any way.

Grains to include in your diet

The best grains to include in your diet include wholegrain breads (with a GI rating of 43–49), soya and flaxseed breads (36-50), grainy sourdough breads (48–54), rolled oats (42) (not instant oats), muesli (34–56), oat bran (55), pearl barley (25), brown rice (66–80), basmati rice (58), wholemeal rye, buckwheat (54) (not a true grain; gluten-free; rich in flavonoids) and millet (because it's alkalising).[31]

Gluten

Gluten is a protein found in grains such as wheat, rye, oats, spelt and barley. It is quite a useful protein because it provides elasticity and strength to bread dough so it helps bread to rise nicely. However, gluten can be hard to digest for some people especially if you were born with coeliac disease.

Coeliac (pronounced *seel*-ee-ak) disease is a medical condition where gluten damages the lining of your intestines.[32] If this occurs it makes it difficult for your body to absorb nutrients so you may experience nutritional deficiencies as well as symptoms such as bloating and skin rashes. If you have coeliac disease, eating something containing gluten, such as a humble sandwich, could leave you feeling anything from mildly tired and bloated to violently ill.

Gluten intolerance can cause a skin condition called dermatitis herpetiformis which has all sorts of annoying symptoms such as blistering skin, itchy rash, small lumps like insect bites and pink scaly patches of skin, or it may appear like hives.

Complete the following questionnaire to see if you have any common gluten-intolerance symptoms.

Coeliac disease questionnaire

Circle any of the following symptoms you experience three
or more times per week:

fatigue, muscle weakness

anaemia that doesn't respond
to treatment

stomach bloating, cramping,
flatulence

diarrhoea or constipation

nausea, vomiting

unexplained weight loss

Less common adult symptoms include:

easy bruising

ulcerations of mouth

infertility, miscarriages

muscle spasms

dermatitis herpetiformis
(as mentioned)

altered mental alertness

bone and joint pains

Common symptoms for children include:

stomach bloating, pain, flatulence

nausea, vomiting

diarrhoea or constipation

large, bulky, foul-smelling stools

poor weight gain

weight loss in older children

tiredness, irritability

anaemia[33]

If you have three or more symptoms then you should speak to your doctor about further testing for coeliac disease. If your results for coeliac disease come back negative, firstly celebrate and then check for gluten intolerance by taking gluten-containing foods out of your diet for one to two months (during the Healthy Skin Diet). Gluten-free recipes are included in Appendix 2. See if a gluten-free diet alleviates symptoms and then check if the negative reactions return after you resume eating wheat breads and pasta.

READER QUESTION

Q 'I've heard gluten is bad for your health. Should I avoid wheat and other gluten-containing products?'

A *Not necessarily. You shouldn't need to avoid gluten-containing products unless you have coeliac disease or symptoms associated with gluten intolerance (see the questionnaire above). If you had digestive symptoms that improve after taking gluten out of your diet, this would be a sign of gluten intolerance and you should continue* to eat gluten free. Gluten-free grains include rice, corn, amaranth, buckwheat, millet and quinoa.

Eat good quality protein

Protein is essential for your health. It's the major building material for muscles, blood, hair, nails and internal organs such as the brain. It's necessary for wound healing and vital for healthy skin. As I've said before, skin sags when you're protein deficient. If your diet lacks sufficient 'complete' protein, your body robs it from your muscles and other tissues. This can leave you with a poorly toned body, thin and brittle hair, and skin conditions that are slow to heal.

On the other hand, if you eat *too much* protein, the excess will either be converted to energy or stored in the body as fat. However, protein will only be converted to energy if there are no carbohydrates or fats available (your body's preferred energy source is carbs).

Do this quick test to see if you have any protein deficiency signs.

Protein questionnaire

Circle any symptom you experience on a regular basis
(three or more times per week):

slow wound healing

oedema (swollen
   hands/feet/abdomen)

wasting/shrinking muscle mass

sagging skin

anaemia

poor digestion

fatty liver (diagnosed by a doctor)

hair loss (not including hereditary
   baldness)

If you have circled or highlighted more than three symptoms then you may not be eating enough protein or you may not be digesting your food properly. If you have poor digestion, you can refer back to Guideline No. 1 as it's designed to improve your gastrointestinal health.

How much protein do you need per day?

Around 65 to 100g of cooked meat such as chicken will provide you with sufficient daily protein, as will two small lean chops, two slices of roast meat or half a breast fillet. An 80 to 120g serve of fish or two eggs will also give you enough protein.

220g of lentils, beans, chickpeas, split peas or soyabeans (edamame) served with carbohydrate will provide your daily protein needs as will 40g of almonds served with breakfast cereal.

Your basic source of food protein should come from produce such as fish, eggs, lean meats, beans and pulses and seeds. However, you need to be aware of the *quality* of protein you are choosing.

Choosing the right proteins

Chicken

Antibiotics are routinely added to the feed of caged and free-range chickens. They are partly used to prevent infections spreading (as the chickens are often in small, cramped cages or barns) and also to speed up a chicken's growth. When you eat this chicken some of the antibiotics may be passed on to you, and since antibiotics kill bacteria they can destroy the healthy bacteria in your gut lining. This may or may not be a problem for our health. However, routinely adding antibiotics to animal feed has long been criticised by doctors who believe that overuse of antibiotics is causing antibiotic-resistant bacteria strains and this will eventually be detrimental to our nation's health.

Don't be a confused consumer: chicken manufacturers will sometimes state on the packaging or advertising that they don't use *growth hormones* – these hormones have been banned so of course they aren't using them! But *antibiotics* are legal and they have a similar growth-promoting effect (and bigger chickens equate to fatter profits). So if a chicken manufacturer doesn't specifically advertise that their chicken is antibiotic-free then their product is likely to have them. However, don't panic: occasionally eating conventional chicken is all right; just keep it to a minimum. Organic poultry are raised free of antibiotics and some free-range chickens are advertised as being 'antibiotic-free' so they are the best choices if you are concerned.

Eggs

The quality of the eggs you choose is also important. Eggs from caged hens are often inferior as they have softer shells and paler yolks. Their shells are weaker because indoor-housed chickens fail to get vitamin D from sunshine and they don't get to roam around and peck in the grass and ingest mineral-rich soil. A paler yolk can indicate a poorer B-vitamin content and bright orange yolks are often seen in omega-3 fortified eggs. Signs that you are buying good-quality eggs include tough shells, bright yellow yolks and good egg white consistency (the whites should *not* be runny like water). Look for eggs that are free-range (or organic), antibiotic-free, and omega-3 enriched.

Red meat

Red meat is allowed on the Healthy Skin Diet as long as it's high quality *lean* meat. Lamb (with all the fat cut off) is the best choice as once digested it produces less acid than beef. Avoid wagyu, mince and ham that has been 'smoked' with nitrate chemicals, and don't eat deli meats as they're processed and usually contain preservatives.

As a general guide when eating red meat, have a portion the size and thickness of the palm of your hand. Stick to a maximum of two servings of red meat per week (lean lamb or organic liver). Liver must be organic only as the liver is the animal's chemical processing organ so it may be excessively high in pesticides if not organic.

Fish

Seafood, especially fish, is high in omega-3 fatty acids, protein, vitamins B12 and B6, and it's low in saturated fats. The Food Standards Agency tells us to eat at least two servings of fish each week, and seafood lovers who consume high omega-3 fish more than twice a week are less likely to suffer from eczema, psoriasis, heart disease and depression.

However, some fish is high in mercury and can therefore be harmful. Mercury occurs in nature; it also leaks into our waterways from industrial pollution and ends up in our seafood, especially the larger fish, which are higher up the food chain (they eat more food thus digesting more mercury from the ocean or waterways).

Avoid larger fish that are high in mercury, including flake (shark), large snapper, swordfish, broadbill, marlin, king mackerel, perch (orange roughy), barramundi, gemfish, ling, and larger tuna (albacore, southern bluefin).

Mercury poisoning occurs over the long term and symptoms include irritability, headaches and memory loss. Mercury toxicity can also cause infertility and miscarriages so if you're planning to have a baby, it's best to avoid high mercury fish. Unborn babies and small children are most at risk of mercury toxicity, so be aware of what you feed your children and avoid the fish listed if you are pregnant. For more information about mercury in fish, go to www.food.gov.uk/multimedia/faq/mercuryfish/.

The health authorities suggest if you eat a serving of high-mercury fish, then avoid eating all seafood for at least two weeks afterwards to counterbalance the effects.

The good news is you can safely enjoy omega-3 rich fish, such as salmon, trout, sardines and herring, which are low in mercury, as is the case with hake, bream, shrimp, flounder, prawns, lobster and oysters to name a few. And you can make a healthy snack with 95 grams of tinned tuna twice a week, as the tinned stuff is sourced from smaller sized tuna.

Vegetarian protein (for meat eaters as well)

When protein is digested properly, it's broken down into amino acids that the body uses to keep us looking and feeling good. There are approximately 22 amino acids needed by the body. Your body can make all but nine of these – these nine are called essential amino acids. It's your job to make sure you get these nine amino acids from your diet by *eating protein every day*. Vegetarian meals can be made higher in protein by combining several different types of vegetarian protein.

If you are a meat eater it's necessary to get protein from a variety of sources, especially vegetarian protein, in order to keep your prostaglandins balanced. There is a simple rule to follow to make second-class protein 'complete':

beans and pulses/seeds/nuts ✚ grains   ▬ complete protein

beans, green beans, peas, lentils   rice, oats, wheat, rye

tofu, tempeh, seeds, pumpkin seeds   barley, corn, amaranth

almonds, brazil nuts, soya   millet

Complete protein: meat such as lamb, beef, pork, chicken, seafood, eggs and dairy products.
Second-class protein (low in one or two essential amino acids): vegetarian sources such as soya and other beans, tofu, tempeh, peas, lentils, nuts and seeds such as flaxseeds, pumpkin seeds and sunflower seeds.

Weekly guide to protein intake

As a general guide when eating protein, have a portion the size and thickness of the palm of your hand. Have a maximum of two servings of red meat per week (lean lamb, beef, organic liver)*, and a maximum of two servings of white meat per week (such as skinless chicken). Eat two to three servings of seafood per week (at least one serve of omega-3 rich fish), and daily servings of vegetarian 'combined' protein.

Make sure you consume some sort of protein every day – preferably in two of your main meals.

* If you suffer with eczema, dermatitis, arthritis, asthma or heart disease then decrease your meat intake to once a week for the duration of the Healthy Skin Diet. If you're pregnant or breastfeeding, avoid fish high in mercury and consult with a nutritionist about protein intake (as you will need to increase it).

Eat MORE anti-ageing foods

Looking good is not all about eating less, you can also eat *more* foods that promote healthy collagen formation and smooth skin. The word collagen comes from the Greek term *kolla*, which means glue. This is because collagen is like the glue that keeps your skin together: if you cut your skin, collagen quickly repairs it with the help of a few other key nutrients. Collagen is an amazing protein structure in the skin that cross-links, so it is extra strong and durable – on a per weight basis collagen is nearly as strong as steel!

More than one-third of collagen is made up of the amino acid glycine, another third is proline and a small proportion consists of lysine and other amino acids. These amino acids are found in protein-containing foods such as fish, eggs, meats, beans, nuts and seeds. Lysine and proline also need co-factors vitamin C, iron and manganese to form strong collagen in the skin, and zinc is also necessary for collagen formation.[34,35,36] If you're deficient in vitamin C, iron, manganese, zinc, glycine or hyaluronan you increase your risk of premature ageing. However, don't get bogged down with remembering the nutrient names, just know that the Healthy Skin Diet is specially designed to be rich in all of them!

What is hyaluronan?

Hyaluronan, formerly known as hyaluronic acid, is the fluid that cushions your important organs like your heart and skin so it reduces the chance of damage to these areas. Hyaluronan is hydrophilic, which means it attracts water and it's also slippery, helping to lubricate your joints and without hyaluronan your body would ache as if you had arthritis.[37,38,39]

Hyaluronan is found in collagen and elastin and it has even been called 'the key to the fountain of youth' because studies have shown that hyaluronan can improve the appearance of wrinkles and assist with healing of scars, fractures, hernias, wounds and damaged cartilage and ligaments.[40,41,42]

Low levels of hyaluronan are associated with premature ageing, osteoarthritis, mitral valve prolapse, poor wound healing and connective tissue irregularities such as cellulite.[43,44] Your genes play a role in how much hyaluronan your body produces. And smoking cigarettes decreases the amount of hyaluronan in your body.[45]

The good news is that you can increase hyaluronan naturally by supplying its main building block glucosamine, which you may have heard of because it's a famous nutrient for treating arthritic joints. Glucosamine works to normalise cartilage and restore joint function (at least partially).[46] Magnesium is also needed to manufacture hyaluronan and studies have shown that deficiencies in zinc and magnesium contribute to skin abnormalities.[47,48]

It's thought that traditional societies who age well do so because their traditional diet, rich in root vegetables, supplies plenty of magnesium and zinc for hyaluronan production.[49]

The village of long life

A small Japanese village called Yuzurihara has been dubbed 'the village of long life' because there are ten times as many people living beyond the age of 85 than anywhere in America. Not only do they live longer but they're also famous for their smooth skin, thick hair and flexible joints, and it's rare to find a local who needs reading glasses according to one of their local doctors, Dr Komori, who has written at least five books about Yuzurihara. He attributes the villagers' good health and great skin to their starchy vegetable-based diet that is low in calories and high in skin-cushioning hyaluronan.[50] The local diet consists of root potatoes similar to sweet potato and white potatoes, buckwheat noodles, millet, rice, red onions, sweetfish and fermented soya that is high in plant oestrogens.[51]

Eat your way to beautiful skin

The Anti-ageing Broth is a liquid stock that contains many of the nutrients needed for healthy collagen production. But I'll be honest with you, this recipe is nothing new; for centuries broths have been prescribed for all sorts of ailments involving the connective tissue (collagen and elastin), including problems with the skin, joints, digestive tract, lungs, muscles and blood.

A well-made broth coats the gut lining, heals digestive complaints and helps you to digest your food better. It's rich in glycine (one of the main amino acids needed for your body to make its own supply of anti-ageing glutathione) and sulphur so it enhances liver detoxification and treats skin complaints such as pimples and eczema.[52] Broth also provides collagen, cartilage, connective tissue-producing amino acids, chondroitin sulfate and hyaluronan, so it lubricates joints (and is therefore suitable for arthritis sufferers). Broth made with chicken meat and bones makes a more flavoursome soup that contains cysteine. Cysteine reduces mucus in the body so it offers relief when you've got the sniffles.

But you've got to know how to make the broth correctly so it can be both a food and a 'medicine'. Broth is made by adding vegetables and bones (that have a little bit of meat, cartilage and tendons left on them) to a pot with plenty of water and then boiling the mixture. The good news is that broth is a really inexpensive meal as you can use a chicken carcass or fish bones left over from last night's meal, or lamb neck and other bits that the local butcher usually discards or sells cheaply. And you can add vegetable scraps such as carrot or sweet potato peel (the vegetable skin is where most of the goodness is).

The broth liquid is reduced during cooking and the longer it simmers, the richer the flavour and the more minerals and other goodies it accumulates. But there is a trick to increasing the mineral content of the broth and the next two steps cannot be skipped. The first tip is you need to *add a decent splash of vinegar to the water* before you begin cooking the bones. This is because vinegar is a weak acid that causes an acid-base chemical reaction; the minerals are the base and the vinegar helps to draw the minerals right out of the bones. The second step in making a therapeutic broth is to boil the bone and veggie liquid for a whole day, adding extra water if necessary so plenty of collagen and nutrients are extracted – this takes time and skimping on the cooking period will result in a broth that is low in minerals and lacking that fabulous broth flavour.

After cooking, strain out the vegetables and bones and when you do this you may want to grab a bone to check out how brittle it has become – it's amazing to see how easily it'll crumble in your fingertips from the loss of minerals. (Maybe chicken osteoporosis is only interesting if you're a kitchen nerd but if you want to look good you'll be pleased to know that you've made a broth that is rich in **calcium and phosphorus, magnesium, potassium, sulfate and fluoride** so the broth is really good for your skin, bones *and* teeth.[53]) See the recipe section for more information.

Let's get practical

Eating healthy food is a lot easier when you follow a diet that offers healthy alternatives so that when you're out with friends at a café you can still order from the menu. Instead of having a sandwich made with white bread, choose grainy or sourdough bread (which has a GI of around 43). These breads are readily available in big city cafés but I have to admit, you might be hard-pressed finding grain breads in small-town eateries and rural cafés. If this is the case then order lean protein such as tuna, skinless chicken, tofu or lean beef with your meal to lower the glycaemic load of your meal. Or better still, order fish and salad when you're out and only eat carbs when you're at home so you can always have your healthy wholegrains.

Combining vegetarian protein: If you eat a Thai dish of rice and vegetables, you may not get enough complete protein. However, if you order your stir-fry with cashew nuts and mange tout then you increase the amount of *usable* protein in your meal. If you have oats for breakfast, add soya or almond milk and ground flaxseeds to increase the protein content.

Key points to remember

- Eating less food increases your night-time melatonin levels, which promotes youthful skin and good quality sleep. Aim to eat 30 per cent less.

- For lunches and dinners: fill half your plate with salad or cooked vegetables as they are low in calories. The other half of your plate is for a moderate serve each of carbohydrate and protein.

- If you're eating a heavy meal (such as pasta and meat) only fill two-thirds of your plate, leaving one third of your plate empty. Better still, only put the pasta on half your plate and have a large side salad.

- Have approximately three (average sized) dinner plates of food each day.

- Snack less. Only have one snack break per day (however, if you have low blood sugar or if you're pregnant you will need two snack breaks per day). Have a supply of almonds and an apple on hand.

- Choose Commitment carbs such as grainy breads, brown rice and rolled oats.

- Have protein every day, in two of your main meals. As a general guide when eating animal protein, have a portion the size and thickness of the palm of your hand. If you're eating a vegetarian meal, you will need to eat *double* that amount in vegetarian (combined) protein.

- Vegetarian protein: beans and pulses/nuts/seeds + grains = complete protein.

- Eat less but don't starve yourself! Your food is your fuel, nothing more and nothing less.

Chapter 6

Guideline No. 4
Be a sleeping beauty

You may thrive on only a little, you may suffer insomnia and toss and turn all night or you might laze in bed all day and take the Sleeping Beauty thing way too far, but I'm sure you'll agree you feel better after a decent night's sleep.

Why is sleep so important?

During sleep, your body releases a whole series of hormones that control some significant functions in your body. One of the most vital hormones triggered by sleep is melatonin, which is secreted by the pineal gland in the brain. Light suppresses the release of melatonin and darkness stimulates it so sleeping at night in a darkened room increases your chances of optimal melatonin production. Melatonin is also made in tiny amounts during the day but it is the 'spike' or sharp increase in melatonin during night sleep that is most beneficial.

Why is melatonin so valuable?

As mentioned in Guideline No. 3, melatonin is essential for good health because it sets your circadian rhythms so your body knows when to sleep, and it helps you to wake up in the morning. Melatonin also influences female reproductive hormones and controls when menstruation begins, how long each period lasts for and it even decides when your menopause should begin. Melatonin also helps to preserve your youthful good looks.[1,2]

Children naturally have high levels of melatonin and as you age, your body's ability to produce melatonin plummets. When this happens you experience the physical symptoms of ageing, including anything from increased wrinkles, difficulty falling asleep at night and waking up in the morning feeling drowsy to having irregular periods or early menopause.

READER QUESTION

Q 'If melatonin inevitably decreases with age, why should getting enough sleep matter as you get older?'

A *As I mentioned before, scientists have discovered a way to influence how much melatonin is released as you age. You can have good melatonin secretions at any age if you simply eat fewer calories and get a good night's sleep on a regular basis. For more on this subject, take another look at Chapter 5.*

Insomnia

Getting a great night's sleep so your body has a better chance of producing a nice big surge of melatonin is all very well, but what if you can't doze off in the first place? Insomnia can be a nightmare (literally) and can affect your appearance in many ways. Sallow skin, bags under the eyes and tell-tale dark circles are just the beginning. Wound healing and skin cell renewal also happens at night so you could be missing out on precious skin rejuvenation time.

What causes insomnia?

Many things. If you're stressed about exams or fear you're not loved or live in an unsafe environment then of course you're going to have trouble sleeping. Maybe you've simply trained yourself to be nocturnal or you go to bed feeling worried that it will be another sleepless night (yes it will be). Substances can also affect your state – foods, drinks and drugs – so be careful what you pop into your mouth. Below are the most common reasons for not getting a good night's rest.

- Eating **acidic foods and drinks such as pork chops, sugar and alcohol** leads to acid storage in body tissues which can cause poor sleep.

- **Coffee, tea (including green tea) and cola soft drinks** can also cause insomnia because caffeine triggers the release of adrenaline which promotes alertness. Tea is less likely to cause problems.

- **Drugs** such as over-the-counter cold and flu decongestants, corticosteroids, antidepressants and bronchodilators used for asthma, as well as prescribed drugs and illegal narcotics can interfere with sleep.

- Habits such as **reading, working or watching TV in bed** train your subconscious mind to associate bedtime with activity rather than sleep.

- **Pain, fever and infections** can make it difficult to sleep.

- **Depression** alters REM (rapid eye movement) sleep – about 40 per cent of sufferers also have insomnia.

- **Trauma, grief and post traumatic stress syndrome** can affect your sleep.

- **Sleep apnoea** (associated with snoring) is known to interfere with a good night's sleep.

- **Reflux** also disrupts sleep.

- **Worry, anxiety and stress** are probably the most common causes of insomnia – they all trigger your body's 'fight or flight' nervous system which releases adrenaline and cortisol. These hormones prevent sleep and give you more zest to either run away from or confront your crisis (even if it's an imaginary one!).

- **Changes in altitude and long flights** lead to disrupted sleep patterns and result in jet lag.

- **Eating a big meal before bed** can lead to indigestion and poor sleep. The body also has difficulty digesting food during sleep so you're more likely to wake up throughout the night.[3,4] 'Don't dine after nine' is a good rule to follow.

Avoid foods and drinks that may inhibit sleep, including:

- **foods and drinks that form acids in the body** such as fruit juice, spirits, wine, beer, soft drink, chocolate, pork and vinegar;

- **spicy meals** before bedtime;

- **ice-cream and other sweet desserts** as they not only increase acidity but they also mess up your night-time blood sugar levels. You may initially fall asleep but as your blood sugar levels change, you may wake up in the middle of the night and not be able to resume sleeping;

- **too much food or alcohol** – you may feel like you're sleeping heavily after a binge but it will be poor quality sleep so you're more likely to wake up feeling lethargic;

- **caffeine,** which increases heart rate, breathing rate, speeds up the nervous system, affects blood sugar levels and triggers the release of stomach acids.[5]

Excellent sleeping habits

It's not just about night-time sleep; you have to start your day right ...

Get a dose of sunshine in the morning. A great night's sleep begins in the morning when you wake up. Choose a wake-up time and religiously stick to it (yes, even after a late night out) and then make sure you get 10 minutes of daylight before 10 a.m. This will help to reset your body clock so you're more likely to wake up feeling refreshed.[6]

Have an active and productive day. Do some vigorous exercise daily, preferably in the morning. Don't exercise too close to bedtime. Also make sure you complete at least two tasks on that imaginary to-do list. If you're worried about something, such as paperwork or tax, then do at least part of it immediately and then schedule time each day to get it completed. Worry and stress can cause insomnia so you need to show your subconscious mind that your problems are dealt with *during the day*. If you don't deal with them now, you'll end up being haunted by them when you should be sleeping. Remember, a dynamic, active day equals a restful night's sleep.

Have a night-time ritual. Either have a warm bath one hour before bed or wash and steam your face (fill a basin with very warm water, wet your cloth, wring and hold over your face for five to ten seconds. Repeat three times). When having a bath, add 1 cup of Epsom salts as they contain magnesium which relaxes your muscles.

Only use your bed for sleep or sex. Your bed is not an office, cinema or a place to read adventure novels. Yes, I know it's nice to lie in bed and read but if you can't sleep you need to strengthen your (subconscious) association between bed and sleep, not bed and reading or bed and TV. Bed is for sleep!

Avoid coffee and other stimulants after 3 p.m.

Don't toss and turn in bed for too long. If you can't sleep and you're in insomniac hell, *get out of bed*. If you've been trying to relax, think peaceful thoughts and breathe calmly and none of these has worked then it's better to get out of bed than to struggle and get frustrated. Your frustration will only keep you awake.

However, you may be getting out of bed *but* this is not the time to catch up on emails, do some paperwork or watch TV. Turning on the lights at 2 a.m. and doing any of these is useful only if you want to train your body for shiftwork. If you don't do shiftwork you *don't* want to associate 2 a.m. with activity.[7]

If you want to train your body to sleep properly you need to get out of bed, keep the lights off and go and sit in the dark. You can sit on the lounge or a cushion on the floor and just sit in an upright position and concentrate on your breathing until you feel sleepy.[8] Sounds hideous? Yes it is, especially if it's a chilly night and the heater's been switched off for hours. This is good. Your body will quickly associate night-time wakefulness as being totally painful. Your body doesn't like pain so it will do anything to avoid it. Eventually your body will link comfort with sleeping in your cosy bed. But in the meantime: no pain, no gain. Keep the lights off, sit in the dark, focus on breathing in and breathing out, get sleepy, then go back to your deliciously cosy bed.

Never overstimulate yourself before bedtime. Sure, it's good to have a productive day but don't overdo it too close to bedtime. Don't do vigorous exercise within three hours of bedtime, don't argue, don't watch tense or scary movies, don't read thrilling novels or watch exciting TV programmes as they can hype you up and this period before bed is the time to wind down and prepare for a restful night's sleep.

By the way ... you are *not* an insomniac. Ban the 'I' word: never label yourself an insomniac unless you really want to be one because you are what you say you are. This may sound a bit wacky but if you want to sleep eight hours a night and wake up refreshed then repeat it to yourself over and over again: I sleep eight hours a night and I wake up refreshed.[9] If you have trouble saying this with a straight face then try: Wouldn't it be nice if I slept eight hours a night and woke up refreshed? And remember to ban the 'I' word.

Let's get practical

Foods that promote a more restful night's sleep include tryptophan-containing foods. Tryptophan is an amino acid that the body uses to make serotonin and melatonin, which are sleep-inducing hormones. Tryptophan-rich foods include milk, cottage cheese and plain yoghurt. However, since the Healthy Skin Diet is dairy-free you can have other tryptophan-rich foods such as soyabean, seafood, turkey, wholegrains, beans, brown rice, hummus, lentils, hazelnuts, eggs and sunflower seeds. Half an hour before bed you could try a glass of warm soya milk with a teaspoon of honey or an hour or two before bed eat muesli with soya milk (up to 30g of muesli).

Key points to remember

- Adequate sleep is important for your skin's appearance.
- Get a ten-minute dose of direct sunlight before 10 a.m. each day to help set your body clock.
- Have an active and productive day.
- Have a night-time ritual that signifies sleep: warm bath, warm face cloth, etc.
- Bed is only for sleep or sex.
- Ban the 'I' word if you're an insomniac – you get eight hours sleep a night and you wake up refreshed.

Chapter 7

Guideline No. 5: Sweat for 15 minutes each day

Have you ever noticed what happens to a bucket of water when it has been left outside for a few weeks? It becomes mosquito infested and putrid. Leave it for a bit longer and slime may appear around the edges. Debris falls in and slowly rots; some microbes die while others excrete wastes, tainting the water. For water to be healthy it needs to have a filtering system; it needs to move – down rivers, through crevices and springs, and past rocks. Movement is nature's filter; it cleans and renews and energises.

It's a similar story with your body. If you're an active person, your lymphatic system and blood keep your body clean. This may not sound significant but this flow keeps you alive and makes it harder for bacteria to proliferate. On the other hand, if you're a couch potato, then your blood circulation relies heavily on your heart to pump it around the body.

Your lymphatic system, however, has no internal pump so without daily activity it will be sluggish and wastes are likely to accumulate at a rapid rate. Dead cells and bacteria produce toxins and these pile up to create an unhealthy internal environment – inside your body – as would rubbish on a footpath if the local council garbos went on strike.

READER QUESTION

Q 'What exactly is the lymphatic system?'

A *The lymphatic system is made up of organs and tissues that produce, store and transport white blood cells. These white blood cells are your 'immunity' cells as they fight infections and disease. The lymphatic system includes the thymus, spleen, bone marrow and lymph nodes. You may have noticed in the past when you've had an infection that two lumps in your neck (just below your jaw) swell up and feel tender or painful. These are lymph nodes.*

There is also a network of thin tubes linking the entire lymphatic system. These tubes branch out like blood vessels into all the tissues of the body. This enables your white blood cells to travel wherever they're needed.

Movement from activities such as power walking, running, cycling and swimming increases the circulation of your lymphatic fluids around the body and as you probably already know, good circulation is vital for healthy skin. A pumping circulation is necessary to carry nutrients and oxygen to your skin so wounds can be repaired and new skin cells can be formed.

On the other hand, poor circulation leaves your skin starved of nutrients, so it has fewer essential fatty acids, antioxidants and oxygen reaching your outer layer. Skin that is starving looks malnourished – it looks dry, cracked, dull and pasty or it heals at a snail's pace. It may also appear greyish (a sign of poor blood supply to the outer parts of the body) or fester with stagnant wastes that clog pores and form cysts. Rosacea, or facial flushing and enlarged facial blood vessels, can also occur as your blood vessels dilate to compensate for the poor oxygen supply to your skin. Exercise has been known to reverse conditions such as rosacea (see Chapter 18, 'Rosacea', for more information).

Exercise research

Scientific research into exercise has uncovered the following interesting facts:

- Scientists have found that exercise can cut the risk of developing skin cancer (well it certainly did for the lab mice they tested). The mice were exposed to UVB radiation over a period of 16 weeks. The sunbaking mice who did not exercise developed skin cancer at a rapid rate , while the sun-loving mice who exercised developed fewer incidences of cancer or took much longer to develop skin cancer.[1] However you still should use sun protection even if you exercise religiously, as exercise does *not* guarantee a cancer-free life.

- Moderate exercise burns up the body's fat stores, which leaves less fat available for inflammatory response (inflammation causes eczema, arthritis, asthma etc.).

- Moderate exercise decreases blood levels of arachidonic acid, an acid from meat and dairy which increases inflammation.[2]

- Excess glucose in the blood can damage blood vessels (as seen in diabetes) and exercise reduces blood glucose levels.

The benefits of exercise

You may be the type of person who doesn't worry about your risk of disease especially if you're in your teens or twenties. And I agree. It's better to not worry about what ifs, but that's no reason to get lazy now. So let's use the following positive benefits to motivate you to sweat.

- When you exercise, you release endorphins, which make you feel happy and relaxed.
- Runners can even experience 'runner's high' which feels absolutely amazing.
- Exercise also gives you energy and increased vitality, and don't underestimate the value of having vitality. People with 'spark' are more attractive to be around as they have more energy to give.
- And let's not forget that exercise is one of the best ways to keep your body looking trim, firm and terrific. It also helps to prevent cellulite and gives your skin a healthy glow so you can look hot more often than not.

What type of exercise should I do?

The kinds of activities you choose really depends on your abilities and tastes. For example, if you have a bad knee then you're not going to take up jogging. You may instead go to the gym and have a trainer design a programme that won't irritate your injury, but will make you sweat all the same. If you love tennis, you can include it in your regime but also choose at least one other type of moderate or high impact exercise.

Exercise options

Exercise falls into several categories, depending on how much sweat it produces and how much energy it burns:

Light energy burners

Light energy burners may not make you sweat enough to be beneficial, unless it's a hot day. Light energy burners include: walking (average pace without stopping), golf, table tennis, stretching, ten-pin bowling, leisurely game of tennis.

Moderate energy burners

Moderate energy burners may promote sweating. These include: fast walking, cycling, volleyball, cricket, horse riding, sailing, dancing, badminton, moderately paced tennis game, Pilates, yoga and aerobics. Household exercises include: vigorous sweeping, scrubbing, vacuuming, pushing a wheelbarrow, building work/lifting, clearing the garden. Slow swimming is also a moderate energy burner.

High energy burners

High energy burners make you sweat. These include: fast walking uphill or carrying a load, soft-sand walking (knees up, fast paced), soft-sand running, sprints, fast-paced yoga such as astanga, interval training, gymnastics, tennis (fast paced), ice skating, rollerskating, fast cycling, football, basketball, rowing (moderate pace), jogging (at a pace of more than 7 km/hr), weight training, squash (moderate pace). Household activities include: very heavy gardening, digging, chopping wood, very heavy building and lifting. Swimming (moderate pace) may not make you visibly sweat but it still counts.

Why is sweat so good for me?

Movement such as exercise causes perspiration which contains lysozyme, an enzyme that fights bacteria and flushes the nasty microbes from the surface of your skin.[3] Sweating also assists with removing waste products from your body so toxic build-up does not occur.

READER QUESTION

Q 'Why sweat for only 15 minutes a day?'

A *You can sweat for longer if you want to but I've set a 15-minute minimum for each day because you only need to briefly sweat to improve your skin health. And besides, from a psychological point of view, 15 minutes is 'do-able'. It doesn't require you give up an hour or two of your day. If you're busy, you have no excuse as it's 'only 15 minutes'. It's the time it takes to leisurely drink a cup of coffee; it's shorter than a TV sitcom and briefer than a phone call to Mum (but just as important). Yes, the 15 minutes you spend sweating daily will give you so much more than a coffee or TV programme ever will because sweat gives you your health.*

Your aim is to exercise four to five times a week – on the other days you can have a sauna, swim in salt water or do a body scrub while having a relaxing, warm bath.

Sweat ideas for busy people

- Do vigorous exercise such as star-jumps mixed with sprints around the house first thing in the morning, to help with bowel movements and clearing toxic build-up.

- Saunas and warm baths promote sweating and they are wonderfully relaxing.

- Swimming in salt water gets your lymphatic fluid moving and salt water is fantastic for healing blemishes and mild rashes (if you have sensitive skin you can rinse off the salt water afterwards and then moisturise).

- Buy a digital clock and a skipping rope and skip for 20 minutes a day. If you need to rest, do so for no longer than 40 seconds each time.

- Buy an aerobics DVD or a professional yoga video.

Exercise tips

- If you have injuries or any medical conditions, seek medical advice before taking up an exercise programme.

- Before exercising you should warm up with gentle stretching or walking.

- Running on hard surfaces such as concrete can hurt your back and knees, so run on softer surfaces like grass and sand. You should not experience sharp pain in any part of the body while exercising.

- Invest in a good quality pair of sports shoes that are suitable for your activities.

- Take care when exercising. Injuries will stop your fitness routine in its tracks, so listen to your body to prevent making a silly mistake.

- Talk to a personal trainer or an expert in the sport you wish to do and ask about tips to prevent injury and techniques to help you excel.

- Learning from a fitness expert is much better than learning from your mistakes and injuries!

- Keep your exercise routine *under two hours* a day – too much exercise can age you prematurely and increase inflammation in the body.

- Find 'incidental' ways to be active: walk up (or down) the escalators instead of standing still, take the stairs instead of the lift and park your car further away from your destination (especially if you're going to work and plan to be sitting down for much of the day).

What does an effective sweat programme look like?

Your exercise and sweat routine could be tailored any way you like: you could keep your routine the same and go jogging five days a week or you could spice it up with variety. The main thing is to *just do it*. Exercise on a regular basis. Grab your diary or planner and schedule in 15 minutes of sweating each day this week. Your aim is to sweat for 15 minutes daily, so you may need to exercise for 20 minutes to give yourself a chance to work up a sweat. Here is an example of an effective exercise routine:

Monday	20 minute cardio workout such as walk/run/sprint.
Incidental exercise	Take the stairs to work.
Tuesday	20–40 minutes of weight training, including core strength exercise (abdominal and back muscles).
Wednesday	Relaxation day: do deep breathing exercises for 5 to 10 minutes.
	Have a 20–30 minute warm bath and exfoliate your skin. You sweat in a warm bath!
Incidental exercise	Walk kids to school; walk up the escalators at the shops.
Thursday	Favourite sport such as dancing, football, netball, swimming.
Incidental exercise	Park car further away from work.
Friday	10 minutes of jogging, 1-minute sprints and 20 minutes' brisk walking (or 30 minutes' jogging with 1-minute sprints every five minutes).
Saturday	Relaxation day: do deep breathing exercises for 5 to 10 minutes.
	15-minute sauna followed by a shower and moisturiser.
Sunday	20-minute swim plus dry skin brushing and a warm bath.
Incidental exercise	Walk to local shop to get newspaper.

If you're a busy mum and find it hard to leave home (and your bub) then your exercise routine may look more like this:

Monday	20 minutes' skipping in the back garden (aim to skip for at least 5 minutes before having a brief break of less than 40 seconds, then continue).
Tuesday	Jog around the house for 20 minutes non-stop.

Wednesday	Walk to the park or shops pushing the pram (at least 20 minutes non-stop).
Thursday	Relaxation day: do deep breathing exercises; have a warm bath and exfoliate your skin.
Friday	Follow a yoga or aerobics DVD in your living room.
Saturday	Go for a long walk with your partner or a friend.
Sunday	Relaxation day: do deep breathing exercises; incidental walking or walk to the park; have a warm bath.

The 'sweat for 15 minutes' programme can be tailored any way you like so it suits your lifestyle. However, if you're truly unwell: rest, rest, rest. Then get back into your routine. A minor setback is never a reason to give up. You'll find that you will recover faster if you give yourself a day to recuperate and you'll more than likely retain some of your previous fitness so you *won't* have to start all over again.

Tip: After sweating, replace lost fluids straightaway. Have a glass of Green Water, mineral water or add a pinch of sea salt to a glass of water for instant hydration. See Chapter 3, 'Guideline No. 1', for more information.

Let's get practical

How to get started

1. Picture what you want. See yourself with beautiful skin and imagine how good you will look and feel.

2. Write a list of sports or activities you'd like to try. If you hate exercise and can't think of something you'd enjoy, ask yourself:

- What exercise *might* I enjoy if I was good at it?

- What sports would I like to be better at?

- I *must* exercise so what should I try first?

- What can I do to make exercise more enjoyable? This is a great question – asking this will help you successfully start your programme and if you come up with some good solutions you'll be more likely to stick to your new routine.

3. While it's fresh in your mind do something proactive today. For example:

- Grab the phone directory or get on the internet and look up your local sports centres, gyms or yoga classes (whatever you have in mind).

- Make that first phone call. Inquire about joining fees, timetables and personal trainers or coaches. If you can't afford a personal trainer every week then think about hiring one for three sessions only. That way you get an effective exercise programme and they can monitor you a few times to make sure you're doing the movements correctly so you don't injure yourself. Then you can continue on your own.

- You could also get some friends together and form an exercise group. And you may be able to negotiate a good deal with a personal trainer if you have enough people committed to getting fit.

- Go to your local park or beach early in the morning on weekends and see if there are any trainers conducting group sessions. This is a good way to pick an exercise coach as you get to see them in action (although always check their qualifications).

- Look for a personal trainer, or go to a Pilates class, to assist you with postural correction, which is essential before you begin training. Bad posture will increase your risk of injury and make it more difficult to breathe deeply and perform well.

- If you're a new mum you could inquire about group exercise classes especially designed for mums, where your child is minded as you exercise. Gyms often have childcare facilities that make it possible to exercise. Or simply put bub in the pram and walk to a hilly area; don't underestimate the sweat you'll produce as you push a stroller up a big hill.

- Go to your local sports shop and buy a skipping rope.

- Buy a yoga DVD and an exercise mat.

Key points to remember

- Your aim is to sweat for 15 minutes each day.

- You can sweat for longer if you want to but don't exercise for more than two hours as over-exercising can age you prematurely.

- Exercise four to five times a week; the other days you can sweat in a sauna or a warm bath.

- If you find yourself making excuses to skip exercising then remind yourself *you don't have to feel like exercising, you just have to do it!* And besides, you only have to do it for 15 minutes so even the busiest person can fit it in.

Chapter 8

Guideline No. 6: Have a good skin-care routine

You wouldn't wash your car with a chemical cleaner that damaged your car's paint job, would you? So why would you want to wash your skin with a product containing ingredients that may damage your skin? You wouldn't? Well, you might be surprised to learn that many skin products such as popular brand cleansers, commercial brand shampoos, bubble bath and dishwashing liquids contain ingredients that the scientific studies referred to in this chapter have deemed 'harmful to our skin' or 'not beneficial'.

You may wonder why, if these ingredients are so bad for your skin, are they in your beauty creams in the first place? Because they are cheap and increase the prettiness of a product. They make a cream smell nice or feel silky, or they make it bubble and foam. Can you believe it? Many skin-care ingredients do nothing for your own gorgeousness!

The name and shame file

Before you find out what's good for your skin, let's first look at additives that you *don't* want on your delicate skin.

Sodium lauryl sulfate (SLS)

Uses: A foaming detergent to make cleansing products bubble and an emulsifier that mixes oil and water so they don't separate.

Problems: *Scientific studies have shown over and over (and over) again that SLS penetrates the skin and damages the skin's protective barrier function. This damage can be seen under a microscope for up to four weeks after the use of SLS (and nine days by the naked eye). Products containing SLS create poor skin barrier function, causing excess water loss from the skin, making it easier for other chemicals, dust mites and bacteria to penetrate the skin.[1,2,3,4] SLS can cause reactions such as rashes, dandruff, hair loss and dry skin (and rebound oily skin and enlarged pores).[5]*

Products: SLS is found in foaming toiletries such as commercial toothpastes, shampoos, cleansers, hand wash and bubble bath. This stuff seems to be in just about everything that foams!

Avoid **all** sulfates. The following additives are similar versions of SLS and although they're milder, they can still cause minor irritations:

- sodium C14-16 olefin sulfate

- sodium laureth sulfate (SLES)

- TEA-lauryl sulfate.

Formaldehyde

This information covers formaldehyde and its derivatives imidazolidinyl urea and DMDM hydantoin.

Uses: Cosmetic and skin-care preservative so the product has a longer shelf life.

Problems: DMDM hydantoin releases formaldehyde, which can irritate the skin and trigger allergic reactions such as skin rashes and heart palpitations, and it may affect your breathing according to the Mayo Clinic (the renowned non-profit medical and research centre based in Minnesota). This additive can also aggravate asthma. DMDM hydantoin has caused birth defects in animal studies (keep in mind that this has not been proven in humans).

Products: Found in shampoos, liquid hand soap, hair products such as gel, cosmetics, nail polish and skin-care products such as body moisturiser.[6]

Mineral oil

Uses: Acts as a barrier to lock in moisture.

Problems: It reportedly coats the skin like cling-wrap so your skin can't release toxins (remember: the skin is a major eliminatory organ). Mineral oil is a cheap skin-care ingredient that interferes with the skin's natural immunity barrier and may increase premature ageing.[7] However, mineral oil is a low allergy oil that makes the skin feel softer (like most moisturisers do). Do not use if you have problem skin and avoid use at night to allow your skin to effectively eliminate wastes. It's also not suitable for babies' delicate skin.

Products: Mineral oil is found in cheap moisturisers and some baby oils.

Fragrance

There are up to 4000 varieties of fragrance, many synthetic.

Uses: To hide undesirable smells.

Problems: May aggravate hand eczema, cause skin irritation or dermatitis of the face. Fragrance may also trigger dizziness and hyper-pigmentation of the skin.[8] Synthetic fragrance is not suitable for children's products as it may cause hyperactivity and irritation. If you suffer from skin pigmentation then check to see if your skin cream or sunscreen contains 'fragrance' or 'parfum', as these ingredients can cause pigmentation.

Products: Unspecified fragrance is found in moisturisers, deodorants, cleansers, hair conditioners, shampoos (including some baby shampoos), perfumes, cosmetics and colognes.

Parabens

Including methylparaben and its derivatives butyl-, ethyl- and propylparaben

Uses: Methylparaben is a synthetic preservative/mould inhibiter.

Problems: Methylparaben can trigger skin and mouth irritation so this preservative certainly wasn't added to your beauty products to help you look good. Parabens in general are infamous because they have been detected in breast tumours. Studies have shown that parabens can mimic the action of the female hormone oestrogen and can drive the growth of human breast tumours.[9,10] An editorial published in the Journal of Applied Toxicology *brought up the point that little is known about the long-term side effects associated with low but consistent exposure to these oestrogenic preservatives.[11] We do know that oestrogen can influence the growth of breast cancer but it is unclear whether parabens, like methylparaben, have anything to do with triggering cancer. The evidence looks coincidental at present. But what experts do know is that thousands of beauty products contain parabens and these parabens can be rapidly absorbed into the skin, especially since many cosmetic preparations contain penetration enhancers.[12,13]*

Scientists also agree that parabens in underarm deodorants and other cosmetics should be investigated further as the findings in tumour samples seem to support the **hypothesis** *that there may be a link between parabens in beauty products and breast cancer.[14] Please note that there is no conclusive evidence that parabens are harmful to humans but more research is underway.*

Products: Parabens are used as a preservative in thousands of cosmetics, food and pharmaceutical products.[15] You'll see them on the ingredient list of exfoliating gels, cleansers, underarm deodorants, antiperspirants, cleansers and moisturisers.

Isopropyl alcohol (isopropanol)

Uses: An anti-bacterial solvent made from petroleum.

Problems: *Drying and irritating to the skin, it strips your skin's natural acid mantle making it vulnerable to bacteria and fungus. Can promote liver spots and pigmentation, and can irritate the eyes and skin.*

Products: *Found in shaving creams and other men's skin-care products such as toners. Not a common ingredient these days as irritation is common.*

DEA and MEA

This includes any ingredient with DEA or MEA in the name such as 'cocamide MEA'.

Uses: An emulsifier used to mix oil and water in products and a foaming agent to make products lather when rubbed.

Problems: *DEA can cause contact allergies such as skin rashes and this irritation can occur if a product has 2 per cent concentration of DEA.[16,17] Many skin-care manufacturers have removed DEA from their products since negative reports (involving cancer) were published by the National Toxicology Programme (NTP) in the U.S. way back in 1998, however some still use DEA! According to the 'Final Report on the Safety Assessment of Cocamide MEA', humans should not inhale MEA vapour as it's highly toxic. This means MEA shouldn't be used in aerosol products but MEA is still found in many topical skin-care products. It also recommended that 'cocamide MEA should not be used as an ingredient in cosmetic products in which N-nitroso compounds are formed'.[18] But how do you know which products form N-nitroso compounds? You can only trust that the product's manufacturers have ensured their products are compatible with MEA and don't chemically interact to make toxic by-products. And if your beauty product contains MEA then maybe you'd be wise to avoid using another product at the same time.*

Products: *Some shampoos still contain lauramide DEA and cocamide DEA. MEA is common in many commercial products such as shampoos.*

You don't need synthetic ingredients that are famous for causing skin irritations in your 'beauty' products, because there are many healthy ingredient alternatives available. See 'Fabulous skin-care ingredients' on the following page for more information.

READER QUESTION

Q **'I've heard that some skin-care ingredients are questionable, but do we even absorb them into our skin?'**

A *YES! As mentioned earlier, many skin-care products contain penetration enhancers. Also consider how nicotine patches work: you get a cigarette craving so you place a clear patch on your arm and nicotine is absorbed through the skin, travelling via your bloodstream until it reaches the nicotine receptor sites on your cells. Your nicotine craving is killed, not by inhaling cigarette smoke but from a patch located on the outside of your body. It's a similar story with birth control patches. A patch is placed on your skin, hormones are released into your bloodstream, this changes your hormonal balance and pregnancy is prevented (in most cases). These patches also expose you to about 60 per cent more oestrogen than the traditional birth control pill so they're very potent.*[19]

So is it reasonable to suggest that skin-care ingredients can be absorbed into your body and influence your health? Yes, of course it is.

Children are at higher risk of adverse effects from chemical products because they are small in weight and their bodies are developing at a rapid rate. If, after applying a skin-care product your skin tingles, feels tight or stings, it's being irritated.

Fabulous skin-care ingredients

According to Paula Begoun, author of *The Beauty Bible*, anti-irritants and anti-inflammatory ingredients can help *protect* the skin from pollution, sun exposure and irritating skin-care ingredients and make-up. These include:

allantoin	gingko biloba
aloe vera	glycyrrhetinic acid
bisabolol	grape seed extract
black tea	green tea
borage	licorice root
burdock root	oat extracts
chamomile	vitamin C
comfrey	white willow
coenzyme Q10	willow bark
dogwood	willowherb[20]
fireweed	

Let's look in further detail at some ingredients that are a must-have in your skin-care products:

Great ingredients in skin-care products

Ingredient	Uses and benefits
Almond oil/ sweet almond oil	**Uses:** Anti-bacterial, contains fatty acids and triglycerides to moisturise the skin. **Benefits:** Moisturising, soothes irritation and dryness. Doesn't clog pores so it's suitable for blemish-prone people.
Alpha hydroxy acid (AHA) and beta hydroxy acid (BHA)	**Uses:** Exfoliates, has an anti-ageing effect. Look for names such as 'glycolic acid', 'lactic acid' and 'malic acid' (at least 8 per cent concentration). BHA – look for 'salicylic acid' (at least 8 per cent concentration). Cosmetic physician Dr Van Huynh-Park says you can only get products containing more than 8 per cent AHA and BHA from a chemist/pharmacy or doctor's surgery. Most products sold in cosmetic department stores have only 4 per cent or less AHA/BHA. **Benefits:** AHAs and BHA improve skin texture by thinning the stratum corneum (via a type of acid exfoliation). They also increase collagen synthesis within the dermis and they don't damage the skin's barrier function.[21,22] **Problems:** They can make the skin temporarily peel, flake and look inflamed.
Apple cider vinegar	**Uses:** Disinfectant and mildly acidic. **Benefits:** The acid restores the skin's pH balance; does not strip the skin of its beneficial oils
Beta glucan	**Uses:** Antioxidant, anti-ageing, moisturising properties. **Benefits:** Extracted from the fermentation process of yeast, it assists in the reduction of wrinkles and helps with skin repair. **Problems:** It's a very expensive ingredient and from what I can tell, scientific evidence is limited.
Blackcurrant seed oil	**Uses:** Anti-inflammatory and moisturising properties. **Benefits:** Contains gamma linolenic acid

(GLA, as in evening primrose oil), making it anti-inflammatory and suitable for reducing skin inflammation, redness and irritation. A superb moisturiser.[23]

Calendula **Uses:** Anti-inflammatory, antiseptic and astringent. **Benefits:** Helps protect against bacteria such as staphylococcus. Contains carotenoids.[24] Reduces skin inflammation, helps with skin regeneration and healing, useful for rashes, varicose veins, and bruising.[25,26]

Carrot seed oil **Uses:** Moisturising properties, provides some free-radical protection. **Benefits:** Antioxidants help protect the skin from sun damage and premature wrinkles. Contains beta-carotene and provitamin A. Often used in natural sun care products.[27] Good for moisturising aged skin.

Chamomile **Uses:** Astringent, cleansing, anti-bacterial, anti-inflammatory. **Benefits:** Contains fatty acids, flavonoids and quercetin and rutin, which are anti-inflammatory.[28] Calms irritated skin, controls excess oiliness and acne.

Coconut oil **Uses:** Moisturising properties, anti-fungal/anti-microbial. **Benefits:** Contains capric acid which is anti-fungal, and lauric acid which is anti-microbial and found in your skin's sebum.[29] Protects the skin from microbes and dryness, a traditional and trusted moisturiser.[30]

Evening primrose oil **Uses:** Anti-inflammatory, as it contains gamma linolenic acid (GLA). **Benefits:** Nourishing and rich in essential fatty acids; protects against free-radical damage to the skin.

Green tea **Uses:** Anti-inflammatory, anti-cancer, rich in antioxidants that protect against free-radical damage. **Benefits:** Animal studies have found that when applied topically, green tea and green tea polyphenols can suppress some forms of UV-induced skin cancers. However, drinking the tea had an even stronger anti-cancer effect.[31,32] **Problems:** Some people are allergic to green tea.

Jojoba oil — **Uses:** humectant (protects skin from water loss), superior moisturising properties. **Benefits:** Hypoallergenic, contains wax esters and fatty acids. Restores skin's natural pH balance, won't block pores (non-comedogenic), similar to your skin's own sebum.[33]

Lecithin (derived from soya) — **Uses:** A natural emulsifier and humectant with moisturising properties. **Benefits:** Attracts moisture to the skin and works like a detergent to disperse oil, so it allows oily ingredients to mix with water-soluble ingredients for a smoother-looking product.

Olive oil (extra-virgin) — **Uses:** Moisturising properties, contains phenolic compounds that protect against free-radical damage. **Benefits:** The antioxidant hydroxytyrosol provides some protection against DNA damage and also contains high squalene concentration, vitamin E and carotenes.[34,35] Olive oil studies have found that topical application has an anti-cancer effect – it greatly reduces tumour frequency from UVB rays but doesn't eliminate risk of cancer from UVA rays.[36] **Problems:** Olive oil can be used on its own, straight from the bottle, however it may leave oily patches on clothes if too much is used.

Rosehip oil — **Uses:** Rich in antioxidants – rosehips are the richest source of vitamin C. Also has a natural vitamin A derivative (trans-retionoic acid), lycopene, carotenoids and essential fatty acids (EFAs)*. **Benefits:** EFAs help to maintain collagen and elastin fibres, and may slightly improve appearance of fine lines and wrinkles.[37] **Problems:** Some rosehip oil products are bleached and colourless so the carotenoids have been removed. Good quality rosehip oil should be a rich amber colour.

Sea buckthorn berry oil — **Uses:** Moisturising properties, antioxidant protection. Traditionally this oil was used for treatment of bruised and battered skin.[38] **Benefits:** High in antioxidants such as vitamins A, C and E. Anti-inflammatory. Unique 1:1 ratio of omega-3 and omega-6 oils*. Omega-3 and omega-6 are essential for healthy skin and antioxidants protect the skin from oxidation caused by UV exposure. Contains 35 per cent palmitoleic acid, a rare and valuable fatty acid which also happens to be a component of our skin's sebum; it supports cell tissues and wound healing, and protects against certain bacteria (known as 'gram-positive' bacteria).[39]

Shea butter   **Uses:** An excellent moisturiser, especially for very dry skin. **Benefits:** Contains fatty acids and natural UV factor. Moisturises dry, damaged and irritated skin, helps improve skin elasticity, healing of irritated skin and small wounds. **Problems:** Not suitable for oily/acne prone skin.

Vitamin A/retinol   **Uses:** A natural preservative.[40] Certain forms of vitamin A have a potent anti-ageing effect. Look for names such a as 'retinol' and 'tretinoin'*. **Benefits:** Topical retinoids, such as tretinoin, have been proven to prevent and repair sun-induced skin ageing, prevent loss of collagen, stimulate new collagen formation.[41] **Problems:** Retinol and tretinoin can irritate the skin, making you look like a sunburn victim with inflamed, red raw skin for up to a week. You need to use sun protection daily after vitamin A use.

Vitamin C (ascorbic acid)   **Uses:** Natural preservative and antioxidant. Some forms of vitamin C have an anti-ageing effect. Look for names such as 'L ascorbic acid' (at least 10-15 per cent concentration), 'ascorbyl palmitate', 'magnesium ascorbyl palmitate'*. **Benefits:** Increases elastin tissue growth and collagen production. Decreases UVA and UVB damage to the skin. **Problems:** May cause skin irritation in sensitive skin. Skin may be more sensitive to light after use so apply sunscreen daily.

Vitamin E (d–alpha tocopherol)	**Uses:** Natural preservative and antioxidant. **Benefits:** Helps protect your skin against sun damage and oxidation, protects against free-radical formation within your skin product. May improve circulation and aid new skin cell formation. **Problems:** 100 per cent vitamin E oil may cause browning of the skin if you use it over scars. Avoid synthetic vitamin E which is identifiable by 'dl' (dl-alpha tocopherol).
Xanthan gum	**Uses:** A natural emulsifier used to keep the texture of a skin-care product uniform and prevent separation.[42] **Benefits:** A healthy alternative to chemical emulsifiers.
Zinc oxide (in sunscreens)	**Uses:** Zinc oxide is a sunscreen ingredient. **Benefits:** Helps protect against sunburn; suitable for reducing skin pigmentation. Look for sunscreen that is 'broad spectrum' with an SPF factor above 20 (SPF 20+) and high zinc oxide content (above 12 per cent)*. **Problems:** Sunscreen can make some skin types look pasty; if this occurs you can use bronzer for a healthy glow. If you have very dry skin, zinc oxide may make your skin feel drier.

* Thanks to cosmetic physician Dr Van Huynh-Park from Concept Cosmetic Medicine (Sydney), and Snezna Kerekovic from Bellaboo (teenage skin care) for supplying ingredient information as indicated.

Sunscreen

Sunscreen should play a starring role in your long-term quest for younger looking skin. When going out in the sun, make sure you apply sunscreen to the parts of your body that age the fastest – your face, neck, décolletage and hands.

UVA rays from sun exposure and tanning beds penetrate the skin and cause free-radical damage that disrupts collagen and elastin fibres, and this leads to wrinkles. However, sunscreens don't adequately protect against UVA so it's necessary to also wear a hat. See 'Guideline No. 7: Become a hat person', for more information.

If choosing a non-zinc-based sunscreen look for one that is formulated for children or toddlers as these products are more likely to be fragrance free and lower in synthetic chemicals. And they are just as effective as adult sunscreens. Always reapply sunscreen every two hours, or after sweating or swimming.

Skin types

You also have to consider what condition your skin is in before you choose a beauty product. There are several basic skin conditions. Some experts call them skin 'types' such as oily, normal and dry, but your skin type can actually change to a more 'normal' condition if you eat the right foods and look after yourself mentally and physically.

- Normal skin: Feels supple and looks hydrated, is not overly sensitive and has even pigmentation. May occasionally get out of balance and have an oily T-zone (forehead, nose, chin), small breakouts or dry patches.

- Dry or mature skin: Has trouble staying hydrated, gets flaky, may peel or feel tight and dry. May have premature ageing or sun damage. Super dry skin requires a non-foaming cream cleanser, plus a heavier moisturiser or barrier cream to relieve discomfort, and regular exfoliation.

- Very dry skin: Nothing seems to soothe this skin type except a thick barrier cream and dietary changes. Weekly exfoliation is also recommended.

- Oily or impure skin: Oily, especially in the T-zone, enlarged or blocked pores, poor circulation, blemishes. Dietary changes are required to normalise skin. In the meantime use lighter-textured products, nothing heavy.

- Sensitive skin: Easily irritated by weather, skin-care products and food allergies. Red, inflamed skin, blotchy, patches of dryness, includes rosacea and eczema. Super-sensitive skin conditions require a basic skin-care routine, with plain cleansers and creams that contain little or no essential oils or harsh chemicals. Exfoliation may not be suitable.

- Combination skin: Oily T-zone (forehead, nose and chin) and normal cheeks. Prone to minor breakouts in T-zone, skin is slightly out of balance; use products that won't aggravate/block pores. Don't exfoliate as it may spread spots.

Choosing a cleanser

A cleanser is a type of skin product that is used to dislodge dirt, pollution and make-up. Some cleansers foam, others are thick and creamy with no bubbles, and some are soaps or soap-free bars. You apply the cleanser directly to your wet face or a damp cloth, wipe the cloth (or wet cotton balls) over your face and neck to remove residues, then wash off the remaining cleanser with water.

Many cleansers such as soaps, soap-free beauty bars and cleansers that are specifically formulated for *oily* skin, contain ingredients that strip the skin's natural oils. I call it the 'squeaky clean effect', as your skin feels tight and dry after use. However, too much of your sebum is cleansed away with these products and this is not ideal because you want some sebum on your skin. Sebum is your skin's best friend as it helps to protect your body from invading bacteria, wind and dry conditions.

If your skin feels tight and dry within a minute after cleansing then the product is too harsh. You *don't* want that 'squeaky clean' feeling. A good cleanser can remove dirt and pollution, and some excess oils, without stripping your skin of *all* of its protective sebum.

Case study

I've always had very dry skin and was only prone to spots during my teenage years. However, in my early thirties I bought a cleanser for oily skin by mistake. The first night I used the cleanser I noticed my skin felt tight and dry immediately afterwards so I applied moisturiser (as usual) and pretty soon my skin felt okay. However, within a week of using the cleanser that was supposed to help oily skin, I had developed oily skin; I broke out in spots and my pores became unusually large! My skin continued to feel unnaturally squeaky clean after cleansing. I threw away the product and bought a cleanser that didn't dry out my skin. My pores quickly returned to their normal size but it took about a month for my skin to normalise and stop getting spots.

Toners

I don't recommend using a toner for your skin as I haven't found any literature that states you *must* use a toner for healthy skin. Toners can often cause skin irritations so they should be particularly avoided if you have sensitive skin. Skip the toner in your beauty routine so you'll have extra money to buy a good antioxidant-rich moisturiser.

Moisturisers

It's important to choose a moisturiser that is right for your current skin type. The only exception is if you have oily, impure and acne prone skin – then you may not need a moisturiser at all or you could use a specific 'normalising' oil to help reduce excess sebum production.

If you have *extremely* sensitive skin then choose a moisturiser with plainer ingredients such as almond oil and steer clear of too many essential oils. Dry and very dry or mature skin needs a heavier moisturiser, especially in winter. Before purchasing a moisturiser check the full ingredient list and, if possible, test it on a patch of skin to see if any irritation occurs.

Make-up

Make-up can also have a place in your skin-care routine (though perhaps not if you're a man). For those who want to use it, it can be useful to cover up a stray blemish, highlight your gorgeous features or give the illusion of fabulous bone structure.

READER QUESTION

Q   'I've had my favourite eye shadows for years, in fact, I think they were originally Mum's from the 90s. Are they still okay to use?'

A   *The answer is a big fat NO! Make-up deteriorates over time. Bacteria from your fingers can contaminate make-up products and when you use them you may end up with adverse reactions such as rashes and bacterially infected blemishes. Hand-me-down make-up, no matter how pretty it is, should never be used in different decades. As a general rule, make-up should be replaced within three years after leaving the factory.*

Make-up use-by dates

Once you have opened a product:

*   Mascara can last for three to six months – it is easily contaminated because of the pumping action of the brush which can push bacteria to the bottom of the container.

*   Moisturiser can last for three to 12 months.

*   Foundation and concealer can last for 12 to 18 months.

*   Powder, eyeliner, lipstick and lip liner can last for about two years.

*   Blusher and eye shadow can last for one to two years.

When a product deteriorates, you may see a change in texture and consistency or it may smell off.

*   Natural products that are free of chemical preservatives (they use natural preservatives such as herbs), generally don't last as long. However, these products usually have package information advising how long they will last after opening.

- Wash make-up brushes and other applicators at least once a week to remove bacteria that can cause skin infections.

- Avoid sharing make-up, especially eye make-up products, as you can spread bacterial infections.

> ## Activity
> *Wash your make-up brushes and sponges today.*

Skin-care routine

Here is an example of a simple skin-care regime, suitable for most people. However, if you have acne, see Chapter 11, 'Acne', for a special skin-care routine.

Morning: Wash hands with a gentle hand wash to remove any bacteria, then rinse off with water. Fill a basin or large bowl with very warm water and splash your face four to six times. (If you cleansed your face the night before, then you don't strictly need to use a cleanser in the morning; in fact I think it's better to avoid over-cleaning your face so that your natural oils can work their magic. However, if you have oily and acne-prone skin you'll need to cleanse now.) You can also cleanse while having a shower.

After patting your skin dry, add a small amount of moisturiser to your finger-tips and *pat* it onto your skin, repeating if necessary until your entire face and neck is lightly covered with lotion. Use moisturisers sparingly. Blot skin with a tissue after applying if necessary. If you're going out in the sun today, apply sunscreen after moisturising.

You may notice that I recommend *patting* the moisturiser onto your skin rather than rubbing. This will help you to use much less product (saving you money and reducing wastage). It's also a more gentle way to handle the skin and this pressing motion helps to relax your facial muscles, which may reduce stress wrinkles.

Night: Wash your hands to remove any bacteria, then fill a basin or bowl with warm water and rinse your face, splashing water onto your face and neck several times. Apply your cleanser of choice – gently rub cleanser onto your face and neck. Then wet two cotton balls or a soft exfoliating cloth and gently wipe off the cleanser, pollution and make-up. Repeat if necessary. Rinse the cleanser off thoroughly with warm water. If you have dry and flaky skin then you may want to also exfoliate now (see 'How to exfoliate your face' on page 115). Apply a suitable moisturiser using patting motions on the face and neck.

Exfoliating your skin

Exfoliating scrubs are creams and gels that contain granules or beads. These microscopic beads 'polish' the skin as you rub them in a circular motion on your face and body. Exfoliating removes dead skin cells that tend to look flaky and dry so your skin will appear more smooth and hydrated after exfoliating. Your skin may be a little red afterwards, especially if you have sensitive skin, but this should only last about five minutes. The best time to exfoliate is at night-time before bed, as any skin redness will subside during sleep and you'll wake up with fresh, hydrated-looking skin.

It's not absolutely essential to exfoliate but if you have dry skin, flaky skin or wrinkles and premature ageing, then a granulated cream or a quick scrub will leave your skin looking and feeling softer and smoother. However, you must take care not to use harsh exfoliators that can scratch the delicate skin on your face. This facial scratching may be visible and unattractive so you really do need to exfoliate with care. Natural exfoliators with gentle ingredients can unfortunately do the most damage because they use natural abrasives such as crushed apricot kernels, which have sharp edges. Choose a facial exfoliator with spherical beads as they're the most gentle and effective. For the body you can use mitts, natural body scrubs or dry skin brushing.

Don't exfoliate your skin if you have acne or broken skin such as wounds, bites or rashes. Also, exfoliating may spread spots.

How to exfoliate your face

As mentioned above, you should use a cream or gel containing gentle spherical beads. After cleansing and rinsing your face with warm water, apply a pea-sized amount of exfoliator to your fingertips and softly rub in a circular motion onto your face and neck (use more exfoliator if necessary). Rinse with warm water. Pat skin dry, then moisturise.

Use an exfoliator once or twice a week or whenever you skin develops flaky patches.

How to use a body exfoliator

Have a quick shower. Then spread a generous amount of scrub onto your damp skin and massage it with circular motions. Start at the feet and work your way up towards the heart (this is also how you use the exfoliator mitts). Then exfoliate from your hands to your shoulders, your chest and as much of your back as possible (a dry-skin brush is useful for exfoliating the back). Rinse thoroughly with water (by showering) and then moisturise. Your body should feel deliciously soft!

A cheap way to exfoliate your body (but not your face) is to use exfoliating mitts or by dry-skin brushing with a long-handled body brush. If you're using an exfoliator mitt or glove (which feels rough like Velcro), wet the mitt first, then apply a natural body wash or gel to the mitt, then exfoliate your damp skin and rinse off the body wash.

You must know this!

Keep in mind that your skin-care routine should suit your lifestyle, your skin type and your budget. Don't ever stress yourself by spending too much money on skin creams, as stress ages you prematurely, which negates any positive effects a miracle cream may have. And besides, you just can't look your best when you're having a panic attack about your finances.

Activity

Check your current skin-care products – your moisturisers, cleanser and even your shampoo and conditioner – and see if you can spot any questionable ingredients.

Key points to remember

- Don't be fooled by product advertising. Check ingredient lists and test the product on your skin before purchase if possible.
- Avoid harmful ingredients such as sodium lauryl sulfate.
- Your skin type can change as your diet changes.
- Don't fuss too much with your skin. Look for 'Fabulous skin care ingredients' and have a gentle and effective skin-care regime.

Chapter 9

Guideline No. 7: Become a hat person

It's common knowledge that excess sun exposure can cause premature skin wrinkling but I read so many alarming statistics about sun damage that during the middle of researching this guideline, I went out and bought a hat even though I've always hated wearing them.[1,2] I have effectively become a hat person and now I wear one practically every day.

> ## Activity
> *Take a look at the skin on your bottom (I'm serious!). If you are in a public place this may have to wait, or alternatively you can look at any part of your body that has not had sun exposure. Is the skin that has never been 'sun kissed' in better condition that the sun exposed areas?*

Skin cancer

Another concern with excess sun exposure, especially if you tend to get sunburnt, is the increased risk of developing skin cancer. Skin cancer is the most common type of cancer in Australia and the United States, and the second most common in the UK. However, through increased medical research and more public awareness from widespread media coverage, skin cancers are being detected earlier so survival rates are remarkably high. This is great news.

According to Cancer Research UK, there are three main types of skin cancers. Melanoma is the most dangerous and results in the majority of deaths.[3]

Melanomas can appear as an existing spot or a new freckle or mole that changes colour, shape and size. Melanomas can also have irregular edges that may vary in colour. They can be found anywhere on the body – even places that have never seen sunlight!

Basal cell carcinomas are the most common but least dangerous type – they look like a lump or scaly patch that is red, pale or pearly and are commonly found on the upper parts of the body such as the head, neck and torso.

Squamous cell carcinomas aren't as deadly as melanomas but can multiply if not treated. They appear as a thickened, red spot that may easily bleed or ulcerate and occur on sun exposed parts of the body.[4]

Some alarming skin cancer facts:

- In the United Kingdom approximately 68,000 people are diagnosed with skin cancer each year, even though the sun is not as harsh in this part of the world.

- Approximately 1 million Americans are diagnosed with skin cancer each year, resulting in 1000 to 2000 deaths.[5]

- More than 382,000 Australians are diagnosed with skin cancer each year; of these cases, approximately 8800 have dangerous melanomas and about 1400 die.[6]

It's no surprise that people with pale skin who freckle and sunburn easily have a higher risk of developing skin cancer from UV radiation; but you may not know that people blessed with gorgeous chocolate skin (and truckloads of natural melanin protection) can still get skin cancer.

What is UV radiation?

UV radiation is basically invisible rays that come from the sun's energy. UV rays are also produced by artificial tanning beds and sun lamps. UV radiation (that reaches our atmosphere and us) is made up of UVA and UVB rays: UVB rays are more likely to cause basal and squamous cell cancers as well as sunburn (FYI: As a reminder, the 'B' in UVB stands for Burning).

UVA rays penetrate deeper into the skin and promote free radicals that age your skin prematurely, but scientists also suspect that UVA can indirectly lead to melanoma. (FYI: As a reminder, the 'A' in UVA stands for Ageing.) Note that sun beds, tanning booths and sun lamps give out higher doses of UVA radiation so they are *not* considered a safe alternative to sunbaking at the beach. The best tanning options are spray-on tans, tanning creams or just loving yourself the way you are.

UV radiation is increased by reflective surfaces such as sand, water, snow and ice, which is why it's easier to get sunburnt during your annual holidays to the snow or beach. UV rays can also penetrate through windows, windshields, clouds and thin clothing. A lifetime of sun exposure, with bouts of getting sunburnt, increases your risk of skin cancer but skin cancers sometimes appear in areas of the skin that are never exposed to UV light (yes, I mean that you can get skin cancers on your bottom). This indicates that UV exposure is not the sole cause of skin cancer. According to the latest research diet, lifestyle and genetics also play a role.[7]

How to decrease your risk of skin cancer

- Apply sunscreen and wear protective clothing and a hat (Remember the slogan: slip, slop, slap).

- Keep out of the sun (as much as humanly possible) between 10 a.m. and 3 p.m. If you need to be out, seek shade when you can. UV levels are at their highest at this time so avoid excess sun exposure during these hours.[8]

- Eat small meals. Don't overeat throughout the day (or night) and never binge. And consume foods that are rich in antioxidants and essential fatty acids.

- If you're stressed, implement relaxation techniques, such as deep breathing exercises, into your daily routine.

- Exercise.[9]

- Don't unnecessarily expose yourself to harsh chemicals because they create extra work for your body and chemicals can trigger mutations. To reduce your chemical load, use natural cleaning products and wash all fruits and vegetables before eating them (see Chapter 3, 'Guideline No. 1').

Caution

Please note that this section focuses on sun exposure and its effects; it is not designed to be prescriptive in any way. Therapeutic treatments for skin cancer should be prescribed by your doctor or skin cancer specialist.

Sunscreen

According to the scientific research, broad spectrum sunscreens offer good protection against UVB rays and can decrease the incidence of certain skin cancers. However, sunscreen's ability to protect against free-radical damage caused by UVA rays seems to be limited.[10]

Even though sunscreens have their faults, they still play an important role in protecting your skin against premature ageing. I've tested a lot of creams during my years of research and I've found that sunscreen is still the best topical treatment for minimising wrinkles.

There are a lot of unnecessary chemicals in cheap sunscreens so choose a hypoallergenic sunscreen formulated for babies or toddlers as they work just as well as the adult formulas and they're kinder to your skin. If you have uneven skin pigmentation, look for a sunscreen that has a high zinc oxide content (review

'Guideline No. 6: Have a good skin-care routine'). And always reapply sunscreen every two hours, or after sweating or swimming.

Clothing

Clothing such as a heavy cotton T-shirt and a wide-brimmed hat may not sound very sexy, but with a bit of styling you can look fab and also protect your delicate skin from cancerous spots. You also get bonus points because sun protection is your best defence against wrinkles and premature ageing. Become a 'hat person' today.

You must know this!

A little bit of sunlight is essential for your health. You need to have small exposures to sun on a regular basis so your skin can produce a form of vitamin D that helps your bones to stay strong. This is highlighted by the fact that children who are covered from head to toe with sunscreen and protective clothing can end up with rickets (causing deformed bones such as bowed legs). This is because their skin never gets a sensible dose of sun. Minimum UV exposure is the key here: about ten minutes of unfiltered sunshine directly on the skin will keep vitamin D deficiency away in healthy individuals. Get your ten minutes of vitamin D-producing sun exposure during the morning or afternoon, outside the hours of 10 a.m. to 3 p.m., when the sun is not too harsh.

Let's get practical

Skin self-examination

Early detection of skin cancer is essential. If you're lucky, someone else may notice a weird-looking spot on your body and mention it to you, but don't count on this happening. Take charge of your own health and regularly examine your skin for suspect moles and spots. You should also ask your partner (or your mum) to check your back, scalp and other areas that can be difficult to self-monitor. Don't be shy: this could save your life!

The best time to examine your skin is after having a shower or bath and during the day when there is plenty of natural light. Use a full-length mirror and a hand-held one so you can see where your moles, birthmarks and other spots are. Check how they look and feel. You may want to take photos of areas of the skin which have a large gathering of spots so you can record their appearance for future reference.[11]

During the skin self-examination you are looking for:

- new skin spots – a new mole that looks different to the other moles, such as a new red mole or dark-coloured mole or a new flesh-coloured firm bump;

- a flaky patch that may be slightly raised or a crusty sore that doesn't heal;

- a small lump which is pale, red or pearly in colour;

- any spot that has changed in size, colour or shape over a period of weeks or months. [12,13]

Check your skin from head to toe. Check your back, scalp, genitals, between your buttocks, between your toes, soles of your feet, toenails and fingernails. [14] Remember that the earlier you report suspect spots to your doctor, the more likely you will live a long and healthy life. Your doctor may do a biopsy to check if a spot is cancerous. You may also want to get a second opinion if you're concerned about the diagnosis. Don't be afraid to ask to be referred to a skin cancer specialist.

Activity
Buy hypoallergenic sunscreen and a hat, and use them daily – when you look in the mirror at age 50 you will be very thankful that you did.

Key points to remember

- Check your skin regularly for unusual spots, moles and freckles (or for any change to spots you already have) and get your skin checked by your doctor if you are unsure what to look for. You may want to check your skin on the first day of every month so you remember.

- Apply sunscreen, protective clothing and a hat if you're spending time in the sun.

- Try to keep out of the sun between 10 a.m. and 3 p.m.

- Avoid getting sunburnt at all costs – a tan is not worth sacrificing your precious skin or your life!

- Become a hat person and wear a hat when outdoors.

- Use a lightweight hypoallergenic sunscreen that is formulated for toddlers or bubs as they have less chemical additives.

- It's important to avoid sunburn, however it's also *essential* for your health to have small daily doses of sunshine. Ten minutes of sun exposure a day is recommended for healthy vitamin D production.

Chapter 10

Guideline No. 8: Relax and make peace with your body

When you relax, you feel good. You don't need a bunch of scientists to tell you this. However if you want to get technical, relaxation is vital for your health in general because it stimulates the 'rest and digest' part of your nervous system. The rest and digest nervous system, as the name suggests, allows you to have a good night's sleep and promotes good digestion. This is important for your skin health in particular because the nutrients extracted from your foods during digestion are necessary for skin repair and maintenance. If you have *poor* digestion then you'll also have decreased absorption of fat-soluble vitamins, which leads to dry, cracked skin and skin conditions such as eczema.

Conditions associated with stress

Stress and similar states such as anxiety, worry, fear and rage all stimulate the 'fight or flight' part of the nervous system, while preventing the release of digestive juices and hormones such as insulin. There's also a decrease in blood supply to your gut, liver and kidneys. This can also occur if you are a chronic shallow breather or running a marathon (physical stress). Your body, during these states, releases adrenaline and increases blood pressure. Chronic stress can result in conditions such as skin inflammation, constipation, insomnia, impotence, low sex drive, dry eyes, dry mouth and digestive complaints such as irritable bowel syndrome.

Relaxed states

On the other hand, relaxation, listening to relaxing music, deep breathing and calm thoughts promote the 'rest and digest' part of the nervous system. Having confidence in yourself, self-love, self-respect and acceptance also encourage relaxed feelings and can suppress the stress response.

Relaxation promotes:

- proper digestion

- good sleep/wake cycles (circadian rhythms)

- calm feelings

- healthy skin

- healthy sex drive

- lower blood pressure.

READER QUESTION

Q 'When I'm stressed I always get dermatitis on my hands; they become red, raw and peel, and it's really painful. Why does this occur?'

A *Stress can affect the skin so dramatically because it causes the release of cortisol hormones, which are associated with dry skin and premature ageing. Stress also blocks some key prostaglandins from being made. (Prostaglandins were discussed in Chapter 4, 'Guideline No. 2: Eat moisturising foods', so this should be familiar to you.) So you get red, hot inflammation in some form or another. Your genetic predisposition means this inflammation is expressed as dermatitis, while other people may get asthma, pimples or psoriasis during times of great stress.*

Chronic stress not only leads to bad skin, it can also make you more vulnerable to serious illnesses.

What is stress?

Stress is not easy to define because, as the saying goes, one person's stress is another's adventure. For example, an afternoon walk along the beach on the English south coast at Whitstable may be considered relaxing by many people. Some people drive for an hour through Sunday traffic to enjoy this walk. However, for others, the walkway might feel too crowded, it makes them feel self-conscious and they experience stress. They become more and more anxious as they have to dodge groups of people who may be blocking the pathway.

Other people may find the process of walking tedious, so they too can experience the biological effects of stress. Hassles or minor difficulties such as annoying drivers on the road, parking tickets and long bank queues may cause major stress for some people yet be a minor annoyance for others. But whether your stress is justified or not, your body cannot tell the difference and experiences a cascade of hormonal changes to help it cope with the 'emergency'. Is your body constantly in the 'fight' or 'run away' state?

Do the stress test below to see if you have any signs of chronic stress.

The Stress Test

	Yes	No
1. Do your shoulders rise up when you breathe in? (Stand in front of a mirror to check if you have shallow breathing.)	5	0
2. Is your sex drive currently lower than is normal for you?	5	0
3. Do you often feel lonely, anxious, misunderstood or isolated?	5	0
4. Do you lash out at others or do you often get angry or upset if things go wrong?	5	0
5. Does your weight fluctuate because of stress?	5	0
6. Do you dislike yourself or suffer from low self-esteem?	10	0
7. Do you worry about your job, income or debts, or are you bothered by daily hassles (bad drivers, bank queues, etc.)?	10	0
8. Are any of your relationships causing you stress?	10	0
9. Do you *need* to be around people to have fun, feel safe or pass the time/does spending time alone make you anxious?	10	0
10. Do you have a psychological disorder or take any medications for stress-related problems?	15	0
11. Have you suffered a major loss recently which caused grief?	20	0

Your score:_____ / 100

If you scored between 50 and 100 then you are likely to be highly stressed or have a decreased ability to relax. In this case, learning to calm your mind for a few moments daily would be a high priority for you. If your score was between 20 and 50 then you may experience moderate amounts of stress, and relaxation would be beneficial for your skin's health and your overall health. If you scored less than 20 then your stress levels are okay.

However, let's clear up something before you read any further: a bit of stress is okay, in fact it may even be good for you. A short burst of stress motivates you to study before exams and it can help you run away or 'fight' if there is real danger. It is the regular or 'chronic' stress that can be harmful to your skin and health in general. The solution is to switch off the stress response for a period of time each day.

How do you do this? You make time to relax. However it's not as simple as it appears. True relaxation is not just slumping on the couch and watching TV, you must also switch off your busy mind for a few moments and you can achieve this with the following ...

Relaxation

Effective ways to relax include: having a warm bath; listening to relaxing music; and deep breathing exercises.

If you want to have fabulous skin the most important thing to do is relax. Have as many relaxing moments as possible during your day. Have a warm bath and enjoy the sensations of the water. Play music that calms you, and breathe in a relaxed manner: in and out, in and out. Note though, that a deep, *tense* breath will not make you relax. A calm, long breath will.

If you are the type of person who makes time to relax and re-energise then it indicates you have a good level of self-love and respect for your health.

Activity

Have a warm bath tonight. For a relaxing bath add 1 cup of Epsom salts, 1 teaspoon of oil such as olive, coconut or almond oil, and five drops of lavender essential oil (caution: oil makes bath surfaces slippery so clean the bath with baking soda afterwards).

Case study

I tend to be a workaholic (and I'm a recovering perfectionist) so I'm usually very busy. However when I'm having one of those manic days and I hear myself saying 'I'll never make this deadline' (as I start to panic), I force myself to stop working. I effectively *ban* myself from continuing. I remind myself of this chapter (and the fact that a stressed person makes more mistakes and works less effectively), and I say to myself 'I'm not allowed to work until I calm down'. Then I'll reluctantly move away from my desk and take a few deep, slow breaths. I'll also either go and make myself a cup of black tea or dandelion tea, or I'll go for a walk outside for five minutes. Quite often this is the time when I come up with a good idea or a solution to a problem.

Make peace with your body

READER QUESTION

Q 'How could I possibly like myself when my skin is so disgusting?'

A *When you greatly dislike your looks, whether it's your skin, your waistline or a facial feature, you create an enormous amount of stress in your body. This is not good for you **and** it won't get you the skin you desire. You cannot hate yourself into* having gorgeous skin! It's just not possible. However, you can choose to like yourself, imperfections and all, while you learn how to create gorgeous skin ...

Making peace with your body is the most important step to getting better looking skin. When you accept yourself and praise yourself for your good qualities then you'll begin to realise you deserve better (better skin/job/lifestyle).

Another positive benefit of liking yourself faults and all is that your body releases endorphins that make you feel good. These chemicals are also released during exercise – it's often referred to as 'runner's high' – and happiness, laughter, smiling and warm hugs all cause the release of endorphins.

When feel-good endorphins are floating around in your system you are more likely to eat healthy food, exercise and breathe deeply. These are all healing activities that are great for the skin.

On the other hand, when you feel bad about your skin and berate yourself, you suppress the feel-good chemicals from being made in your body. As you deny yourself love and self-care you deny yourself endorphin pleasure. You also block healing from occurring so your skin conditions stay with you. It is a vicious cycle. If you focus on what you hate about yourself, such as your skin problems, then you inadvertently keep your skin looking bad.

It's **absurd** to think you can hate yourself into having beautiful skin.

Activity

Right now: stand up and go over to a mirror (take this book with you) and look at your reflection. Focus on a part of your skin that you're not happy with, such as a pimple or wrinkles. Then tell yourself out loud (or in your head, if there are people nearby), the following: 'My skin looks disgusting and I'm so ugly!'

Say it again and put lots of emotion into it. Screw up your face, frown and cross your arms for extra effect: 'My skin looks disgusting and I'm so ugly!'

Now, how bad do you feel? I can guarantee you don't feel good. This is the feeling of stress chemicals flooding into your bloodstream. Did you also feel a sinking feeling in your chest area? Self-hate literally hurts your heart.

Now change your focus and look at a part of your body that has beautiful skin. Then stand up tall, smile a big warm smile and say with enthusiasm: 'I have such beautiful skin!' Okay, I realise you may feel a bit silly doing this and it sounds like a sappy positive affirmation but it's purely an exercise to teach you a very valuable lesson.

Now say it again as if you mean it: 'I have such beautiful skin, I'm so lucky!'

> *Now use your whole body to show your excitement; stand up tall and smile even wider: 'My skin is so gorgeous, I'm so lucky!'*
>
> *How do you feel? If you did this activity with enthusiasm then you have just created an endorphin rush that is good for your whole body. So, what's the lesson? You **do** have control over how good you feel, even if only for a few fabulous seconds.*

Eight ways to feel good in an instant

If you're experiencing stress, anxiety or depression it can be impossible to just 'get happy'. You can't simply tell yourself to cheer up and suddenly you're better. And what if you've just gone bankrupt or your marriage has ended: how do you get an endorphin rush then? A long-term solution may be difficult to find but there are plenty of short-term ways to make yourself feel good. You can create your own natural endorphins with the following eight ideas.

1. Self-compliments

If you feel uncomfortable about praising yourself for every little thing you do right, then this activity is the one for you. And if you're the type of person who thinks it's better to wait and hope that you'll receive praise from someone else this activity should hopefully wake you up from your delusions.

In reality, it's no use waiting for someone else to lavish you with kind words. People may or may not oblige but, quite frankly, expecting a compliment from others is like trying to control the weather. You can't turn on the rain by command or force a person to be nice to you. However, self-compliments are always reliable. You can make them exactly what you want to hear and they are available at a moment's notice.

I have such gorgeous skin!

I am so lucky!

I look so good in this dress!

My eyebrows are the best!

I am so caring and generous!

I am so clever and fine and one of a kind!

You get the message (and the endorphin rush).

If you have trouble praising yourself, begin by listing your strengths on a piece of paper and then read them out aloud, with enthusiasm. You need to put energy and emotion into your words so you can feel the rush of positive chemicals. Doing a bland old affirmation won't make you feel much better. It is the *emotion* you attach to the compliments that will release healing endorphins.

Activity

*Grab a pen and piece of paper or your diary/planner and list your personal strengths. For example, if your sister is great at playing tennis and you are good at writing stories, **don't** pine about being a bad tennis player. Instead, praise your good fortune and talents as a writer. You may also be excellent at remembering song lyrics or people's names. List these and anything else you can think of. When you focus on your strengths and compliment yourself, it is **impossible** to feel anxious at the same time.*

2. Listen to your favourite music

Music can elevate your feelings in a split second. Play your favourite song, turn it up loud and relax for a few minutes. Choose your music wisely, however. If you tend to be depressed and negative, you may naturally gravitate to sad ballads or thrash music that resonates with your mood. You want to rise above your negative feelings so choose music that improves your feelings. If you have to do a task you find annoying, such as cleaning the house, then you can listen to music while you work to make the job more pleasant. You'll have great company and a few extra endorphins to boost your energy.

Activity

Play your favourite CD today. Stand up and look for this CD (or your iPod) right now and if you can't listen to a song right away, leave it in a prominent spot so you remember to listen later.

3. Engage in your favourite hobby

Is there an activity that always makes you feel good? Whether it is painting, kicking a ball, window shopping or designing shoes, you can elevate your mood with a positive activity that is either creative or involves movement. Steer clear of destructive hobbies like gambling, spending too much money and binge drinking as they can lead to problems with your finances and your health. You don't want an even bigger reason to be stressed. Choose something fun. Take football lessons, round up some friends and do a fun form of exercise or join a club.

4. Smile and laugh a lot

Smiling and a good old belly laugh instantly releases feel-good chemicals in your body – but how do you get more laughs into your day? The easiest way is to watch funny movies. Ditch the news, miss the dramas and skip the cat fights caught on camera and divert your attention to comedies. Do this daily and laughing will become second nature.

Smile when you are not laughing and you will continue to feel good. You don't even have to find anything to smile about as studies have found just the act of smiling a big, crinkle-eyed grin is enough to release endorphins. Smile and feel good in a flash.

> ## Activity
> *Pause from reading this book for a moment and smile for 30 seconds right now.*

5. Deep-breathing exercises

Increase your oxygen intake in an instant with deep-breathing exercises. Breathing exercises can also switch off your 'fight or flight' nervous system and change your body into 'rest and digest' mode *without* you having to suddenly change your view of the big, bad world. Learn how to relax with breathing exercises in Chapter 19, 'Beauty breathing'.

6. Gratitude

Some people appear to have everything – money, fame, good looks and a great house – but they're still not happy. I could name a few people in the tabloids right now who are rich and famous but they are destroying their lives with drugs and alcohol, and the next stop will be rehab (again). Why do people who appear to have everything still seem unhappy? According to happiness expert and motivational speaker Anthony Robbins, it's because they're not grateful.

He says, when you're grateful you feel rich. When you're ungrateful and looking at what's missing in your life, you feel poor and stressed and you end up doing crazy things to try to get 'that good feeling' back. A prime example is resorting to drugs, binge drinking and other addictions.[1] The quickest way to get health problems, bad skin and low energy is to focus on what you *don't* have in your life. It encourages you to make bad choices. When you put a spotlight on your problems, your negative feelings intensify and your judgement is clouded. It's okay to define a problem but it's important to focus on a solution or if there is nothing you can do to change a situation then to look for the 'lesson' or move on, rather than dwelling on what you cannot change.

When you *shift* your focus and list all the things you're grateful for, your positive feelings are magnified. Now you are less likely to eat junk food or binge and you'll be more likely to exercise and go to bed on time because you're more relaxed. It is not quite that simple, but this is a good start to being healthier and happier.

When you focus on the good things in your life and say a heartfelt thank you it's impossible to feel bad in that moment. This may only make you feel good for 60 seconds but that minute will be a beautiful one. Feel grateful for a few moments every day.

Activity

Grab your diary or planner and schedule in five minutes of gratitude each day. In fact, right now is a good time to list ten things you're grateful for. Here are some questions to get you started:

- *Are you grateful your home keeps you dry when it rains?*
- *Are you grateful you have a TV?*
- *Are you grateful for your loved ones? What are the specific things you appreciate about them?*

Now read out what you have written, with emotion and intensity (as if you mean it) and you will get an endorphin rush. For example:

- *I'm so grateful I have a roof over my head and I live in a beautiful house.*
- *I'm so lucky I get to eat delicious food.*
- *I am loved.*
- *I have a great family and I really appreciate everything they do. My mum is so wonderful because she is caring and kind, my dad loves me and my sister is such a ray of sunshine.*

*You don't have to only be grateful for what has actually happened; you can also elevate you mood by **imagining** that what you want has already occurred. Have fun with it.*

7. Observe beauty

Have you ever noticed how you feel when you appreciate a beautiful sunset or a pretty picture or anything you consider beautiful? You feel good. You can't help it because the appreciation of beauty causes a release of endorphins inside you.

On the other hand, if you view something you consider beautiful but then reject it or criticise it, you don't get any good feelings whatsoever. Say a beautiful woman (or man) walked into the room and you felt jealous or threatened. You would instantly feel tense, on guard or uncomfortable in some way as your body is flooded with stress hormones. You may call it fear, jealousy or an inferiority complex but they all cause the same internal disturbance. Jealousy is a quick way to suppress your good health and an instantaneous way to disregard your self-confidence!

If you want to feel good then don't reject beauty and the feel-good rush you receive from accepting it. Whether it is a beautiful person, a book, a painting, a view or a trinket, just observe it for a moment and be thankful that there is so much beauty in the world. As you observe beauty and accept and appreciate it, you feel good. Read Chapter 20, 'How to be beautiful,' for more information.

8. Throw a tantrum!

Anxiety can arise when you feel powerless. A quick remedy for feeling powerless is to throw a tantrum. This is usually more appropriate when you are alone. So take a moment to be by yourself and then stamp your feet and say to yourself 'I deserve better!' Look at the sky with determination and imagine you are yelling 'I deserve a promotion!' or 'I deserve to be treated with love and respect!' A power 'tantie', when enjoyed in private, can stop an anxiety attack in its tracks simply because it feels good to say what you really want. Say it with conviction and you will feel much better.

Can you relax and make peace with your body?

While it may not be possible to feel good all the time, it's fun to indulge in endorphin-creating activities so you can at least feel fantastic sometimes. The 'eight ways to feel good in an instant' really work. They're also scientifically valid but you don't need a researcher to tell you that gratitude and listening to the right music elevate your mood, because when you do them you *feel* good. You can feel the endorphin rush. You may not say 'Oooh, that endorphin rush was nice', but it has still occurred.

Key points to remember

- Relaxation helps you to digest your food properly and sleep better at night.
- A person who prioritises relaxation time is more likely to have great skin.
- A bit of stress in your life is okay; in fact it can be a good motivator.
- Chronic, long-term stress can lead to serious health issues.

- You can decrease your negative feelings of stress in an instant.

- If you are the type of person who makes time to relax and re-energise then it indicates you have a good level of self-love and respect for your health.

- Compliment yourself often (no one else need know, so do it with enthusiasm).

- Listen to your favourite music. Make sure it is relaxing and elevates your mood.

- Enjoy your favourite hobbies. Do at least one a week.

- Smile and laugh a lot. Watch funny movies or positive, uplifting TV programmes.

- Do deep breathing exercises (see Chapter 19, 'Beauty breathing').

- Be grateful for everything you currently possess. This makes you feel fabulous, even if it's only for a moment.

- Appreciate beauty; don't attack it.

- To unwind after a long day at work, have a relaxing warm bath.

Review of the Eight Guidelines for Healthy Skin

I hope you enjoyed the Eight Guidelines for Healthy Skin. As you implement each guideline into your life, expect that you are creating beautiful skin. Remember, it takes four to six weeks for new skin cells to form and come to the surface so it won't take very long to see positive results.

Let's quickly recount the guidelines so you know the main points to remember. You may notice that I have excluded what to avoid doing. This is because you don't want to focus on what *not* to do; you only need to remember what you *can* do to create gorgeous skin and long-term health and vitality.

Guideline No. 1: Think green and friendly

- Hydrate yourself with eight to ten glasses of fluids daily OR one to two bottles of Green Water.
- Eat alkalising foods daily: salad, cooked and raw vegetables, avocado, almonds, banana, and use fresh lemon, lime and apple cider vinegar.
- Eat two handfuls of dark leafy green vegetables every day.

Guideline No. 2: Eat moisturising foods

- Moisturising foods are the healthy fats, namely omega-3, EPA and DHA from oily fish and flaxseed, and GLA from sources such as evening primrose oil.
- Have 1 to 2 tablespoons of ground flaxseeds or flaxseed oil per day.
- Have 1 tablespoon of lecithin granules daily to help you digest the moisturising oils properly.
- Eat fish two to three times per week (trout and sardines are the best choices as they are lower in acid).
- If you have dry skin, psoriasis, rosacea, dandruff or wrinkles and premature ageing, take an omega-3 fish oil supplement or flaxseed oil if you're vegetarian.

Guideline No. 3: Eat less!

- Sensible calorie restriction (of no more than 30 per cent) promotes youthful skin and good quality sleep.
- For lunches and dinners: fill half your plate with salad or vegetables as they are low in calories. The other half of your plate is reserved for carbohydrates and protein.

- Have approximately three average-sized dinner plates of food each day.

- Choose 'Commitment carbs' – grainy or wholegrain breads, brown rice, rolled oats and wholemeal pasta.

- Have protein every day. As a general guide when eating animal protein, have a portion the size and thickness of the palm of your hand.

- Eat *more* foods that are great for the skin. From the recipe section of the book these include: Tasty Antioxidant Salad; Marinated Whole Steamed Trout; Anti-ageing Broth; Flaxseed Lemon Drink; Skin Firming Drink, etc.

- Eat less but don't starve yourself! Excessive dieting is bad for the skin so be sensible and never skip a meal. Your food is your fuel, nothing more and nothing less, and if you choose mostly healthy foods and eat a sensible amount, your body will look and feel great.

Guideline No. 4: Be a sleeping beauty

- Adequate sleep is essential for gorgeous skin.

- Get a ten-minute dose of direct daylight in the morning (before 10 a.m.) to help set your body clock and boost your vitamin D levels.

- Have a night-time ritual that signifies sleep: warm bath, warm face cloth, etc.

Guideline No. 5: Sweat for 15 minutes each day

- Your aim is to sweat for 15 minutes a day but you can sweat for longer if you want to (keep exercise under two hours).

Guideline No. 6: Have a good skin-care routine

- When choosing a beauty product, check the ingredient list and test the product on your skin.

Guideline No. 7: Become a hat person

- Wear a hat and apply sunscreen if you're spending time in the sun.

Guideline No. 8: Relax and make peace with your body

- A person who prioritises relaxation for a few moments each day is more likely to have great skin.

- Make peace with your body by complimenting yourself often.

Part 3

Specialised programmes

Chapter 11

Acne

Acne vulgaris can appear as tender red bumps, small white nodules, blackheads and deep, painful pus-filled cysts that can lead to scarring. The face, back, chest and shoulders are the major problem spots and sufferers can experience embarrassment, poor self-esteem, anxiety and depression as a result of their appearance.[1,2,3,4]

According to studies, acne has been clinically diagnosed in children as young as four years old; and as many as 93 per cent of students aged between 16 and 18 years can experience acne, with one in four of these students also having acne scars. However, acne is not just reserved for the young: approximately 13 per cent of Australian adults experience some form of acne vulgaris.[5,6] In the United States, approximately 85 per cent of 12- to 24-year-olds have acne.[7]

Suffering from a serious skin condition can be depressing. It can cause social phobias, missed employment opportunities and, if not treated, in very severe cases it can lead to suicidal tendencies. In the *Journal of Paediatrics and Child Health*, a study was conducted on 10,000 high school students in New Zealand and the results showed a strong link between severe skin problems and depression and suicide. The findings were very disturbing: one in three teenagers with severe acne had suicidal thoughts and more than one in ten had tried to kill themselves.[8]

Many people turn to drug therapies to treat their acne. However, treating acne with medications can not only be ineffective but also a potential health hazard with all sorts of side effects such as severe depression. The drug Accutane (also known as Roaccutane, and with the generic name isotretinoin) is often prescribed for chronic acne; however the US Food and Drug Administration ranks it as one of the top ten drugs that can *cause* depression and lead to suicide attempts.[9]

Antibiotics are often prescribed for acne vulgaris as they suppress acne-related bacterial infections (known as propionibacterium acnes). Antibiotics can be ineffective, however, due to emerging antibiotic-resistant strains.[10] Antibiotics also wipe out the good gut bacteria that are necessary for a healthy gastrointestinal tract, and negative side effects, such as candida albicans (a yeast infection), and future skin problems can result. So, as you can see drugs are clearly not the answer.

Management plan

Acne can be treated effectively with *natural* methods that are not only good for your entire body but also free of harmful side effects. Step one is the management plan and step two is the Anti-acne Programme, which teaches you the true cause of acne and offers scientific ways to prevent your skin from breaking out. For your convenience, this whole programme has been divided into five steps.

Let's assess what may be contributing to your acne problem. Do you relate to any of the following factors that contribute to acne?

- poor diet
- high dairy product consumption
- hormonal changes
- oral contraceptives
- steroid medications
- trauma and emotional stress
- overuse of cosmetics
- irritation from tight clothing
- harsh cleansers and soaps.

What can aggravate acne?

- harsh cleansing of skin and using the wrong skin products
- scrubbing or exfoliating your skin
- touching your face with unclean hands (bacteria on hands).

Step one: Have a suitable skin-care routine

If you have acne you need an extra gentle skin-care routine. You want to soothe the inflammation, minimise bacteria and keep your skin clean without stripping all of its protective oils. When choosing a skin product for acne remember the following:

- Avoid using overly drying cleansers and soaps – if your face feels 'squeaky clean' or overly dry immediately after cleansing then this product is wrong for you.
- Avoid irritating ingredients such as sodium lauryl sulfate (unfortunately this

synthetic foaming agent is in most cleansers).

- Read Chapter 8, 'Guideline No. 6' for information on suitable cleansers and ingredients.

How to cleanse acne-prone skin

1. Unwashed hands may harbour bacteria so you need to clean them before touching your face. After washing your hands thoroughly, fill a small basin with warm water.

2. Splash your face with water and apply to your fingertips, one to two pea-sized drops of cleanser. Gently apply cleanser to your face and neck.

3. You can use an exfoliating cleansing cloth (one specifically for acne) to remove the cleanser or you can wet two cotton balls/pads, wring them out and then gently wipe off the cleanser with them. You may need to repeat this process to remove make-up and excess oils.

4. Rinse your face with water at least six times to thoroughly remove cleanser.

5. Softly pat dry your skin with a clean towel.

Do you use toners on acne-prone skin?

No. See 'Guideline No 6: Have a good skin-care routine', for more information.

Do you moisturise acne-prone skin?

If you're not using any medicated treatments for your acne and if your skin is excessively oily then you may not need a moisturiser at all. However, if you want to normalise your skin, a good moisturiser, with the right ingredients, can help you do this. According to Dr Hauschka Skin Care, acne sufferers can use a 'normalising' oil or skin product during the day and skip the moisturiser at night. Wearing no face product at night allows the skin to remove metabolic wastes as you sleep.

Look for moisturisers containing the following ingredients:

- sweet almond oil
- apricot kernel oil
- chamomile
- tea tree oil
- St John's Wort (hypericum perforatum)

- vitamin E, d-alpha tocopherol
- calendula
- neem oil
- jojoba seed oil
- sea buckthorn berry oil
- macadamia seed/nut oil
- alpha hydroxy acid (AHA)
- beta hydroxy acid (BHA).

AHA and BHA have an exfoliating effect that helps to remove dead skin cells without damaging the skin (see 'Guideline No. 6: Have a good skin-care routine').

How to apply moisturiser to acne-prone skin

1. If you have spots or inflamed skin then, after cleansing and drying your skin, apply a pea-sized amount of moisturiser to your fingertips.

2. Apply moisturiser to your acne-free skin first, to limit the risk of cross contamination. Pat moisturiser lightly onto your skin.

3. Then apply it to the rest of your face and neck. Repeat the process if necessary.

4. If you have applied too much moisturiser, blot with a tissue (however, using the patting method should help prevent excess application of skin-care products and minimise the risk of blocking pores).

Do you apply sunscreen on acne-prone skin?

This is a tough one ... Applying sunscreen over acne or on acne-prone skin can often make it worse or cause new breakouts. If this is true for you, then I suggest you become a hat person. It's so important to protect your sensitive acne-ravaged skin from UV rays as excess sun exposure may contribute to acne scarring. Once your skin normalises (after the Healthy Skin Diet), you may find that you can use sunscreen without suffering any negative reactions.

When you have acne, light moisturisers that also contain an SPF factor are less likely to trigger breakouts than sunscreen products. Do a patch test first.

Caution

If you're currently taking Roaccutane you may already know that it's absolutely vital to stay out of the sun or wear protective clothing such as a wide-brimmed hat, as the skin becomes highly sensitive to light. If you are taking this drug and concerned about the effects, then it's best to ask the advice of your doctor or specialist for more information.

READER QUESTION

Q   'How come I always get a spot just before I go out on a date and what can I do to clear it up quickly?'

A   *The universe seems to have a wacky unwritten law which states that you must get a spot before a hot date, school dance, formal occasion or much-anticipated night out. Special events can stir up stress chemicals in the body, which can trigger the appearance of a stray spot or three. If this occurs you may need to manage your stress a little better. Chapter 19, 'Beauty breathing' can give you techniques to help you relax without you having to suddenly get a new perspective or change how you react to the world around you. However, if the spot has already reared its ugly head you could try the following ...*

    Swim in salt water. Swimming in the sea has a reputation for clearing up spots. The natural salt water seems to initiate healing as if by magic. This is because salt water has mild anti-bacterial qualities and it's also alkaline, so it helps to normalise sebum production (your skin has an acid mantle but your blood and tissues should be slightly alkaline). If possible, go for a swim in the sea, dunking your whole body under the surface at least three times. Don't wash off the salt water for about half an hour after your swim, if at all. If you don't live near the sea, you can go swimming in a saltwater pool or make your own Saltwater Face Bath at home (see below).

Saltwater Face Bath

- Wash your hands and make sure your face is clean and free of make-up. Then fill a bowl with warm water, add ½ a cup of natural sea salt and mix until dissolved (to speed up the dissolving process, add the salt to a cup of boiling water, stir and disperse in lukewarm water).

- Splash your face with salt water or hold face under, on and off, for a few seconds each time. This should take about one minute, then wash off salt with fresh water and moisturise.

- You can re-use this salt bath twice. To re-heat it, just add some boiling water or *briefly* heat it up on your stove. Always test the temperature before use: it should be pleasant.

Other quick spot treatments include tea tree oil dabbed on the blemish, or products containing benzoyl peroxide or salicylic acid.

Studies have found that topical use of tea tree oil (at 5 per cent strength) can be an effective treatment for mild to moderate spots (but not severe acne). Tea tree oil has anti-inflammatory and broad spectrum antibacterial and antifungal properties.[11] Dab a tiny amount directly onto to your spot and allow it to dry. Do not moisturise over the top.

Benzoyl peroxide (BP) is a strong chemical ingredient used in commercial acne creams. BP works by destroying the bacteria associated with acne. It acts as an antiseptic and reduces the number of blocked pores. However, it is a very harsh ingredient that has temporary side effects such as mild to major skin dryness, severe irritation and redness.

Salicylic acid is a mild acid ingredient used in some over-the-counter acne treatments. It dissolves dead skin cells and helps to prevent clogged pores, whiteheads and blackheads. When using salicylic acid, don't use any other medicated creams containing BP or sulphur. Salicylic acid may sting on application and cause redness and irritation.

Natural antiseptics such as sweat and salt water can be just as effective as BP and salicylic acid when managing acne symptoms (and kinder to your face).

The Anti-acne Programme

Let's get stuck into the fantastic Anti-acne Programme that clears up blemished skin from the inside out. This programme addresses the true causes of acne and goes beyond treating the surface symptoms.

What causes acne?

I am sick of hearing 'There's no known cause for acne', 'Acne is *not* caused by diet' and 'Acne is caused by the sebaceous glands producing too much oil'. For starters, a lot *is* known about the causes of acne: acne *can* be caused by diet; some people do have breakouts after eating chocolate (or is it just me?); and the sebaceous glands are not the *cause* of acne – excess oil production is a *symptom* of something deeper happening in the body (or from something simple such as using the wrong cleanser to wash your skin).

Let's look at the basic *symptom* of acne, without confusing it with the cause. Acne is inflammation of the skin's oil glands. When you have acne, the glands grow unnaturally large and produce too much sebum, which appears oily. This oily layer then mixes with the skin's natural bacteria and dead skin cells and this liquid becomes thicker, like pancake batter, which blocks the skin's pores and leads to acne.

- Sebum is a mix of fats, proteins, cholesterol, salts and pheromones (FYI: pheromones are your sexual attraction hormones so you don't want to cleanse them away!).

- Sebum is your skin's best friend. It keeps the skin soft, prevents excessive water loss and helps inhibit bacteria growth on the skin.

- Sebum coats the surface of your hair to prevent it from becoming dry and brittle.[12]

Standard acne topical creams and cleansers treat the surface symptoms such as bacterial infection and excess sebum, but remember that these symptoms are never the *cause* of your acne; they have been triggered by something.

Step two: Help your liver remove excess hormones

Why aren't the skin's sebaceous glands behaving like normal glands? There are several reasons; one involves hormonal changes in the body. During puberty, a surge in hormones, such as androgenic or sex hormones, occurs. Boys and girls both have androgens such as testosterone but boys usually have more. These androgens tell your sebaceous glands how much oil to produce, and too many hormones give too many signals saying 'More oil, more oil!' so your oil glands grow bigger in order to fill the 'more oil' command. As I said before, this excess oil then mixes with dead skin cells and bacteria, and this blocks your pores.

Your hormones regulate most of your body functions – hormones dictate your growth cycles, sleep cycles, muscle production and how much fat you store or burn up. Androgenic hormones trigger the development of sex organs, they can initiate sex drive and increase muscle and bone mass (which is a good thing) so your hormones aren't the enemy.[13]
Women can break out with spots when menstruating because of a temporary increase in hormones.

But if all teenagers get a surge in hormones why do only some get acne? When a teenager's body is overflowing with excess androgens, their liver should quickly deactivate and remove excess hormones from the blood. So if your liver function is strong then you won't experience acne. However, if your liver is overworked from poor diet and not-so-good lifestyle habits then your blood stays loaded with toxins and hormones.

Adult acne

Hormone production should normalise by your early twenties but skin breakouts can still be experienced in adulthood. With adult acne you have fewer androgenic hormones being released but if your liver detoxification system isn't efficient then higher amounts of hormones remain in the blood, sending out the 'more oil' message to your oil glands. The liver's detoxification system slows down if it doesn't have enough of the right nutrients (helpers) to deactivate androgenic hormones. The right nutrients are supplied by healthy food so acne *can* be caused by poor diet along with several other key factors.

According to ARL Pathology, specialists in liver detoxification pathways, there are several key nutrients needed to safely remove sex (androgenic) hormones from your system. They are: essential fatty acids (especially omega-3/DHA/EPA); zinc; magnesium; vitamin B complex (this includes B1, B2, B3, B5, B6, biotin, folic acid, B12); and calcium saccharate (formerly known as calcium d-glucarate), which helps to remove excess oestrogens from the body (this is a specific type of calcium and other forms of calcium won't do the same task).[14]

Liver detoxification supplement

You can remove excess hormones from your body with a good liver detoxification product. If you're over the age of 15, look for a liver detoxification or cleansing supplement that contains zinc, magnesium, chromium, glycine, taurine, vitamin A, vitamin C, selenium and B vitamins (B1, B2, B3, B5, B6, biotin, folic acid and B12), milk thistle (St Mary's thistle/ silybum marianum). If you're female, also look for calcium saccharate in the ingredients list, however this nutrient is not available in most supplements. Take a liver detoxification supplement for two to four weeks.

CAUTION

Don't take a liver cleansing supplement or high-dose vitamin A if you're pregnant or breastfeeding. If you're pregnant, take a multivitamin/mineral supplement that is specific for pregnancy as it should contain the liver nutrients zinc, magnesium, vitamin C and B vitamins including folic acid/folate.

Step three: Control your oil production

Acne is synonymous with excess sebum but you can literally control how much oil your skin produces when you ingest nutrients that alter your prostaglandins. Prostaglandins are a lot like 'project managers' in the body – they transfer messages from your cells and they give these messages to your hormones so they can cause modifications in your body. Your prostaglandins alter sebaceous gland secretions so they control how much oil is produced in the skin.[15] Prostaglandins regulate hormones, inflammation, pain, temperature and fat metabolism.[16] 'Good' prostaglandins eliminate inflammation and promote clear skin, while 'bad' prostaglandins can promote inflammation and excess oil production.[17]

How do you get 'good' prostaglandins so your hormones get the right management? There are good and bad 'project managers' out there – you've probably heard at least one horror story about a bad builder who hired a dodgy plumber or botched the flooring on a home renovation. It's the same with your prostaglandins – some give out undesirable instructions to hormones so inflammation and skin breakouts occur. So, no doubt, you want to hire the 'good' prostaglandins to make your skin look as healthy as possible. You can do this simply by modifying your diet.

'Good' prostaglandins are made when you eat very specific healthy foods and have a balanced life, which includes relaxation and learning how to cope with daily stress. 'Bad' prostaglandins are manufactured by the body from foods containing saturated fats, fried foods (which have damaged fats or trans fats). Stress, anxiety and high GI foods (such as pastries and other white flour products) also trigger a reaction that causes the production of 'bad' prostaglandins (see Chapter 4, 'Guideline No. 2' for more information).

Omega-3

It's not always possible to eat a perfect diet and be relaxed and stress-free but you can begin to be healthy by eating the main ingredient for good prostaglandins – an essential fatty acid called omega-3. Omega-3 was discussed in more detail in Chapter 4, 'Guideline No. 2', but here are the basics again:

- Unsaturated fatty acids such as omega-3 are anti-inflammatory.
- Omega-3 provides anti-bacterial substances for healthy sebum production.[18]
- Omega-3 has to be converted to EPA and DHA in the body, which are then used to make the good prostaglandins and beautiful skin.
- EPA and DHA are readily available in fish and fish oil supplements.

If you're eating fish such as salmon, trout or sardines at least twice a week and having flaxseeds or flaxseed oil then you should be getting enough omega-3 from your diet. However, if you don't eat enough fish or flaxseeds, or if you have poor digestion, you may not be getting enough omega-3 so you should consider taking an essential fatty acid supplement. Refer to Chapter 4, 'Guideline No. 2', for more details on omega-3 and correct dosages.

Zinc

Zinc is another nutrient vital for acne-free skin. Zinc helps to convert the fats found in nuts and seeds (omega-6) into good prostaglandins. Zinc is needed to manufacture (and release) many hormones, including the sex hormones, insulin and growth hormones. Oil gland activity is also regulated by zinc so zinc supplementation is very specific for treating acne.

Zinc is vital for teenagers. During your teenage years you develop at a rapid rate and this requires lots of zinc. Growth spurts can lead to zinc deficiency, which is bad news as the skin is the first to suffer when your body doesn't have enough of this mineral. This is because the skin is low on the body's priority list when your zinc is depleted – what little zinc you have is used for more important jobs such as DNA replication and fertility.

See if you have any signs of zinc deficiency by taking the zinc deficiency questionnaire below.

Zinc deficiency questionnaire

Circle any lifestyle habits or symptoms you experience on a regular basis (three or more times per week):

acne/spots	'frizzy' hair or hair loss
stretch marks	poor wound healing
white coated tongue	poor sense of taste
white spots on fingernails	poor sense of smell
impotence	testicular atrophy
infertility	drinking alcohol every week
frequent infections	

If you circled more than three symptoms then you may have a zinc deficiency. However, it's best to also do a zinc taste test, to confirm if you have a true deficiency. Speak to your GP, a naturopath or nutritionist at your local health food

Continued overleaf

shop about doing a zinc taste test. All you do is have a measured dose of liquid zinc and hold it in your mouth for a few seconds before swallowing it. Your taste buds will indicate the degree of need for zinc supplementation: if you have a deficiency, the mixture will taste like water, be pleasant tasting or leave a furry feeling in the mouth. If you do not have a deficiency, the liquid will taste metallic or foul and you'll probably want to spit it out.

Causes of zinc deficiency

Zinc deficiency is very common and it can be caused by the following:

- High calcium and salt intake. Canned food is high in salt and dairy products are rich in calcium and too much of either can create a zinc deficiency. Zinc, sodium and calcium compete with each other for absorption. Iron deficiency is also common from having too much dairy, and copper deficiency can also occur.

- Zinc is needed to detoxify alcohol, so drinking alcoholic beverages is probably the fastest way to diminish zinc stores.

- Zinc is also depleted by stress, coffee, tea, high fibre diets, menstruation and ejaculation (semen contains approximately 1–3mg of zinc per ejaculation).

Getting enough zinc

Good food sources of zinc include: oysters (a serving of six medium oysters contains a whopping 76.4 mg of zinc), wheat germ, watercress salad, roasted soyabeans (edamame), bran flakes, rolled oats, chickpeas and red meat such as lamb's fry.

There is good scientific evidence that zinc supplementation is effective at eliminating acne.[19] A group of scientists who treated acne sufferers with zinc oral supplementation found at the end of the four-week study that, of the group who took zinc sulfate, 85 per cent were acne-free.[20,21] This is a great result!

Adults (over the age of 15 years) who are suffering with acne require 12–20mg of zinc per day and should have zinc-containing foods. Children between nine and 15 years of age with acne should have 8–11mg of zinc per day, plus food sources. Children four to eight years old with acne need to have 5mg of zinc per day, plus zinc from food sources. Note that fibre-rich foods and other supplements containing calcium, iron and phosphorus can pre-

> **CAUTION**
>
> Do not take zinc supplements if you have copper deficiency or if you're taking tetracycline (a drug for infections) as zinc competes for absorption with copper and may make your medical treatment less effective. Do not exceed the prescribed dosage.

vent zinc supplements from being adequately absorbed so have your zinc supplement two hours apart from these substances. Take zinc for at least two months. Once your acne clears, stop taking the zinc supplement and continue to eat zinc-rich foods.

Dairy products

Milk and other dairy products are associated with acne outbreaks. Researchers from one particular study said that dairy consumption increased the risk of acne, and this may have been due to the animal hormones and bioactive molecules found in milk products.[22]

Dairy products also contain small amounts of arachidonic acid, which is the main building material for 'bad' prostaglandins that increase oil gland activity. Dairy is also an acid-forming food group (see Chapter 3, 'Guideline No. 1', for more information, and pay particular attention to this information as it's really relevant to your skin). And dairy products exert an insulin response, and foods that trigger excessive insulin are linked with acne and premature ageing.[23,24] So removing dairy from the diet, for a minimum of two months, helps to eliminate acne quickly.

READER QUESTION

Q 'I always have a red, bumpy chin; the bumps look like blind spots and they seem to get worse when I'm trying to be healthy. What can I do to get rid of them?'

A *I inquired about this reader's diet when she said she was trying to be healthy and she told me she was making fruit and protein smoothies (having close to a litre of light milk a day) and eating diet yogurt and cottage cheese (with salad and rye bread). The skin problems are likely to be linked with her dairy consumption as milkshake or smoothie addictions and red chins seem to go hand in hand. Look for other signs of dairy sensitivity such as a runny nose (post nasal drip), fatigue, fluid retention and skin rashes.*

If you have acne, avoid dairy for at least two months during the Healthy Skin Diet (which is dairy free). After your acne has cleared up, dairy products can be consumed in moderate amounts. Plain yogurt, that contains healthy live bacteria such as acidophilus, is the best dairy option. After you complete the Healthy Skin Diet you can have one serving a day each of plain yogurt, milk in coffee/tea and ricotta cheese on grainy bread. Also get your calcium from non-dairy sources such as tahini, almonds and dark leafy greens such as watercress. Read Chapter 4, 'Guideline No. 2', for a full list of non-dairy calcium sources.

Chromium

If you suffer from acne, you may be deficient in the mineral chromium. Chromium is essential for the metabolism of glucose; without chromium in your diet you can end up with too much glucose floating around in your blood and this may lead to skin breakouts and more serious conditions such as type II diabetes and associated skin ulcers. For more information, go back to Chapter 5, 'Guideline No. 3', and do the chromium deficiency questionnaire to see if you need a chromium supplement.

Vitamin A

Vitamin A is also important for healthy, acne-free skin as it helps to reduce oil production if your glands are overstimulated. However, scientific studies have shown that zinc is more effective in eliminating acne than vitamin A supplementation.[25] So, get your vitamin A or its precursor beta-carotene from your diet (see 'Let's get practical' at the end of this chapter).

Activity

Control your oil gland production by supplementing with zinc for the duration of the Healthy Skin Diet (eight weeks). Commence taking these supplements after you have taken a liver detoxification supplement for two weeks. This is partly for the convenience of not taking too many supplements all at once and also so you don't double up on zinc intake.

Step four: Improve your bowel health

Bowel health is essential for clear skin. If your gut is slow to remove waste products then your skin will have to help 'put out the garbage', so to speak. Remember, your skin is one of the body's major eliminatory organs so you don't want it to have to compensate for poor waste elimination, constipation or microbe overgrowth. Poor bowel health can also cause smelly wind, abdominal discomfort, bloating, food allergies and sensitivities.

It's very important to eat the right foods for good bowel health. These foods include:

1. Insoluble fibre from fibre-rich carbohydrates and vegetables. A high-fibre diet is essential for clearing up acne. Fibre binds to and removes toxins from the colon and promotes healthy bacteria in the gastrointestinal tract, also minimising the bad bacteria and fungus that can cause undesirable skin conditions. Eat whole-

grain products such as brown rice, grainy bread, wholemeal pasta, dark leafy green vegetables, sweet potatoes and other vegetables.

2. Soluble fibre from apples and pears. Apples and pears contain pectin, which promotes healthy bowel movements and beneficial gut flora.

3. Also remember to drink plenty of water, exercise and relax (and be confident) as stress causes all sorts of gastrointestinal disturbances, such as ulcers and irritable bowel syndrome.

4. Take a liquid chlorophyll supplement. Liquid chlorophyll contains magnesium and chromium and it not only helps to prevent constipation, it also has a deodorising effect on the body and helps to cleanse the liver. Drink one bottle of Green Water daily. See Chapter 3, 'Guideline No. 1', for more information about chlorophyll – pay particular attention to the Three Day Alkalising Cleanse as this cleansing programme is great for improving acne. And you'll find out how to make pleasant-tasting Green Water in the recipe section.

Step five: Exercise and sweat

Although I am a nutritionist I must say that you shouldn't rely solely on diet and supplements to make all your spots disappear because true 'holistic' health comes from having a balanced life. For fantastic skin and long-term health I recommend you also exercise and sweat because, when done on a regular basis, exercise will change your health like nothing else and it will enable you to have clear skin *without* having to have a perfect diet. The three main points to remember about exercise and sweat are:

- moderate exercise decreases skin inflammation;
- sweat is anti-bacterial; and
- exercise promotes healthy bowels and elimination of wastes.

Read Chapter 7, 'Guideline No. 5', for more information on exercise and sweat.

Let's get practical

To get more omega-3 in your diet: eat fish (salmon, trout, sardines, mackerel, herring) at least twice a week and eat omega-3 rich eggs, walnuts and flaxseeds on a regular basis. Recipes from Appendix 2 include Salmon Steaks with Peas and Mash; Rainbow Trout with Honey Roasted Vegetables; Salmon and Salad Sandwich; Marinated Whole Steamed Trout and Salmon, Smoked Salmon and Eggs.

If you don't eat fish or you want to have some fish-free days you can add 1–2 tablespoons of flaxseeds to your food or use flaxseed oil in one of the skin drinks. Try one of the following recipes: Flaxseed Lemon Drink; Berry Beauty Smoothie and B Muesli with flaxseeds (many of these recipes are also high in B vitamins). Also eat lots of bright red and orange vegetables as they're rich in beta-carotene which is converted to oil-reducing vitamin A.

To get more zinc and magnesium in your diet: have sardines on grainy bread for breakfast; pepitas and almonds for snacks and enjoy a few oysters at your next social function. Remember that alcohol *rapidly* depletes zinc and magnesium so it's best to avoid alcohol during the Healthy Skin Diet. Recipes to increase zinc and magnesium intake include Roasted Sweet Potato Salad; Designer Muesli; Gluten-free Muesli and Vitamin E Muesli. Chlorophyll is rich in magnesium so drink 1–2 bottles of Green Water per day.

Swap dairy for other high protein foods such as free-range chicken (antibiotic free), free-range eggs, fish, beans and chickpeas and small servings of red meat. Get your daily requirement of calcium from the Anti-ageing Broth, Almond Milk (naturally high in calcium), Calcium-rich Smoothie, tahini spreads, sesame seeds, almonds and dark leafy green vegetables such as watercress. Try the Sweet Raspberry, Avocado and Watercress Salad.

Remember to drink enough fluids – water, Green Water, Spot-free Skin Juice, herbal teas, fresh vegetable juices, mineral water with freshly squeezed lemon. Also do the Three Day Alkalising Cleanse and the Healthy Skin Diet.

Key points to remember

Step one: Have a suitable skin-care routine

- Make sure your skin-care products are suitable for your skin.
- Swim in the ocean or use a Saltwater Face Bath (see page 140).

Step two: Control your hormones

- Take a liver detoxification/cleansing supplement for two weeks (see Resources).

Step three: Control your oil production

- Avoid dairy products and decrease saturated fat intake (limit meat and butter, avoid pork and deli meats).
- Avoid fried foods, trans fats and margarine. Use avocado, tahini and extra-virgin olive oil instead (in moderation).

- Increase omega-3 intake by eating salmon, trout, tuna, sardines, omega-3 forti-fied eggs, flaxseed oil and flaxseeds. If necessary, supplement with omega-3 (from week 3 to week 8 of the Healthy Skin Diet). Add lecithin granules to your diet so you digest and eliminate fats correctly.

- Take a zinc supplement during weeks 3 to 8 of the Healthy Skin Diet.

Step four: Improve your bowel health

- Ditch the white bread, white flour and white sugar and switch to wholegrains and honey or agave nectar (which can be bought in health food stores).

- Do the questionnaires in Chapter 3, 'Guideline No. 1', and complete the Three Day Alkalising Cleanse (necessary for *all* acne sufferers) and the Healthy Skin Diet.

- Think green! Eat salads *every day* (with either lunch or dinner) and have more fresh, fibre-rich vegetables, especially the bright red and orange ones. Ensure you have five servings of veggies and two servings of fruit every day.

- Drink one to two bottles of Green Water per day (1.5 litre bottles).

Step five: Exercise and sweat

- Sweat every day and exercise four days a week (see Chapter 7, 'Guideline No. 5').

Chapter 12

Cellulite

Cellulite is a fancy name for dimpled skin that resembles the texture of orange peel (if you're lucky); however, if you're not so fortunate you may look in the mirror some days and wonder who super-glued the cottage cheese to your behind. It's no practical joke though; having cellulite can cause distress. The good news is that you don't have to worry about your dimples any longer because a solution is at hand. You probably won't like the answer to your problem, however, because it's not a quick-fix miracle and it involves effort and patience. Lots of it. Read on if you want to know more.

READER QUESTION

Q 'What is cellulite? I've heard it is not caused by being overweight.'

A *Cellulite is found in the fatty layers of your skin but cellulite is **not** normal body fat, or unique to overweight people as even slim women can get it. This hail damage effect is commonly found on the thighs, hips, bottom and stomach. It afflicts women more often that men because men have a genetic tendency for stronger connective tissue in the dermis layer.[1] Unfortunately, women are more likely to have irregular connective tissue immediately below the skin, making us more prone to getting disorderly connective tissue fibres that lose flexibility and movement, similar to when an old swimsuit loses its elasticity and no longer fits snugly. This tissue weakness allows the fatty layer (the subcutaneous layer) just below the skin's deep dermis layer to **protrude** into the dermis, which makes the skin look lumpy.*

Although cellulite occurs in varying degrees in as many as 85 per cent of women, not all women get cellulite and it's from these ladies that we can gain hope and also a bit of insight into how to avoid cellulite in future. However, don't get me wrong: cellulite is not necessarily a bad thing. It's quite a common 'cosmetic' condition that can naturally happen as you age and there's certainly nothing wrong with learning to love yourself lumps, bumps and all.

What can cause cellulite?

* genetics and hormones
* poor circulation
* sedentary lifestyle

- diets high in dairy products and sugar
- environmental pollution, chemicals, toxins
- nutritional deficiencies
- stress (running around looking after everyone else's needs but not your own, being too busy, worrying, having an anxious disposition).

Coincidentally, weight problems are caused by many of the same issues and as a result being overweight is often associated with cellulite. In reality, they are two separate symptoms caused by very similar genetic, diet and lifestyle factors.

Internal influences on cellulite

The two internal factors that can cause the appearance of cellulite are: irregular connective tissue in the dermis layer of the skin; and the fatty layer intruding into the dermis, making skin appear lumpy.

Irregular connective tissue in the dermis layer of the skin

You wouldn't want your liver to dislodge and squash an artery, blocking off your valuable blood supply, would you? Luckily you have connective tissue, which is a fibrous material that literally connects your muscles and organs to one another so they can't aimlessly move around the body. This 'cellular glue' also helps bring nutrients to the tissues and gives tissues form and strength. Without good connective tissue the skin becomes fragile and sags.

Connective tissue is where you find the famous beauty materials collagen and elastin: both provide the skin with strength, the ability to stretch and the capacity to return to its original shape after extension (this is the ideal scenario). If the connective tissue *doesn't* return to its normal shape it becomes irregular and cellulite can occur. Connective tissue can also tear if it hasn't been supplied the right skin nutrients (such as the mineral zinc), causing stretch marks to appear.

Many factors are involved in poor connective tissue quality such as stress, environmental pollution, poor diet and genetics. Stress burns up valuable nutrients that could have otherwise been used to repair connective tissue. Toxins from pollution and cigarette smoke are absorbed into the body and can become lodged around connective tissues. If you eat a poor diet that doesn't supply enough protein, connective tissue loses strength and your skin eventually sags. This is often seen when overweight people follow poorly designed diets that consist of nothing but salads and soups. Poor digestion can also hamper protein supply to the skin. If your body can't digest protein properly and 'pluck' out the amino acids needed to make collagen and elastin then you'll end up with connective tissue dysfunction. Fluctuating oestrogen levels (the hormone that's generally higher in women) can also play a part in weakening connective tissue.[2]

The fatty layer intruding into the dermis, making skin appear lumpy

Another structural problem seen with cellulite is lumpiness caused by the fat layer pushing into the dermis, which can be caused by faulty fat cells.

Inside your body, billions of tiny cells sit together, side by side, and layer by layer they form your skin and the rest of you, and your connective tissue keeps them all in place. Remember that when cellulite occurs, your fatty (subcutaneous) layer starts pushing into your skin layer, making it look bumpy – this fatty layer is mostly made up of fat cells. The health of your fat cells determines just how good your skin looks on the outside.

Your fat cells have three main functions: storage, insulation and protection. Fat cells insulate and protect valuable organs such as the skin and they provide protective padding on the bottom and thighs (apparently this cushioning is a 'must' during childbirth). Your body also thinks that your fat cells are a good spot to store unwanted toxins, such as acid, that would be harmful if left floating around in the blood. Your fat cells are trying to do the right thing for your health and wellbeing but they leave your skin looking less than perfect in the process.

Leaky cells contribute to cellulite

When your fat cells store chemicals and acids (toxins) they can get damaged and become leaky. Imagine a cell is like a balloon filled with water, and over time wear and tear has caused little pin-prick holes to appear in the balloon membrane, causing fluid to seep into surrounding tissue. If this leaked fluid builds up enough you can see it: it's what we call fluid retention or oedema. Swollen ankles, puffy eyelids and cellulite all have 'problem water' hanging out where it's not supposed to.[3]

In the case of cellulite, the water may have been drawn there because the body wanted to use the fluid to dilute acids or it may have been from leaky cells that cannot adequately hold on to water but it's impossible to tell which is the case, so anti-cellulite treatment should involve addressing both of these issues.

Why might your cell walls be leaking fluids?

Your cell membranes are largely made up of fat (lipids) but the types of fat used to build your cell walls will help determine how resistant they are to leakage. You choose what types of fats your cell membranes are built with every time you eat a meal: saturated fats from meat and dairy can make rigid cells and essential fatty acids (EFAs) from nuts, seeds and fish oils contribute to more flexible, resilient cells.

Cell membranes can be prone to damage if they're not continually repaired and the best patching materials for leaky cells are EFAs, such as omega-3. EFAs also work to draw water ('problem water') from outside the cell back into the cell. This means EFAs help to keep fluid in the right place so you have hydrated cells and healthy looking skin.

Your cell membranes are also made up of lecithin (phosphatidylcholine). Lecithin sits in the cell walls and helps to determine what enters and leaves your cells.[4] A shortage of lecithin equals faulty cell membranes that can leak fluids into your subcutaneous layer. Lecithin helps to break up cholesterol and promotes proper digestion of fats; it helps cleanse the liver; maintain a healthy nervous system and it promotes healthy weight loss.[5] Your body doesn't produce enough lecithin of its own so you need to eat foods that contain it (which will be covered in step two of the Anti-cellulite Programme).

Management plan

The management plan is your first step to feeling more comfortable in your skin. This section details topical treatments and camouflage ideas. The Anti-cellulite Programme follows and it's a diet and lifestyle programme that will improve and even eliminate your cellulite. In all there are five steps to follow.

Step one: Use massage oils

Everybody loves a topical treatment, but most commercial cellulite creams are loaded with chemicals and additives, such as artificial fragrance, that contribute to your body's toxic load. To treat cellulite you want to decrease your skin's waste burden, increase toxin removal and improve local circulation. Massage oils – containing no artificial ingredients and with the addition of natural essential oils – specific for cellulite are your best option (refer to Chapter 8, 'Guideline No. 6', for more information on artificial chemicals found in beauty products).

When choosing an anti-cellulite oil look for the following two ingredients. **Birch oil** is extracted from the plant betula alba, it contains salicylic acid and it is astringent so it helps to tone the skin. Birch oil also improves circulation, increases toxin removal and has a mild diuretic effect. **Rosemary oil** increases circulation to the skin and assists with elimination of toxins. Do not use this oil on its own – it can be found in anti-cellulite massage oil formulas or mix it in with almond and birch oil.

How to apply anti-cellulite oil

Have a shower or a bath as usual and then pat your skin dry. To apply your anti-cellulite oil of choice, tip a small amount (about the size of a large coin) into the palm of your hand, then rub your hands together to warm the oil. Apply the mixture where necessary (thighs, bottom, stomach, arms), using more oil as necessary. Then give yourself a slow massage, working in a circular motion from the legs to the heart (to help your lymphatic system remove toxins).

Tip: Apply oil to affected skin twice a day. Ideally, use anti-cellulite oil in the morning and at night (it's not essential to bathe beforehand). Also remember to moisturise the rest of your skin with a suitable natural-based moisturiser (see Chapter 8, 'Guideline No. 6').

> **CAUTION**
>
> Do not use rosemary oil during pregnancy or if you have epilepsy or high blood pressure. Other suitable ingredients include apricot kernel oil, almond oil, jojoba seed oil, wheat germ oil, vitamin E, limonene, grapefruit extract, calendula/marigold, carrot oil, fennel extract, rosehip oil, and kelp/seaweed.

> **CAUTION**
>
> Never use a cellulite cream or oil without the addition of exercise. Anti-cellulite products can mobilise toxins and these chemicals may deposit somewhere else in the body if you don't exert yourself and sweat.

READER QUESTION

Q 'What are toxins?'

A *'Toxin' is a general term for a substance that has no positive use in the body, such as chemicals from cleaning products, pesticides, artificial food additives and the pollution you've inhaled. Toxins are also waste products generated by your cells. Your body has several ways of removing toxins, including the lymphatic and blood circulatory systems, sweating and not forgetting the waste you dump when you go to the toilet.*

Since cellulite can be caused by fluid and toxins becoming trapped in the subcutaneous layer of skin, you can help to reverse this accumulation by reducing your toxin load. The first thing you can do is swap those stinky chemical cleaners for natural ones (see Appendix 3) and cut down on packaged goodies such as crisps, biscuits and soft drinks. You can also take a liver detoxification supplement to speed up toxin elimination in the body.

Toxins and hormones that can contribute to cellulite formation include: pesticide residues found on fruits and veggies; artificial additives such as preservatives; pollution and cigarette smoke; excess hormones such as oestrogen; chemical cleaning products; and beauty products containing artificial chemicals.

Model's Cellulite Treatment

It is claimed that this treatment is used by supermodels but I haven't heard of anyone famous owning up to it. However, this remedy was often talked about within the modelling industry in the 1990s but I have to warn you: it's only a temporary skin tightener and it may only work on the genetically blessed.

The natural compounds in coffee are said to marginally tighten the skin. Seaweed is also considered to have a toning effect when applied to the skin, which is why it's often an ingredient in anti-cellulite treatments and creams.

30g (1oz) warm used ground coffee (preferably organic) or organic instant coffee
60ml (2fl oz) cup extra-virgin olive oil (can infuse it with rosemary or birch oil)
4 soaked kombu (seaweed) strips
cling wrap

Method: Mix coffee and oil in a glass bowl. Line the floor or shower with newspaper (some of the coffee mixture is bound to fall off), then massage the mixture in a circular motion over cellulite-affected thighs for 1 minute.
Wrap the area with kombu, wash hands and then apply cling wrap around each affected area to hold the mixture in place. Leave on for 10 minutes then have a shower to rinse off. Repeat this once a day for at least two weeks as results take two to four weeks to appear.

READER QUESTION

Q   'I'm going on a beach holiday with friends and I need to know how I can hide my cellulite. Can you help me?'

A   *If you want to instantly make your skin look better you can camouflage cellulite with fake tan products. Spray-on tans, applied by trained professionals, can give you a wonderful natural tan that lasts up to a week but you can still use a home-applied fake tan bought from a chemist or department store. But I have to tell you that fake tans are full of chemicals that are readily absorbed into your skin. Chemicals can contribute to connective tissue damage and lead to cellulite, so you could make your skin condition worse with regular fake tan abuse. To be on the safe side, keep the tan-in-a-can use to a bare minimum. And after five days, when it starts to go patchy, have a good body exfoliator on hand.*

If you're still panicking about being seen on the beach you may want to try the following:

- *Buy a gorgeous sarong that complements the colour of your swimsuit.*
- *Buy a swimsuit that draws the eye towards your best assets.*

Self-confidence is very attractive so take time to work on your self-esteem. In the meantime you could go to the beach and pretend not to care what anyone else thinks. Basically 'fake it til you make it'. Walk tall, all the way to the water's edge and enjoy the water, the sand and the sunshine, just like everyone else. The more you step out of your comfort zone, the sooner you'll feel what it's like to be truly confident.

And remember, you are so much more than just a pair of wobbly thighs! Remind yourself about your strengths and positive attributes, and then have fun at the beach because you deserve to be there as much as anyone else.

Now let's get to work on the Anti-cellulite Programme.

Step two: Consume nutrients to repair tissues and cells

Nutrients for healthy cells

As you've read, your cells leak fluids when they don't have the right nutrients such as omega-3 and lecithin for maintenance and repair. You can get these nutrients along with their little helpers (antioxidants) from the meals and special drink recipes of the Healthy Skin Diet, such as the Skin Firming Drink which has been specifically designed to reduce the appearance of cellulite. As mentioned earlier, omega-3 is found in oily fish (trout, sardines, salmon, tuna), as well as flaxseeds, flaxseed oil and in small amounts in dark green vegetables. Lecithin is found in egg yolk, liver, nuts, soya products, corn and you can also buy soya lecithin granules.[6]

Dosage: Adults with cellulite should take 2000–4000mg of lecithin per day. Note that 1 tablespoon of soya lecithin granules contains approximately 1700mg of lecithin, so have 1.5 to 2 tablespoons of lecithin daily.[7] Add lecithin granules to the Skin Firming Drink or muesli.

Nutrients for healthy connective tissues

Collagen and elastin are made up of amino acids such as glycine and proline and a substance called hyaluronic acid, which has recently been renamed 'hyaluronan'.[8,9] I discussed hyaluronan and its essential role in healthy skin in some detail in Chapter 5. Remember that its main building block is glucosamine, which normalises cartilage and restores joint function. Magnesium is also needed to manufacture hyaluronan and studies have shown that deficiencies in zinc and magnesium contribute to hyaluronan abnormalities.[10,11] Supplements with glucosamine, glycine, proline, vitamin C, copper, manganese, magnesium and zinc can help to restore elasticity and strength to connective tissue (these nutrients can be found in some glucosamine complex supplements, available in most health food shops).

Dosage: Adults should take 1200mg (1.2g) of glucosamine sulfate OR glucosamine hydrochloride (HCL) per day, with either food or the Skin Firming Drink. Make sure your glucosamine supplement also contains magnesium, zinc, vitamin C, copper and manganese.

Step three: Exercise and improve your circulation

Your circulation plays an important role in having smooth, evenly textured skin. Circulation of blood is essential for health but it's also the lymphatic circulation that will help to keep your skin looking fabulous.

If you want to get rid of your cellulite you *must exercise*. You don't have to like exercise or be good at it, you just need to prioritise at least 15 minutes a day to get some good lymph-pumping movement. Some experts claim that exercise won't get rid of cellulite but you just have to watch the Olympic Games and look at the average female athlete, with her firm, toned body to know that exercise does a good job at preventing cellulite.

You may be surprised to know that there is another way you can pump your lymphatic fluid around your body – by breathing deeply. When you breathe correctly, you utilise the diaphragm, a muscle found below your lungs, which causes movement of your lymphatic fluid, enabling it to collect cellular garbage and 'problem water'. When you breathe well, your lymphatic vessels drain 'problem water' from tissue spaces and this helps to prevent fluid retention. Read Chapter 19, 'Beauty breathing', to learn about a breathing technique that can help improve exercise stamina so you can feel like an athlete as you power up those stairs!

Boost your circulation with the following:

- dry-skin brushing (see Chapter 8, 'Guideline No. 6: Have a good skin-care routine');
- have a shower and alternate from wonderfully warm water to chilly cold water, then exfoliate your skin with a granulated gel or cream (see caution box overleaf);
- massage your skin with an exfoliation glove;
- get a lymphatic massage from a qualified masseuse;
- gently self-massage cellulite-prone areas with natural anti-cellulite oils;

- do breathing exercises (in Chapter 19) ;
- make sure you exercise and move daily (see Chapter 7, 'Guideline No. 5' for information and inspiration).

CAUTION

If you suffer from any kind of medical problem, such as a heart condition or diabetes, please have a chat with your doctor before trying to improve your circulation as some treatments such as high impact exercise, and warm and cold water therapy, may not be suitable for you.

Activity

*For severe cellulite I suggest doing heart-pumping activity for **at least** 15 minutes. (If you aren't able to do high impact exercise, combine walking with other forms of exercise – see 'Let's get practical' below.) Do 15 minutes of continuous high impact exercise **today**, then over the following weeks, work up to a 30- to 60-minute routine. A personal trainer could also work wonders for you!*

Step four: Avoid dairy products and sugar

Just as there are foods that strengthen connective tissue and cell walls for gorgeous skin, there are also foods that can promote the onset of cellulite. The main offenders are dairy and sugar.

Dairy products can increase your risk of cellulite because they are mucus forming. To demonstrate this, the next time you have a cold or flu, drink a glass of milk and see if you suddenly have an increase in phlegm/mucus production. Naturopaths say that dairy products make your lymphatic fluid thicker so it has a harder time travelling around your body. A sluggish lymphatic system can't remove cellular waste fast enough so it builds up. These cellular toxins can be harmful if they are floating in your blood so they are quickly relocated to be safely stored in your fat – especially on your lovely soft thighs.

Dairy also supplies saturated fat and arachidonic acid, which your body can use to make rigid cell walls that are prone to leaking. I find that eliminating dairy products out of the diet is essential to reducing the appearance of cellulite. This dietary change works better than any other treatment because it quickly enhances lymphatic health and it allows better absorption of other minerals such as zinc, copper and magnesium, which are essential for firm and toned skin.

Eating too much sugar can also increase your risk of cellulite. This occurs because sweets, junk foods and processed 'white' carbohydrates such as white bread, pastries and cakes increase acid in the body and they also affect your blood sugar levels. This surge in glucose in the blood uses up lots of vitamin C and may therefore cause low levels of this important antioxidant. Excess glucose in the blood can also cause blood vessel damage, which may hamper circulation to cellulite-prone areas.

Vitamin C is essential for strong, healthy blood vessels and low levels of vitamin C can lead to poor blood vessel strength and varicose veins, which are often associated with cellulite. Vitamin C is also important for cell membrane health and may help prevent leaky cells because of its role in recycling vitamin E.

Foods and drinks to avoid include:

- dairy – milk, milkshakes, cheese, yogurt, ice-cream, creamy spreads and butter;
- pastries, cakes, doughnuts, biscuits, muesli bars, white bread, white rice (basmati is okay), sweets, white flour pancakes and crisps;
- soft drink, diet soft drink, fruit juice and alcohol;
- margarine.

For more information on non-dairy calcium-rich alternatives, read the 'Calcium' section in Chapter 4.

Case study

I had mild cellulite in my late teens; maybe it was because I must have been the laziest teenager on the planet. I hated exercise, I would sit in my room and write and draw all day and I'd only take breaks to have milkshakes and mountains of toast made with white bread. I used to drink a litre of milk, and eat a bowl of yogurt and ice-cream every day. However, my dimply butt miraculously firmed up when I ditched the dairy. After I made dietary changes I also had a lot more energy and my skin was less prone to rashes. Now I'm older and I've had a baby, dietary changes alone are not enough. I also need to jog on soft sand several times a week and sweat, and use massage oils to keep my skin firm.

Step five: Promote good bowel health

Good bowel health is essential for healthy looking skin. Poor bowel health can result in constipation, allowing toxins from your poo to be reabsorbed by your body which slowly poisons your whole system. If you have constipation or any other bowel complaints then it's essential that you seek treatment before your bowels harm your health. See Chapter 3, 'Guideline No. 1', for more information about constipation and gut health.

Hydration

It's important to drink enough fluids each day to prevent dehydration and a sluggish lymphatic system. Dehydration can also damage your cells, and cause constipation and poor bowel function.

Cellulite can be impossible to get rid of in a select few people. However please never, ever dislike yourself because you have cellulite. Self-hate and self-criticism can damage your self-confidence; ruin your motivation and suppress your ability to make healthy improvements. Remember that it's your self-confidence that ultimately makes you attractive because you walk taller and give off an air of being relaxed and loveable. Other people adore being around someone who is confident and relaxed in their skin, because it helps them to feel at ease too (don't underestimate this power).

Love the body you're in and focus on your best assets – the parts of your personality and your body that you love – and make them stand out with the right clothes and accessories. If you want to work on your cellulite then go for it; you can get rid of dimpled skin one way or another but don't hate yourself along the way as it will be a slow and arduous mountain to climb if you do. Also remember that Olympic athletes don't get fit overnight; it takes time and effort for them to reach competition standard. Cellulite removal is kind of the same: you can't get rid of it overnight, or in a week or two. It takes time, effort and truckloads of patience. Great results may be seen in two to six months and earlier than this if your cellulite is mild.

Let's get practical

The best anti-cellulite exercises include soft sand jogging, fast-paced soft sand walking (keeping your knees high), running, swimming, cycling and running up lots and lots of stairs. (Be warned: you'll miss your knees if you damage them so remember to avoid movements that trigger sharp pain and be kind to your body by running on soft surfaces only [sand, grass, carpet]. Also wear good quality running shoes during workouts.) One of the very best exercises to help you get rid of cellulite is sprinting. Sprinters have the most amazing bodies and it is from them that we can gain inspiration to be cellulite-free: If you are a walker and are able to do so, combine walking with 30-second sprints, every 5 minutes. For example, 'power' walk for 5 minutes, then sprint as fast as you can for 30 seconds, then briskly walk for 5 minutes and again sprint as fast as you can for 30 seconds or more (up to 1 minute) and so on. Do this routine for at least 20 minutes. If you are a jogger, combine slow jogging with 30-second sprints in a similar manner to the walking routine.

To reduce the appearance of cellulite from the inside out: have the Anti-ageing Broth which is rich in glycine, calcium, magnesium and natural collagen. Also have the Skin Firming Drink on a daily basis – you'll need to buy a powdered glucosamine supplement (one that contains some or all of the following: glucosamine sulfate, glucosamine hydrochloride, vitamin C, magnesium, copper, zinc and manganese).

To get more omega-3 and lecithin in your diet: try recipes such as Skin Firming Drink; Flaxseed Lemon Drink; Salmon and Salad Sandwich; Perfect Poached Eggs; Egg Soldiers; Creamy Mayonnaise; Salmon Steaks with Peas and Mash; Rainbow Trout with Honey Roasted Vegetables; Smoked Salmon and Eggs; and Tuna and Avocado Wrap. To get more zinc in your diet eat fresh oysters when out socialising or try the recipes for Oysters with Dipping Sauce and Lamb's Fry in Rich Tomato.

To get a good dose of magnesium: the Green Water drink is the best choice as it's rich in magnesium. Drink one to two bottles of Green Water per day. Also have the following: Buckwheat Crepes (with the topping of your choice); Creamy Chickpea Curry with brown rice; Roasted Sweet Potato Salad; Designer Muesli; Vitamin E Muesli; Gluten-free Muesli; and snack on a small handful of hazelnuts and pumpkin seeds. All of these recipes contain a rich variety of antioxidants.

Key points to remember

Step one: Use massage oils

- Massage your skin using anti-cellulite oils containing all-natural ingredients.

Step two: Consume nutrients to repair tissues and cells

- Eat healthy food rich in omega-3, lecithin and antioxidants.

- Make the Skin Firming Drink daily and have Anti-ageing Broth and Green Water.

Step three: Exercise and improve your circulation

- Exercise and sweat daily.

- Improve your circulation in as many different ways as possible.

Step four: Avoid dairy products and sugar

- Avoid dairy products for two months (while on the Healthy Skin Diet) and stop adding sugar to your foods and drinks.

Step five: Promote good bowel health

- Drink enough water.

- Avoid constipation (see page 278 for the Three Day Alkalising Cleanse).

Chapter 13

Dandruff

You look gorgeous in that black dress but what's with the white flecks on your shoulders? On closer inspection of your scalp it's dandruff, a combination of inflammation, flaking skin, lumps and crusts.[1] But don't freak out, just exchange your little black frock for a cream one and try not to scratch because dandruff can be as itchy as an infestation of head lice.

Seborrheic dermatitis, the technical term for dandruff, can commonly occur on the scalp, face and middle of the chest, but (if you're extra unlucky) it may manifest anywhere on the body. Newborn bubs may develop cradle cap, which shows up as thick yellow crusts on the scalp.[2] See the next chapter for more information.

Management plan

The dandruff management plan includes identifying possible triggers and applying topical treatments to eliminate dandruff as quickly as possible.

Factors that can trigger dandruff include:

- chemicals
- climate (especially winter)
- emotional or physical stress
- fungal/yeast infection
- psoriasis (dandruff can appear during or after psoriasis)
- sodium lauryl sulfate (SLS)
- excess use of hairspray or gel
- hair dyes
- excess sugar and starch in diet
- infrequent shampooing
- inadequate rinsing of hair after washing
- overly dry scalp *or* excessively oily/greasy scalp

- diets high in saturated fats
- deficiency of essential fatty acids, especially omega-3.

Circle anything in the list above that you suspect may have triggered your dandruff.

Dandruff can simply occur when you are run down, overworked or stressed and it can occur in conjunction with psoriasis. Anti-dandruff shampoos address none of these factors.

Step one: Check your hair-care products

Maybe your shampoo is to blame? Sodium lauryl sulfate (SLS) is a synthetic detergent commonly added to commercial brand shampoos, liquid hand soaps and cleansers to make them lather up nicely. SLS also adds the froth and bubbles to bath products. This lathering effect is what we've come to expect when using cleaning liquids but the SLS additive is one of the most irritating chemicals found in hair and skin products today. SLS use can trigger inflammation, dandruff, skin rashes and exacerbate existing scalp flaking. SLS also strips your scalp's natural sebum, which is supposed to protect your skin from invading fungus and bacteria.[3,4]

There are a number of shampoo ingredients that are ideal if you have dandruff. They are either anti-fungal, anti-microbial or anti-inflammatory, and include: tea tree oil*, licorice root, gotu kola, vitamin E, chamomile, calendula, manuka honey, panthenol (vitamin B5), olive leaf extract, citrus seed extract **.

* In a study, 126 patients with dandruff were given either 5 per cent tea tree oil shampoo or a placebo shampoo. They were told to wash their hair daily, leaving the shampoo on for three minutes before rinsing. At the end of four weeks scalp lesions were significantly lower and less itching seen in the tea tree oil shampoo users.[5] The cure rate was low, however, so use tea tree oil shampoo in conjunction with other remedies. Daily shampooing can also help reduce the appearance of dandruff.

** Citrus seed extract/grape seed extract is a potent anti-fungicide and antibiotic, inhibiting many different types of fungus, bacteria and parasites. Citrus seed is good for drying damp conditions such as oily scalp – an oily scalp promotes fungus-related dandruff.[6]

Activity

Read Chapter 8, 'Guideline No. 6', taking note of the ingredients to avoid. Then look at the ingredient panel on your shampoo bottle: does it look like a chemical cocktail that only a biochemist could decipher? If so, get rid of your shampoo today and buy one with beneficial ingredients from a health food shop.

Anti-dandruff recipes and home remedies

If your dandruff is of the dry variety or appeared in conjunction with psoriasis then this olive oil treatment can be very effective.

Olive Oil Treatment

60ml (2fl oz) extra-virgin olive oil
plastic bag to cover hair

> **Method:** Put the oil into a glass then place the glass in a small tub of hot water to heat the oil. Do not make the oil too hot. Then wet your hair and shampoo it, rinse then apply the oil to your scalp and massage with fingers. Cover your hair with a plastic bag and leave the mixture on for 3 to 5 minutes then rinse with warm water. Shampoo twice to remove excess oil, then use a gentle conditioner. If your hair is still greasy you might want to wash it again the next day.

Natural Anti-fungal Treatment

This recipe is designed to exfoliate flakes, soothe dry skin and balance the pH of your scalp so your head is not so appealing to fungi (ingredients for 1–2 treatments):

120ml (4fl oz) grape seed oil
2 tablespoons cornmeal
1 tablespoon apple cider vinegar
plastic bag to cover hair

> **Method:** Mix the grape seed oil with the cornmeal and vinegar. Stir well. Rinse your hair with warm water and shampoo it with a gentle shampoo. Then rub a tablespoon of the oil mixture in between your palms to warm the oil, and apply to scalp. Rub in with your fingertips. Repeat until you have applied the mixture to your entire scalp. Cover your hair with a plastic bag. Leave mixture on for ½ hour. Rinse thoroughly and shampoo as normal.[7]

Home remedies from the grapevine

ACV Remedy (apple cider vinegar): If you don't mind briefly smelling like a salad then this remedy could be for you. Shampoo your hair, then rinse scalp with quality apple cider vinegar. Leave on for 3 minutes then rinse off and apply conditioner if necessary. This will offer relief from itching and may even clear up your dandruff. For severe dandruff, leave on for 30 minutes before rinsing. This remedy may be best for oily dandruff caused by fungus.

White vinegar: See reader question below.

Wash your hair more often: If your flakes are mild, you may simply need to wash your hair more often, with a SLS-free shampoo, finishing with a suitable conditioner.

Olive oil + sunlight: This works brilliantly for psoriasis and it can also work for dandruff related to psoriasis. Shampoo your hair and apply extra-virgin olive oil to your scalp. Gently massage in, then hop out of the shower (get dry and dressed) and sit in direct sunlight for 5 to 10 minutes. See the psoriasis chapter for more information.

- If you're trying a 'home remedy from the grapevine', I recommend you try the vinegar remedies for at least three consecutive days and the oil treatments once or twice a week for a couple of weeks. Best results are likely to be seen after one to two weeks.

Case study

A 28-year-old woman developed an itchy, flaking scalp after her psoriasis cleared up. For her dandruff she was prescribed EPA/DHA (omega-3) supplements, which she took three times a day, a biotin supplement once a day and 10 minutes of relaxation exercises daily. Once a week she was to massage her scalp with olive oil and she switched to a natural shampoo and conditioner. After her second application of olive oil she stopped experiencing itchiness and no flakes were detected. Five months later she continues to be 100 per cent dandruff free.

READER QUESTION

Q   'My scalp is so oily and itchy that it distracts me from my studies and I'm always scratching my head in class. I don't have a lot of money for expensive treatments. What can I do to stop this embarrassing itching?'

A   *Use white vinegar to treat oily dandruff and reduce scalp itching. This is the cheapie version of the ACV remedy: Fill a spray bottle with no-name brand white vinegar, spray onto scalp and leave it to dry overnight. If there's no smell, you may not need to wash it out the next day. Or you can dilute 120ml vinegar with 120ml filtered water and apply to your scalp. This may sting a bit but try to leave it on for half an hour before rinsing. Use this remedy for three days in a row for best results.[8] If your itching continues, do the Anti-dandruff Programme.*

The Anti-dandruff Programme

Some people love using medicated shampoos but unfortunately the research suggests that your **dandruff is likely to return time and time again when using medicated anti-dandruff shampoos as the only treatment.** This is not surprising, as shampoos can't eliminate the underlying cause of the dandruff. Don't get me wrong, anti-dandruff shampoos and home remedies are great for treating existing fungus and washing away scales but you must fix up your lazy (sick, suppressed) immune system to win the war against dandruff. So let's move on to step two.

Step two: Look after your immune system

Your immune system normally guards your skin from invading bacteria and yeasts but when you're run down, stressed or sick your immune system can let its guard down. A common yeast called pityrosporum lives on your scalp and your immune system ensures that this freeloader doesn't multiply or claim too much territory. Pityrosporum yeasts can be found on everyone but they only cause dandruff in approximately 20 per cent of people.

If your immune system fails to do its job, pityrosporum's offspring, cousins, aunts and uncles take over your head and inflame your skin. Common dandruff treatments, such as medicated shampoos, work by killing this pesky fungi but these treatments don't usually have a long-term beneficial effect because they don't address the underlying cause/s, and not all dandruff is accompanied by pityrosporum.

The first thing you need to do is assess your diet and lifestyle to see if you're pushing your immune system to its limits.

Immune system questionnaire

Circle any of the following that best describes you:

I eat sugar every day (a dash of sugar in coffee or tea, jam, cake, biscuits, soft drinks, ice-cream, etc.).

I have sugar cravings.

I crave dairy products/I eat a lot of dairy.

I eat white bread, I crave processed carbohydrates.

I avoid garlic and onions.

I prefer not to exercise/I exercise less than twice a week.

I'm stressed, anxious or a 'worry-wart' – life is tough for me!

I often get less than seven hours' sleep a night (three or more nights a week).

I take antibiotics when I'm sick (within the last six months).

I'm on the birth control pill.

I'm taking cortisone medicines.

I drink alcohol more than twice a week or I binge drink.

I have been exposed to a high dose of chemicals (pesticides, harsh cleaning products such as oven cleaner/bleach, etc.).

I know my diet should be better (it can't get any worse!).

If you've circled three or more diet and lifestyle factors that promote a poor immune system then you may have found the underlying cause of your dandruff.

The following are six ways you can strengthen your immune system.

Get plenty of rest and relaxation

Quality sleep is essential for a strong immune system. When you sleep, your body goes into repair mode and your immune system recharges its batteries. To have quality sleep, get to bed before 10.30 p.m. and get eight hours' sleep (but no more than eight hours as too much sleep can leave you feeling foggy). Read Chapter 6, 'Guideline No. 4', for more information.

Relaxing breathing exercises

It can be hard to suddenly change from being stressed and anxious into a calm person but you don't need to quit your life or get a lobotomy (just yet) to feel relaxed; you can simply take the first positive step by learning some breathing exercises. Good quality breathing techniques instantly switch your nervous system from stressed 'fight or flight' responses into 'rest and digest' mode. Check out Chapter 19, 'Beauty breathing', for more information.

Ditch the stress addiction

You may fret about not getting enough sleep; you could agonise about losing that job; worry about what other people might think; lose sleep when other people gossip about you; and be concerned about bank queues, traffic, the safety of your family or the state of the economy. Yes, these are all super good reasons to worry but I'll give you one more: you are ruining your health! Being a worrier (the opposite of a warrior) will make your body's main defence system less effective and this is bad for your whole body, not just your scalp's health.

Does worry really cause dandruff? Well, worry is another form of stress and it's easier for me to describe worry as opposed to the highly subjective state of stress. In fact, stress is really worry or fear in disguise: when you feel stressed, the underlying thought process is that you are *worried* about your ability to cope or manage the situation at hand.

You may not consciously think 'Gosh I'm worried' but the next time you feel stressed, experiment by telling yourself something positive and strong. For example, stand up straight with good posture and stick your nose in the air as if you're posh, then shout (or think to yourself in an assertive manner): 'Of course I'm strong enough to get through this problem! I'm clever and capable, I will survive this!' *And mean every word of it.* I guarantee that for a split second or two you won't feel any stress or anxiety.

So why is stress, and its close cousins anxiety and worry, so bad for you and your dandruff? According to Chinese physiology, anxiety and worry can cause 'damp' excess in the body, which promotes fungus overgrowth.[9] Western health and science researchers may have different reasoning to our Chinese neighbours but all health practitioners agree that chronic anxiety, worry and stress are bad for your health.

Have less sugar, dairy and alcohol

The sad fact is that fungus loves sugar and milk sugars. Fungus literally can't live without them. If you have a fungus problem, whether it is dandruff or candida albicans, then you will most likely crave sugar and/or carbohydrates such as breads and pastries. And this 'addiction' is often so strong that when you have one sugar-free day you wind up feeling crabby, tired and you may even want to lash out at others. But this addiction is a fungus-triggered craving because the fungi are dying and they need a sugar hit to live. Processed carbohydrates such as white bread, white rice and white flour products all supply your body with a big dose of sweet glucose so your yeast freeloaders stay well fed. Fungi also love dairy and thrive off the milk sugar.

Alcohol is simply another form of sugar and one that rapidly depletes the vitamins and minerals needed for a healthy body and strong immune system. Zinc and B vitamins are rapidly lost when you drink alcohol and as a consequence they are not available to keep your immune system functioning properly or your skin clear. You cannot look and feel good when your body is depleted of zinc and B vitamins.

How much sugar is too much?

Some experts say you have to avoid all sugar, even fruit sugars, to kill off out-of-control fungi but it's quite possible to get them under control without having to avoid all forms of sugar (which is very good news). You see, if you're a relaxed person, who is great at managing stress, gets plenty of sleep and eats garlic regularly then you can still have small amounts of sugar, fruit and moderately drink alcohol without your immune system being affected. On the other hand, if you're a stress-head, a worrywart, an insomniac or you have immune suppression, you'll probably have to strictly avoid sugar, fruit and alcohol for at least three months. Trust me: learning how to relax is a much easier option.

If you are a relaxed type (or a new fan of relaxation) this is how you can eliminate yeast infestations:

- Eat no more than one piece of fruit daily (no fruit leather or fruit juices other than fresh lemon juice).

- Avoid or only drink alcohol once a week (no binge drinking).

- You can eat wholegrain bread and wholegrain products.

- You can have a sweet treat occasionally (but not every day). To do this successfully, give yourself strict guidelines such as 'Sunday is sweets day'.

- Substitute sugar with the natural herb agave nectar to sweeten your food and drinks. Honey is also a better choice than sugar as it contains minerals.

- Eat protein with every meal (fish, eggs, skinless chicken, beans and pulses and lean red meat); eat lots of fresh vegetables and drink plenty of water (or just follow the Healthy Skin Diet).

- Liquid chlorophyll and apple cider vinegar, which are used in the Healthy Skin Diet, also work to prevent microbe overgrowth.

Tip: If you have sugar cravings, add cinnamon to your meals and take a chromium supplement. Chromium and cinnamon help to keep your blood sugar levels normal so there's less sugar floating around in the bloodstream so your fungi starve quickly. There is information about chromium in Chapter 5 on page 76.

Counteract the negative effects of medications

Drug medications such as corticosteroids, birth control pills and antibiotics suppress the immune system, allowing fungi to multiply rapidly. Antibiotics are administered to kill a bacterial infection but they also kill your 'good' bacteria so they annihilate a vital part of your defence system. Most antibiotics don't kill fungi so they soon have free rein of your skin and bowels. If you've taken a course of antibiotics in the last six months it's important to take a probiotic supplement to replace the good gut flora and win the war against dandruff.

What has taking probiotics got to do with fixing the dandruff on your head?

Everything. Probiotics take the load off an overworked immune system by offering a helping hand – it's like having a million tiny 'bouncers' making sure fungus and bacteria don't shack up in too many areas of your body. For more information on the right probiotic for you refer to Chapter 3, 'Guideline No. 1'.

Step three: Exercise and improve scalp circulation

Being a couch potato can be so much fun, especially on a rainy day when you can sit in front of the TV watching your favourite action movie and munching on popcorn. But couch potatoes are more likely to have dandruff, and dandruff is not a bucket of fun, so when it stops raining you need to move out the door and into a park or gym for some of your own blood-pumping action.

Busy people may not be couch potatoes but they suffer from the same type of dandruff because they can either have poor circulation from lack of exercise or a poor immune system from overworking. Yes, the people who suffer from the 'busy flu' (an insidious disease that prevents them from looking after their own body), can end up with 'busy' fungi on their scalp.

Exercise junkies, on the other hand, should be praised for their motivation – they put their body first all the way and everything else comes a poor second. Four hours of exercise is not a problem for the gym bandit but for some reason their immune system eventually shuts down in protest. No, over-exercising is not the answer to good health either (if you're a professional athlete you're exempt of course, as you're probably getting super health advice from experts to minimise the risk of burnout). Moderate exercise *is* good for your immune system. Moderate exercise basically means to exercise but not overdo it. Overdoing it would be exercising for more than two hours without specialised coaching, or running a marathon. Fifteen to 30 minutes of high-impact exercise can be beneficial; or one hour of walking or a similar low- to medium-impact workout would be good for your immune system. Your aim is to improve circulation to your scalp without depleting your immunity.

You can also improve circulation to your scalp by doing headstands (but go to a yoga class to learn how to do it correctly).

Activity
Grab your diary or planner right now and book in 15 minutes of exercise for today or tomorrow. Find out more about moderate exercise routines in Chapter 7, 'Guideline No. 5'.

Step four: Eat moisturising foods

The Healthy Skin Diet can help you eliminate dandruff but you don't have to go overboard with dietary changes; you can simply add some fabulous foods to your existing diet. Look for the recipes that contain the following ingredients and use at least one anti-fungal ingredient each day:

Salmon, trout, sardines, mackerel. Oily fish are a great source of omega-3 fatty acids which are vital for healthy, flake-free skin.

Ground flaxseeds and flaxseed oil are also a good source of omega-3. Have them on the days you don't eat fish. Make the Flaxseed Lemon Drink at least three days a week as it is specific for immune system health.

Garlic, onions, avocado, basil and radishes have anti-fungal properties. There are plenty of snack and lunch recipes containing avocado; also try the Anti-ageing Broth or Therapeutic Chicken Soup recipes as they naturally boost the immune system.

Horseradish and ginger have antiseptic properties and they're also good for the immune system.

Raw salt-free sauerkraut is a natural probiotic.

You can also take certain supplements to help prevent dandruff:

- Omega-3 fish oils, which are high in DHA and EPA (see Chapter 4, 'Guideline No. 2' for more information).

- B vitamins especially vitamin B6 and biotin. There is a biotin deficiency questionnaire in Chapter 15, 'Eczema/dermatitis'.

- As mentioned earlier, take a suitable probiotic supplement (not all probiotics treat low immunity so look up the correct one for your needs in Chapter 3, 'Guideline No. 1').

Other considerations:

- Avoid using a hair dryer if your scalp is overly dry and flaking.

- If your dandruff was triggered by chemical exposure or psoriasis then you should take a liver detoxification supplement for two weeks. Refer to Chapter 17, 'Psoriasis', for information on liver detoxification.

Let's get practical

Grab your diary/planner and schedule in some time to learn the breathing exercises from Chapter 19, 'Beauty breathing', as they reduce stress.

To get more omega-3 in your diet: add flaxseeds, flaxseed oil, fish and omega-3 fortified eggs to your diet. Suitable recipes include Flaxseed Lemon Drink (have it three times a week); Designer Muesli; Gluten-free Muesli; Vitamin E Muesli; Mango and Buckwheat Crepes; Smoked Salmon and Eggs; Tuna and Avocado Wrap; Salmon Steaks with Peas and Mash; Marinated Whole Steamed Trout; Rainbow Trout with Honey Roasted Vegetables.

Fresh oysters contain lots of zinc so have half a dozen at your next social function, and biotin is found in egg yolk so make Creamy Mayonnaise. To boost your immune system make the Anti-ageing Broth or Therapeutic Chicken Soup every week until your dandruff clears up.

Key points to remember

Step one: Check your hair-care products

- Wash your hair regularly with a natural shampoo and conditioner and avoid using hairspray or gel products. Read Chapter 8, 'Guideline No. 6: Have a good skin-care routine'.

Step two: Look after your immune system

- Learn how to relax. Refer to Chapter 10, 'Guideline No. 8: Relax and make peace with your body', and Chapter 19, 'Beauty breathing'.

- Drink Green Water and have the Flaxseed Lemon Drink three times a week.

- Eat anti-fungal foods such as garlic, sauerkraut (salt-free) and onion, and have the Anti-ageing Broth and Therapeutic Chicken Soup.

Step three: Exercise and improve scalp circulation

- Improve circulation to the scalp with moderate exercise and hair brushing. See Chapter 7, 'Guideline No. 5' for more detailed information.

Step four: Eat moisturising foods

- Eat a healthy diet (follow the Healthy Skin Diet in Chapter 21).
- Increase omega-3 in your diet (read Chapter 4, 'Guideline No. 2').

Chapter 14

Cradle cap

As you may already know, cradle cap is not a cute bonnet made to match that twin set and booties Grandma sent last Christmas; it's a skin condition that looks like a 'cap' (apparently) and it consists of thick, yellow crusts and scales on your bub's sweet little head. Your baby might not even notice (or care) about his or her musty mop top, although it may become a tad itchy and affect your child's sleep.

Below is a simple management plan for you to follow in caring for your baby's skin condition.

Step one: Use natural and gentle skin care

1. **Find a natural baby shampoo that is free of sodium lauryl sulfate.** This is not so easy – you'd be surprised at how many commercial baby shampoos contain SLS or its close cousin sodium laureth sulfate. Be suspicious if your childrens' products foam and bubble on cue! Also avoid brightly coloured products containing synthetic dyes and fragrances. You might need to visit your local health food shop to find a decent, gentle shampoo, although still check the ingredients as some health food shops stock 'natural' and 'gentle' products that contain synthetic chemicals. Also avoid baby shampoos that contain diethanolamine (DEA) and triethanolamine (TEA) as they can cause skin irritations and your bub doesn't need a chemical cocktail on his or her delicate noggin.

Babies don't need bubbly, coloured bath products. They can be adequately cleaned with water and a soft cloth. There is a list of natural baby products on my website (www.healthbeforebeauty.com).

2. **Shampoo your bub's hair and scalp often.** Three times a week is ideal. Your bub does not need to be bathed every day. While shampooing, massage the head, be gentle and thoughtful and your little one will just adore the extra attention.

3. **Use oil to massage your baby's head.** Rub a natural oil such as olive oil or rosehip oil into the cradle cap two to three times a week (you can do this when you're bathing him/her). Then loosen the crusts by brushing the scalp, in a circular motion, with a very soft toothbrush (or you can gently use a fine tooth comb). Shampoo afterwards to remove some (not all) of the oil.

Suitable moisturising ingredients

If your child's scalp needs moisturising, gently massage the scalp with a suitable oil product that contains any of the following ingredients:

- calendula
- extra-virgin olive oil
- rosehip oil
- sweet almond oil*
- vitamin E
- apricot kernel oil
- manuka oil
- evening primrose oil
- flaxseed oil.

*Caution: as this is a nut oil, do not use if you know your baby has a nut allergy or if there is a family history of nut allergy.

Step two: Feed your child moisturising foods

Your child may need essential fatty acids such as omega-3 to moisturise the skin from the inside out. If you are bottle-feeding your baby make sure the infant formula contains omega-3 (EPA and DHA). Omega-3 may also be written as 'alpha-linolenic acid'.

If you're breastfeeding your child, you can increase omega-3 in your own diet as some of the essential fatty acids will end up in your breast milk and be passed on to your child. This will help to moisturise the skin from the inside out. Also read the 'Children's Clear Skin Programme' as your child may need to have a probiotic supplement to enhance immune system development.

Key points to remember

Step one: Use natural and gentle skin care

- Only use gentle skin and bath products on your baby's delicate skin.

- Gently remove crusting and moisturise your bub's scalp.

Step two: Feed your child moisturising foods

- Choose an infant formula with added omega-3 (EPA and DHA) or if you're breast-feeding you can consume omega-3 to increase the amount of essential fatty acids in your breast milk.

- Read 'Children's Clear Skin Programme' for suitable supplements and dosages.

Chapter 15

Eczema/dermatitis

Eczema (pronounced *ex*-ma) is also known as atopic dermatitis and its distinguishing feature is its maddening itch – an itch that begs for scratching if only for a moment's relief. Other symptoms include dry red patches and cracked skin. In severe cases, weeping, bleeding and crusts may form in the elbow creases and behind the ears and knees, and bacterial infections can occur. Having a family history of eczema, hay fever or asthma increases your chances of inheriting eczema and a mighty flare-up can be triggered by stress, anxiety, chemicals, food intolerances and allergens such as dust mites.[1,2]

- Approximately 15 million Americans suffer from eczema at any given time.[3]
- Around 6 million Australians at some time in their life will suffer from eczema.[4]
- In the UK one in five children and one in 12 adults have eczema.[5]
- In developed countries, atopic eczema affects more than one in ten children.

Management plan

The management plan is Part 1 of your programme. This section shows you how to identify triggers and irritants that may be contributing to your condition. It also gives you information on allergy testing and how to soothe your skin with topical treatments. Most conventional eczema treatments prescribed by specialists end here. Part 2 is the Anti-eczema Programme, which details the other vital steps that can actually prevent eczema from occurring. To make this routine simple to follow, Parts 1 and 2 have been divided further into six steps. **Note:** There is a lot of information listed in the eczema management plan but you don't have to follow every bit of advice. Decide what's relevant to your condition and keep it simple and as 'doable' as possible. It is the Anti-eczema Programme that is most important to follow (steps 4, 5 and 6).

Step one: Identify triggers and irritants

Your genetics play a major role in whether you'll end up with an inflammatory condition or two. If you have a family history of hay fever, asthma, sinusitis or arthritis and both parents have had eczema at some point in their life then you have an 80 per cent chance of developing eczema.[6]

Common triggers of inflammatory conditions such as eczema include:

- high chemical exposure
- illness
- food intolerances and allergies
- drugs such as aspirin
- dietary deficiencies
- eating excess saturated fats
- eating too many processed vegetable oils
- ageing
- carbohydrates with a high GI rating
- chronic stress.[7,8,9,10]

High chemical exposure

Pest control sprays, household cleaning products, perfumes, hairdressing chemicals and crop spray exposure can cause toxic build-up in the body. When you breathe in or ingest too many chemicals they can block enzyme reactions and lead to eczema. A chemical trigger could be caused by something as simple as cleaning the oven with a heavy-duty chemical cleaner or not ventilating your house for a few weeks during winter. Furnishings and carpets give off mild gases that can build up in your home over the weeks so open the windows daily to keep your chemical exposure low.

Illness

Bacterial and viral infections, such as glandular fever, or fungal infections such as candida albicans can deplete the body of nutrients and weaken the immune system. This can trigger hypersensitivity to 'harmless' substances, causing an increased incidence of allergies and intolerances.

Food intolerances and allergies

Allergies and intolerances/sensitivities can cause an inflammatory response in the body. Food intolerances generally occur when either you have a weakened immune system (from illness or poor diet) or digestive disturbances so these factors must be addressed.

Drugs such as aspirin

Aspirin is a type of salicylate that can block an enzyme reaction in the body called cyclooxygenase. This causes an excess of leukotrienes, the 'pathway' in the body that makes eczema.

Dietary deficiencies

Omega-3, vitamin C, vitamin B complex (including biotin), zinc and magnesium are all needed for eczema-free skin.[11] These nutrients work as little 'helpers' to assist enzyme reactions needed for clear skin (series 1 and 3 prostaglandins). Prostaglandins are very relevant to your condition and were clearly described in Chapter 4, 'Guideline No. 2', which you can review for more information.

Eating excess saturated fats

Saturated fats from meat and dairy products supply arachidonic acid, the building block for inflammation (series 2 prostaglandins).[12]

Eating too many processed vegetable oils

Trans fatty acids, heated or burnt vegetable oils and foods that are fried or deep-fried in oil contain damaged fats. Trans fats are found in margarines, shortenings, and partially hydrogenated cooking oils and these damaged fats can only make damaged prostaglandins so they cannot promote healthy cell function. One study found that children who consumed margarine had an increased risk of eczema or allergic sensitisation (such as hay fever).[13]

Ageing

As you get older, your body produces fewer enzymes, especially digestive enzymes and this can lead to poor digestion and nutritional deficiencies, causing drier skin and increased risk of inflammatory conditions.

Carbohydrates with a high GI rating

High GI foods such as white bread, jasmine rice, biscuits, pastries and alcoholic drinks rapidly break down into glucose. This influx causes losses in vitamin C and prevents utilisation of essential fatty acids, so high GI foods can indirectly cause skin inflammation. See Chapter 5, 'Guideline No. 3', for more information on GI (look for the 'Commitment carbs' section).

Chronic stress

Chronic stress can be caused by many things including grief, emotional breakdown, a busy life coupled with not enough relaxation or a negative disposition (focusing on the bad in your life more often than appreciating the good). Chronic stress is incredibly harmful to your health. It blocks valuable enzyme reactions in the body (such as series 1 prostaglandins) so you are more likely to suffer from skin inflammation, dry skin, irritability, poor sleep and anxiety. You will have a heightened sense of pain when you are stressed.

When did your eczema first appear?

If your eczema appeared during adulthood then it's a good idea to figure out what may have triggered it (keeping in mind that eczema is usually hereditary so you're literally trying to figure out what may have 'switched on' your eczema gene).

It's beneficial to work out what triggered the appearance of your eczema so you can make sure you're not still exposing yourself to it.

Activity

Think back to when your eczema first appeared – what was going on in your life at the time? For example, were you exposed to a new chemical or food? Did you move house? Did you renovate or put in new carpets in your home? Was your home or office sprayed for pests or were the carpets chemically cleaned? Were you under great financial or personal pressure? Were you feeling rundown from a virus?

Or if you have a child with eczema: Did your baby start drinking formula or milk just before the rash appeared? Did your baby start on solids or did your child go to a birthday party and eat brightly coloured party foods, flavoured crisps or sweets?

Sometimes it's just not possible to work out the exact trigger for your condition. If this is the case, don't worry as the Anti-eczema Programme is designed to address all the triggers of eczema.

What can aggravate eczema?

Now that you've looked at the triggers of eczema, you need to work out what may be aggravating your current condition. Not all of these aggravating factors will apply to you so you may want to circle the relevant ones.

External factors that may aggravate eczema:

air-conditioning	overheating
chlorinated water/pools	pet allergy (cat/dog/bird)
dust mites	sand
nickel (if allergy present)	soaps, shampoos, washing powders

some cosmetics and toiletries

some synthetic and woollen material

some grasses, moulds and pollens

stress

tobacco smoke

weather conditions
(hot/humid/cold/dry/season
changes)

Internal factors that may aggravate eczema:

alcoholic drinks

chemical food additives

citrus fruits

dairy products

eggs (if allergy present)

food colourings (esp. red and yellow)

food preservatives

nut allergy or rancid nuts

salicylates and MSG

seafood (if allergy present)

stress

wheat products

nitrates (in ham/bacon)[14,15]

Foods that can cause/contribute to eczema flare-ups:*
(The possible reasons for irritation are listed in brackets.)

avocado (v.h.s.)

chocolate (caffeine, dairy, amines)

oranges/citrus fruit (salicylates)

dairy (acid producing, lactose)

dried fruits (preservatives)

grapes (v.h.s., MSG)

sultanas/raisins (salicylates, MSG)

kiwi fruit (v.h.s.)

stone fruit – plum, apricot, peach
(v.h.s)

tomato (v.h.s., MSG)

soy sauce/tamari (MSG)

food spreads/Vegemite (additives)

honey/jam (v.h.s.)

wine, especially red (v. h. s., MSG,
preservatives)

broccoli, spinach (v. h. s., MSG)

mushrooms (v. h. s., MSG)

prune juice (v. h. s., MSG)[16]

*According to my own research and client feedback

v. h. s. = very high in salicylates

MSG = monosodium glutamate (occurs naturally in the plant, not the chemical additive)

Short-term relief

If you are suffering with severe eczema, there are many short-term activities you can do to help minimise your discomfort:

Wear 100 per cent cotton clothing

Avoid wearing synthetic or woollen fabrics

Avoid using soap and foaming cleansers

Avoid bubble baths and normal shampoos

Avoid fragranced toiletries and perfume

Use lukewarm water for showering and bathing

Use gentle, non-chemical bath oils

Avoid stress and overtiredness

Find a gentle, non-irritating skin cream

Avoid stuffed toys (they harbour dust mites)

Use rubber gloves with cotton lining

Take off tags from clothing

Use 100 per cent cotton bedding

Avoid using heavy duvets (overheating)

Use cotton sheets and woollen, breathable blankets in winter

Change bed linen weekly

Avoid feather-filled pillows

Vacuum carpets regularly

Avoid cigarette smoke

Use washing powder for sensitive skin

Use natural cosmetics if necessary

Keep away from freshly cut grass

Keep the house well ventilated

Avoid using electric heating (dries skin)

Apply moisturiser up to five times a day

Avoid artificial chemicals/additives*

(See a doctor if your rash becomes infected.[17])

*An important part of the management plan is to reduce your chemical load and avoid problematic food additives. This is necessary as additives and chemicals can not only trigger the onset of eczema but can also aggravate eczema on a daily basis. If your eczema is only mild or occasional, then reducing the chemical load in your body, as a step on its own, may clear up your skin condition. See Appendix 1, for a list of additives to avoid.

READER QUESTION

Q   'I went on holidays and my rash cleared up, but within weeks of returning home it reappeared. Why is this so?

A   *You may notice your skin clears up when you go on holidays to sunnier, more tropical climates. This can also occur when you simply get out of the big city and go somewhere quieter and slower. Eczema can improve in certain climates but the reason is more likely to be exposure to cleaner air, away from pollution and industrial zones. There is also evidence that salt water baths and swimming in the ocean can reduce eczema symptoms, especially if your rash is oozing or infected. This may be because sea water is a weak antiseptic and promotes healing.[18] Swimming in salt water and exposure to sunshine (ultraviolet light) can also have a therapeutic effect but your eczema may also clear up simply because when you're on holidays, you stop stressing and actually relax!*

Step two: Identify allergies

Studies done on childhood eczema have found the most common food allergies are:

eggs (71% of study participants)   sesame seed (18%)

peanut (65%)   wheat (13%)

milk/dairy products (38%)   soya (4%).[19]

other nuts (34%)

You may already know if you are allergic or sensitive to something, especially if it causes physical reactions such as swelling or redness of the skin. However if you're unsure, you can speak to your general practitioner about allergy testing. Your doctor can refer you for a skin prick test. This test involves an allergy specialist putting onto your forearm about a dozen little dots of liquid samples containing potential allergens. Then the specialist pricks your skin where each dot of liquid sits. This test can help to identify if you're allergic to cats, dogs, dust mites, dust, certain nuts, dairy, soya and so on.

The skin prick test or 'scratch' test is useful but it only tests a small number of potential allergens and it only measures immediate IgE reactions or histamine reactions (involving skin swelling and redness), not sensitivity reactions (which can take hours to show up). The skin prick is also not 100 per cent reliable so you need to trust your instincts. For example, if you feel unwell after eating a food (a couple of times in a row) or if you get a flare-up when you eat a food, then listen to your body and stop consuming it for a couple of months.

READER QUESTION

Q **'I have eczema and I was told to avoid salicylates. What are they?'**

A *Salicylates are found in many fruits and vegetables, and products such as sauces and gravies. Salicylates occur naturally in plant foods and they function as a pesticide and preservative offering the plant some protection from insects and spoilage. So salicylates are beneficial for plant survival and help to keep fruits and vegetables fresher for longer.*

Salicylates don't usually pose a problem to our health; in fact many wonderful cancer and heart-protective foods such as blueberries and spinach contain salicylates. However, salicylates can cause problems if your liver doesn't process these chemicals quickly enough. If your liver already has a high chemical load to deal with (from high chemical exposure) or if your liver has low phase II detoxification, then salicylates and other chemicals are able to build up in your system.[20] Your diet may contain up to 200mg of salicylates or the equivalent of one aspirin tablet per day.[21] And if you have aspirin sensitivity then you can bet you have salicylate sensitivity.

Symptoms or conditions associated with salicylate sensitivity include:

eczema and other skin rashes	rheumatoid arthritis
irritability	asthma
hyperactivity disorders (ADD, ADHD)	anxiety
behavioural problems	depression
migraines, frequent headaches	insomnia, poor sleep
irritable bowel syndrome	fatigue[22]

If you have eczema, psoriasis, rosacea, contact dermatitis or chemical sensitivity then you are more than likely to have salicylate sensitivity (or similar chemical sensitivities). Salicylate sensitivity can be detected by a saliva test.

Salicylate sensitivity can be greatly decreased and even eliminated with very specific nutritional supplementation. See step four of the Anti-eczema Programme for more information.

Step three: Soothe your skin with topical treatments

Topical treatments such as creams and ointments are used to temporarily soothe flaky, irritated skin and reduce the itch. Oil-based moisturisers are especially useful as the lipids and fatty acids supply nutrients and trap moisture. This helps to keep out unwanted bacteria, irritants and allergens, and can restore the skin's barrier function which allows healing to occur.[23,24]

Your topical treatment options include: ointments; creams and lotions; bath treatments; medicated creams; wet bandaging.

Ointments

Ointments are thick and greasy. They are useful for scaly skin and extremely dry patches and may temporarily soothe itchy skin. Ointments can also protect your skin from stinging when you go for a swim in the ocean or chlorinated pool if a thick coat is applied beforehand. However, ointments can also stain your clothes if not used sparingly.

Creams and lotions

These are much thinner in consistency and soak into the skin better than an ointment. On the down side, creams and lotions wash off faster so they need to be reapplied more often (two to four times per day, or more if necessary). Lotions are even thinner than creams in consistency so they may not offer enough moisture for severely dry and itchy skin.

There are many eczema creams on the market and there are two basic types to choose from. First, there are conventional creams containing synthetic and natural ingredients designed to coat the skin and trap moisture with as little irritation as possible. And second, the more natural oil and herb-based products provide nourishment and anti-inflammatory ingredients to help heal the skin.

Through talking with my clients who had eczema, I have found that they all have differing opinions about what types of creams soothed their eczema and what creams irritated their condition. Positive feedback related to: the calendula-based creams; zinc-based creams; pawpaw-based ointments; ointments containing grape seed oil; oatmeal-based creams and emu oil; sorbolene cream; almond oil and creams containing evening primrose oil and licorice root. There were also *negative* reports about sorbolene creams; oatmeal-based creams; and creams containing alcohol or too many herbs. However, it does not matter what other people think of a moisturising product because you must find one that is right for you. Both categories of moisturisers have their good and bad points. Allergic reactions can occur with any product from either group and the only way you can figure out which cream is right for you (or your child) is to try them one by one. If you find a cream that soothes the inflammation and offers relief, then stick with it. I have a list of reviewed eczema products on my website.

Bath treatments

Bath oils coat the skin and lock in moisture; however, keep the bath lukewarm and brief so you don't dry your skin out further. After bathing, pat skin semi-dry with a soft towel then apply a suitable moisturiser over your irritated skin.[25] Apply your moisturiser when your skin is still a bit wet.

When choosing a bath oil look for these ingredients: sweet almond/almond oil; emu oil; olive oil; coconut oil; apricot kernel oil; jojoba oil; vitamin E; borage oil; evening primrose oil.

Q 'The bubble bath and soap products I buy claim to be gentle on babies' skin so why does my child's skin break out in a rash after I bathe her with these products?'

A *There are many reasons why a cleansing or beauty product can cause skin rashes. Some products alter the skin's pH level, others contain synthetic chemicals that irritate the skin and products can also have substances that trigger allergic responses in sensitive people.*

Studies show that soap can break down the skin's valuable barrier function. In fact, normal skin should have a pH of 5.5 but after soap use the skin's pH increases to more than 7.5, which can leave you vulnerable to irritants and allergens.[26] Soap-free washes are not a good substitute to soaps as they can also mess with the body's pH balance and leave your skin vulnerable to microbes.

Also be wary if your cleansing product bubbles and foams with ease. It probably contains a synthetic ingredient called sodium lauryl sulfate (SLS) or one of its 'close cousins' such as sodium laureth sulfate (which is milder but still problematic in sensitive individuals). Studies have shown that SLS damages the skin barrier function for up to a month after use.[27,28,29] So avoid cleansers, soap-free washes, shampoos and bubble bath containing SLS. After SLS damage has occurred, you can use a moisturiser containing natural oils to speed up the healing process.[30]

Tip: If you want to have a bath, limit your soaking time to less than 15 minutes as bathing can strip the natural oils from your skin (which is already far too dry). To replace lost oil, add a teaspoon or two of your oil of choice to bath water.

Moisturising Bath Recipe

Mix a teaspoon of oil (olive, coconut or almond) with a teaspoon of your favourite moisturiser and then disperse it into the bath – this helps the oil to diffuse easier.

Healing Bath Recipe

Add 120ml of apple cider vinegar and 6 to 8 drops of rose oil to warm bath water. A budget version is to substitute apple cider vinegar with plain white vinegar and skip the scented oils. Vinegar, especially apple cider vinegar, promotes healing of inflammation and helps to restore the skin's acidic pH. Pat your skin semi-dry and moisturise your skin immediately afterwards. CAUTION: apple cider vinegar may increase itchiness in some individuals; if this occurs, use 35g of baking soda in new bath water to relieve the itch.

READER QUESTION

Q 'My daughter has severe eczema and my doctor prescribed cortisone cream for her. However I've heard steroids are bad so I feel guilty using it on her. Is it bad for her?'

A *I know how awful it is to see your child itching madly and crying from the pain of eczema so don't feel guilty when using medicated creams. You need to help minimise your child's discomfort and topical steroids are an acceptable short-term treatment.*

Medicated creams

Cortisone creams/topical steroids. It's important to know the good and bad points before using a medicated treatment. On the up side, topical steroids temporarily suppress surface inflammation and can offer relief for children (and adults) who have severe eczema. Short-term use of topical steroids shouldn't cause any long-term side effects. Use only in severe cases where temporary relief is necessary, apply sparingly and follow your medical practitioner's instructions.

However, long-term use of topical steroids can damage collagen protein, which reduces skin elasticity and thins the skin. Steroids can also cause increased susceptibility to skin and blood vessel damage (similar symptoms to premature ageing).[31] I learnt this the hard way after years of using cortisone on my face during my teenage years: now my skin has thinned and the underlying blood vessels are more visible. My skin is also extra sensitive to sunlight and prone to sun damage so I have to take extra special care of it.

Corticosteroids also increase urinary losses of chromium. Steroids reduce the beneficial effects of vitamin C and reduce vitamin D absorption. You may worry about these factors if you continue to rely solely on steroid creams for your management of eczema. However, you can look at it this way: use the medicated creams for a short period of time while the Anti-eczema Programme takes effect, and each week halve the amount of steroids used. By the fourth week you shouldn't need to use medicated creams at all.

Anti-fungal creams. These creams can be prescribed by your doctor for eczema that is infected with candida albicans, a fungus that can inhabit the skin. However, long-term use is not recommended as resistance to treatment can eventually occur. Also try colloidal silver: when applied topically it has a similar anti-fungal effect (however, only use colloidal silver externally and you should only need it for up to four weeks).

Wet bandaging

In severe cases, medical bandages can offer relief from severe itchiness and help heal lesions. Wet bandaging is often used on children with severe eczema who persistently scratch until they bleed. Speak to your doctor or pharmacist for more information.

READER QUESTION

Q **'I've tried eczema creams before and they always sting my skin. How do I know if a skin product is right for me?'**

A *Patch testing emollients. When testing a product, if your skin swells, burns or feels hot, tingly or slightly more irritated ON UNDAMAGED SKIN, then the moisturiser is not right for you. If a reaction occurs then wash the product off and apply something soothing such as a plain ointment.*

    *If no reaction occurs then apply a small amount of moisturiser to your eczema. As your skin is damaged, this is likely to sting. Stinging shouldn't last longer than three minutes (usually between one and three minutes) and you should stop reacting to a cream **within** three applications. For example, if you apply the moisturiser twice a day then by the end of the second day your skin shouldn't sting at all. If your skin continues to hurt after the fourth application then you might be reacting to an additive in the product and you should wash the cream off and discontinue use.*[32]

Applying a topical product

It is a good idea to apply a moisturiser when your skin is still damp to trap extra moisture within your skin. If you don't want to have a shower or a bath, you can always gently apply lukewarm water to your skin with a quick splash or by patting it on with a wet cotton cloth before moisturising.

When applying a moisturiser to damaged skin there is a very specific method according to Professor Hywel C. Williams from The British Association of Dermatologists: don't rub it on in a circular motion as you would a normal emollient; apply the moisturiser in one direction only by wiping it onto your skin in the same direction as the hair growth.[33] Professor Williams says this can help to prevent your hair follicles from clogging and becoming infected.

Moisturisers can be very useful for managing the symptoms of eczema. Studies have shown that the damaged barrier function, as seen in eczema, can be restored or partially healed with oil-based creams and ointments.[34] When choosing a moisturiser or eczema cream look for the following ingredients:

calendula	rosehip oil
sweet almond oil/almond oil	vitamin E
beeswax	apricot kernel oil
evening primrose oil	extra-virgin coconut oil
GLA	zinc oxide

licorice root	rosemary*
shea butter	aloe vera*
cocoa butter	manuka honey*
chamomile*	borage oil[35,36]

*May cause irritation or allergic reaction in some individuals.

READER QUESTION:

Q 'I always get rough, dry hands after gardening; they also peel and it takes ages for them to soften. What can I apply to help speed up the healing process?'

A *If you have dry and rough hands, then there are several great hand scrubs on the market. Look for one that contains natural ingredients such as sea salts, sodium bicarbonate, and oils such as apricot seed, grape seed and rosemary.*

Hand Scrub Recipe

You can make a basic scrub by mixing a small amount of *finely* ground sea salt (less than ¼ teaspoon) with two teaspoons of olive oil. Then apply a teaspoon of the mixture to your hands and rub gently. Rinse and dry your hands. This exfoliates dry skin and moisturises at the same time. Afterwards you can add extra moisturiser to protect your skin from dehydration.

Note: Don't make the scrub with too much salt or it will be too rough. Begin with less salt and you can apply more if you need to. Don't use this remedy on raw and sensitive skin, open sores or weeping skin (ouch!).

READER QUESTION

Q 'When my eczema flares up I get unbearably itchy. What can I do to stop the itch?'

A *If you're having an itch attack there are several remedies you can try.*

- *Fill a plastic bag with ice cubes and hold it next to the skin.*
- *Add 35g of bicarb of soda to a lukewarm bath and soak in it.*
- *Immediately after bathing, pat skin semi-dry then apply moisturiser to your entire body plus a thick ointment over the itchy areas.*

The Anti-eczema Programme

The Anti-eczema Programme shows you how to eliminate atopic dermatitis from the inside out. It details effective supplements and lifestyle changes and this unique and exciting programme can allow you to have normal life, free of eczema. This programme also strengthens your body to the point where you may stop getting minor allergies and intolerances so you can eventually eat a wider variety of foods if you wish.

Note: The Anti-eczema Programme eliminates eczema symptoms, however I cannot claim to *permanently* cure eczema. It will disappear on the Healthy Skin Diet but eczema can reappear if you don't look after your wellbeing in the future. If you have a genetic tendency for eczema it can be re-triggered by poor health, poor diet, high chemical exposure or a severe bout of stress. Ongoing nutritional supplementation may be required to sustain clear skin.

Treating children with eczema

Please note that step four is specifically for adults. Don't give adult supplements to children or babies and speak to a nutritionist or naturopath before buying a supplement for your child. You will find the 'Children's Clear Skin Programme', starting on page 204, which discusses suitable foods and supplements for children with eczema.

Step four: Take anti-eczema supplements

This is a very important step towards ridding yourself of eczema. This step can also prevent food sensitivities from occurring so you can eat a more varied diet after the eight-week Healthy Skin Diet programme.

The appropriate supplements for adults with eczema include:

- glycine (taken during weeks 1 to 8 of the Healthy Skin Diet)
- liver detoxification product – this is optional (taken during weeks 1 and 2)
- probiotics (weeks 1 to 8)
- liquid chlorophyll and/or apple cider vinegar (from week 3 onwards)
- biotin – optional, if you have deficiency signs.

Glycine

The most wonderful news I found while doing eczema research was that there is an amino acid called glycine which helps the body to eliminate salicylates safely and effectively. Amino acids are the main components of protein foods and glycine is classed as a non-essential amino acid, as the body is supposed to be able to manufacture its own supply. However in the case of eczema and salicylate sensitivity, this may not occur.

Aspirin is a famous salicylate. Medical studies have shown that glycine is effective at treating aspirin overdose. In hospitals glycine is also used in combination with activated charcoal to treat aspirin overdose.[37,38] The liver should store a supply of glycine and use it for chemical detoxification as necessary. For example, when you eat salicylate-rich fruit such as oranges, strawberries or kiwi fruit, your liver uses glycine to detoxify and remove the salicylate portion through a process called glycination (a liver detoxifying pathway). Glycine deficiency can be caused by inadequate digestion of protein, poor diet, genetics and/or high chemical exposure. And without adequate reserves of glycine (plus vitamin B6 and magnesium), glycination cannot occur. You then get a flare-up.[39] So the salicylates stay in your body; they can cause skin rashes and even hyperactivity in some people, especially kids. Too many salicylates can also trigger an asthma attack. However, salicylates aren't the bad guys – it is a deficiency in glycine and other liver detoxification 'helpers' that is the underlying problem.

If you have good glycination then your body can effectively process and remove salicylates, benzoates (food preservatives) and phenylacetic acid (found in nuts and cigarettes). Glycine supplementation can effectively reduce salicylate sensitivity in eczema sufferers.

Dosage: 2000–5000mg per day (2 to 5g)[40]. See caution box below. Take glycine for eight weeks. It may be necessary to supplement with glycine on a long-term basis, at a reduced dosage.

CAUTION

Do not take glycine if you are on blood thinning medications such as aspirin as glycine will reduce the effects of aspirin. If you have any condition and are taking medications, seek medical advice before taking liver detoxification supplements.

Other nutrients that help the liver process salicylates

Vitamin B6, also known as pyridoxine, is another nutrient which is useful in reducing salicylate and monosodium glutamate (MGS) sensitivity.

Magnesium is a mineral known as 'the great relaxer' as it relieves muscle tension. Magnesium helps to prevent inflammation so it's a valuable mineral for the treatment of eczema. This mineral is also a vital component of your bones; in fact, calcium can't make strong bones without magnesium's presence. Magnesium is also another component needed for glycination in the liver. You will get enough magnesium in your diet if you drink Green Water daily as chlorophyll is a rich source of magnesium.

Calcium carbonate can also counteract a salicylate reaction. Since the Healthy Skin Diet is a dairy-free programme, look for a soya milk alternative that is fortified with calcium carbonate.

Q 'I'm so sensitive to chemicals! I can't even use furniture polish without feeling dizzy and ill, and perfumes make me sneeze. I'm also sensitive to salicylate so I can't eat tomato, citrus, soy sauce or strawberries without getting a flare-up. Is there anything I can do to feel well and have a more normal life?'

A *Yes, you can take a liver cleansing supplement that contains a therapeutic dose of glycine.*

Liver detoxification product

If you have chemical sensitivity (such as an aversion to perfumes, chemical household cleaning products, amines, MSG or food additives) and/or salicylate sensitivity then I highly recommend taking a specific liver detoxification supplement. Two weeks of taking a liver detox product can assist your liver with clearing out excess chemicals so you can handle them better in future. This works wonders but the detox supplement *must* include magnesium, vitamin B6 and a therapeutic dose of glycine. (Note: a therapeutic dose is the recommended dose for a particular supplement and taking a lower dosage may not have the desired effect.) If your liver detox supplement does not have a therapeutic amount of glycine then you can take an extra dose of glycine separately. A liver detox/cleansing supplement should only be necessary for two weeks.

If you have chemical or salicylate sensitivity then look for a good detoxification or cleansing supplement that includes amino acids such as glycine, cysteine, glutamine and taurine; vitamins such as vitamin B6, vitamin B2, vitamin B12, folic acid, biotin and vitamin C; and minerals such as magnesium, calcium saccharate (glucarate), zinc and selenium. St Mary's thistle (milk thistle, silybum marianum) is a useful liver detoxification herb, however it contains salicylates so it must be used with 1–2 grams of glycine to help process the salicylates.

> **CAUTION**
>
> Don't take liver cleansing supplements if you are pregnant or breastfeeding. Alternatively you can take a multivitamin/mineral supplement formulated for pregnant women and you can take glycine separately (1g per day in divided doses).

Tip: When finding a detox/cleansing supplement for eczema, choose one with fewer herbs (and fewer salicylates) and favour one that contains more amino acids (especially glycine), vitamins and minerals. (See Resources on page 371.)

Probiotics

Microscopic bacteria that are *beneficial* to health are found in the gastrointestinal tract of healthy people. This 'friendly' flora works by adhering to your gut wall and 'policing' the bad microbes so they can't multiply and thrive. However, studies have found that this is not always the case. People who have eczema are more likely to have an uneven balance of friendly bacteria and harmful microbes, with an increase in bad bugs and a near absence of good bacteria.

Probiotic supplements supply a dose of friendly bacteria needed for healthy bowels. Common types of probiotics that you've probably seen on television commercials include acidophilus and bifidus. You can read Chapter 3, 'Guideline No. 1' for the full details about how probiotics work.

READER QUESTION

Q 'I've heard probiotics are good for eczema but I tried one and it didn't work. Did I choose the wrong supplement?'

A *You may have chosen the incorrect supplement because not all probiotics are specific for treating eczema …*

In the Journal of the Australian Traditional-Medicine Society, *Naturopath Jason Hawrelak compared the scientific research on probiotic supplements. He found the benefits you get from probiotics are strain-specific: this means they don't all treat the same conditions.[41] Probiotics can be used therapeutically for treating eczema but you need to know the* **specific** *strain that has been scientifically proven to suit your needs.*

The 'key' probiotics proven to reduce the severity of eczema include:

- *Bifidobacterium lactis Bb12 (it's now called Bifidobacterium animalis)*
- *L. fermentum PCC*
- *L. rhamnosus GG or Lactobacillus GG (it must be the GG variety)*
- *L. paracasei shirota.[42]*

Well, now the answer for eczema is as clear as mud! To remove confusion Hawrelak also listed where to find the specific strains of good bacteria. However, product companies can change their supplement formulas so I have listed the specific brands on my website so this information can be updated if necessary.

Tip: If your local pharmacy or health food shop tries to convince you to buy another brand or strain of probiotic then politely say 'no thanks' and keep looking for the 'key' probiotics.

Dosage: Take one capsule, three times a day on an empty stomach. For example have your capsule 15 minutes before breakfast, lunch and dinner. Probiotics should be ingested with room temperature water, or lukewarm rice milk/soya milk. Avoid having probiotics with excessively cold or hot drinks as extreme temperatures may damage the beneficial bacteria. It is essential to take a probiotic supplement for the duration of the Healthy Skin Diet.

Liquid chlorophyll and/or apple cider vinegar

As mentioned in Guideline No. 1, green vegetables are about the only foods that contain chlorophyll, a substance that appears as a green pigment. Chlorophyll is plant energy, converted from sunshine in a process called photosynthesis and this plant pigment is available in a liquid supplement that has an alkalising effect when you consume it. It is this alkalising effect that is especially important because people with eczema tend to have an incorrect acid and alkaline balance.

This acid and alkaline imbalance can be caused by: inflammation (eczema); genetics; eating too many acid-producing foods and not enough alkalising vegetables; not coping well with stress or not looking after your wellbeing; not getting enough sleep and rest; medical drugs; chemicals; over-exercising as well as a lack of exercise. An acid–alkaline imbalance in the body can also result in inflammatory conditions.

The Green Water recipes in the recipe chapter will help you to restore your acid and alkaline balance. I recommend making up a 1.5-litre bottle of water, adding liquid chlorophyll (start with the lowest dose) and a therapeutic amount of glycine and sip it throughout the day. Do this on an ongoing basis from week 3 of the Healthy Skin Diet. Apple cider vinegar (ACV) also has an alkalising effect in the body so it can be useful for treating eczema. Add ACV to salad dressings (see 'Let's get practical' at the end of this chapter for suitable salad recipes).

Since liquid chlorophyll and apple cider vinegar are high in salicylates, use them after the glycine and probiotic supplementation has taken effect. This should be by week 3 of the Healthy Skin Diet. Chlorophyll and ACV are also a great addition to your diet after you have completed the eight-week programme as they will help you to keep the correct acid and alkaline balance and stay free from eczema. Read Chapter 3, 'Guideline No. 1', for dosages and cautions.

Biotin

Q 'I've had dermatitis and dry skin for a while but recently my skin has started looking greyish and I'm tired all the time. What is wrong with me?'

A *It sounds like you may have biotin deficiency. Biotin is a B vitamin that is essential for rash-free skin. The first signs of biotin deficiency include scaly dermatitis and dry skin.[43] A biotin deficiency can be caused by: excessive alcohol intake; frequent use of antibiotics; smoking; low calorie diets; excessive junk-food intake; a lack of friendly bacteria in the gut; egg white injury.[44]*

   Biotin can be manufactured by friendly bacteria in healthy intestines (as with many of the B vitamins); however this bacteria can easily be destroyed by antibiotics, including the second-hand antibiotics you get from eating chicken and other non-organic meats that are fed antibiotics. Friendly bacteria can also be wiped out if you have a bout of diarrhoea or illness, or if you have a poor diet.

What is egg white injury?

Regularly eating raw egg whites can cause 'egg white injury', which is a biotin deficiency. Raw egg whites contain a protein called avidin which latches onto biotin, making it too large for absorption in the body. The more raw egg white you consume, the more biotin you need to avoid deficiency symptoms.

Raw egg white is found in certain food products but you won't always know you're eating your way to a deficiency. For example, if you order a sandwich or fish burger made with mayonnaise then you could be eating raw egg white as it's often used in 'whole egg' mayonnaise. If you're eating party dips such as baba ganoush or tuna dip then you could be eating raw egg white. Hollandaise sauce on eggs Benedict, chocolate mousse and icing on traditional wedding cakes also contain raw egg white.

Occasionally having raw egg white won't give you a biotin deficiency. However it's a good idea to avoid raw egg white or limit it to once a month if you have eczema. Once you limit eating raw egg white your body will absorb biotin better.

The good news is that when egg whites are cooked the avidin is 'deactivated' so it does not affect biotin, making cooked eggs a healthy option. Egg yolks are also a rich source of biotin so they are generally good for eczema.

Do the following questionnaire to see if you have any biotin deficiency signs.

Biotin deficiency questionnaire

Circle any symptoms you have on a regular basis
(three or more times per week):

scaly dermatitis/eczema*

dry skin*

greyish skin*

rash around the mouth and nose

redness and hardening around
the eyes

dandruff

muscular pain

lack of energy

depression

hair loss (not including hereditary
baldness)[45]

If you have more than three symptoms and two of them are marked with an
asterisk, then you may have a biotin deficiency.

Dosage: Adults require approximately 100–300mcg (micrograms) per day (there is no official RDI). A therapeutic dose for adults with biotin deficiency is 1–5mg (milligrams) per day for four to five days only.[46] Then reduce the dosage to 100mcg per day for the duration of the Healthy Skin Diet. If you cannot get high-dose biotin, just take 100mcg per day until your symptoms cease (speak to your doctor if symptoms persist).

CAUTION

As with all B vitamins, if you are taking biotin for longer than a few weeks it should be taken with all the B vitamins (in a B complex supplement) to avoid causing other B vitamin deficiencies. If you are on medication, speak to your doctor before taking B vitamins.

Step five: Eat moisturising foods

When eczema occurs, it's partly due to the fact that your cells can't hold fluids properly – they leak – and as a result the skin barrier becomes dry, cracked and inflamed. Omega-3 is anti-inflammatory and it can reduce pain and inflammation when combined with an anti-inflammatory diet.[47,48,49,50] Omega-3 also literally draws fluid back into your cells so they remain hydrated. You can read more about this in Chapter 12, 'Cellulite', and in Chapter 4, 'Guideline No. 2'. You can literally moisturise your body from the inside out with the right types of foods. See 'Let's get practical' at the end of this chapter for recipe ideas.

Step six: Go on an elimination diet

As mentioned earlier, if you suffer with eczema you need to avoid or limit certain foods that can exacerbate your condition. Having eczema means you will be more prone to food chemical sensitivity and dairy products will contribute to inflammation whether you have an allergy to them or not. In fact, the most dramatic results I see when treating eczema patients are when dairy is eliminated from their diets. This is why I now include this step for everyone with eczema.

The following is a very basic elimination diet that only needs to be followed for two months as your eczema should clear up within this time (although you should continue to avoid consuming artificial additives, margarine and preservatives).

Foods and drinks to AVOID

food colourings (esp. red and yellow)

food preservatives, bread preservatives (no. 282)

nitrates (ham, bacon)

chemical food additives (see 'Additives to avoid', page 303)

dairy products

chocolate (contains dairy and sugar)

citrus (oranges, mandarins, limes)

dried fruits (preservatives)

kiwi fruit

strawberries

stone fruit – plums, apricots, peaches, etc.

tomatoes

grapes, sultanas, raisins

avocados

soy sauce/tamari/oyster sauce

anything containing raw egg white

alcohol, especially red wine

margarine

some saturated fats (including milk, cream, cheese, fatty meats, pork/ham/bacon, many desserts, doughnuts, fried eggs and anything deep fried)

Food and drinks to LIMIT

mushrooms

prunes

red meat

sauces

certain vegetable oils (including safflower, sunflower, corn, rapeseed (canola), soya and sesame oils because they contain omega-6 which can convert to arachidonic acid and cause inflammation – see Chapter 4 for the facts)[51]

READER QUESTION

Q 'When do I reintroduce these foods back into my diet?'

A *Two weeks after your eczema clears up you can to begin to reintroduce these foods.*

*When reintroducing foods or drinks, do it **gradually** and only **when you are relaxed**, as a bout of stress will make you more likely to react negatively to these foods.*

I find that eczema sufferers, once their eczema has cleared up, can go back to eating the 'Foods to avoid' as long as they don't overindulge in them. For example, having a dairy milkshake, cheese and a creamy dessert all in one day may cause itchiness, however one serving of plain yogurt or milk in your coffee should be fine.

READER QUESTION

Q 'My eczema first appeared when I took on a stressful job minding four children. The eczema practically covers my whole body now and I constantly overheat and feel uncomfortable. I'm also very busy so I need simple ways to get rid of my eczema, what can I do?'

A *If stress is your trigger then you need to implement good relaxation techniques and also look after yourself a bit better. I understand this may not be so simple, especially if you believe it's not possible to slow down and be good to yourself. But remember that chronic stress is harmful to your health. You can't work or look after a family effectively if you become sick and debilitated through lack of self care.*

Daily relaxation is vital for your health. All you have to do is spend 15 minutes at the end of your day (or in the middle of the day if that's when you're most stressed) relaxing with one of the recommended techniques. The relaxation techniques for eczema sufferers include breathing exercises and taking lukewarm baths with natural bath oils (if bathing is not too uncomfortable for you). Spend 15 minutes indulging in relaxation each day and you will be more likely to cope with daily stress such as screaming children, bad traffic and bank queues. Stress is covered in Chapter 10, 'Guideline No. 8'. Breathing exercises are covered in Chapter 19, 'Beauty breathing'.

Exercise is another way to decrease the effects of stress, and you get a double bonus as moderate exercise decreases blood levels of arachidonic acid (AA) so it may help prevent eczema.[52] Exercise also induces sweating which has a mild anti-bacterial effect on the skin and helps to release toxins from the body. You literally sweat them out. As you can imagine, this can initially make your complexion look worse but this is only temporary. Your skin will soon improve after the toxin load in your body has decreased. Trust me, it's worth the wait. I recommend you sweat for at least 15 minutes each day for beautiful, clear skin. The key is consistency. You must sweat nearly every day to change your health status. See Chapter 7, 'Guideline No. 5' for further information.

Let's get practical

Increase your glycine intake naturally. As I mentioned earlier, glycine is an amino acid that occurs naturally in protein foods such as fish, eggs, chicken, red meat, beans and pulses, although you need to be able to digest your food properly to get a dose of glycine from these foods. If you're on medication (or have poor digestion) then you can get a daily dose of glycine simply by drinking the Anti-ageing Broth (see recipe section). This broth is a rich source of glycine so sip one to two cups of it per day during the eight weeks of the Healthy Skin Diet. Chamomile tea also increases glycine stores in the liver, however be cautious as chamomile may initially irritate your eczema because it is high in salicylate (and chamomile allergy is possible).

Familiarise yourself with the foods to avoid and the foods to limit on page 199, including additives and preservatives, and anything containing raw egg white. Be aware of which foods you should steer clear of when you are eating out.

A note on alcohol: If you want to drink alcohol during the Healthy Skin Diet, avoid all wines and beer, and favour vodka and lemonade (unpreserved lemonade), whisky and soda or gin and soda/lemonade (a splash of *fresh* lemon would be okay). Vodka, whisky and gin (and soda) are all very low in food chemicals such as salicylates but they're still alcohol so they need to be limited during the Healthy Skin Diet.

Eczema sufferers need to get adequate amounts of omega-3 from food sources. You don't need to take a fish oil supplement if you eat enough fish (especially salmon, trout and sardines, and tinned tuna is okay). Other food sources rich in omega-3 include flaxseeds and omega-3 fortified eggs. (I have reversed eczema without using fish oil supplements but I find it is important for eczema sufferers to consume food sources of omega-3 such as flaxseed oil or flaxseed meal daily and eat oily/deep sea fish.) Omega-3 rich recipes to include in your diet: Pear Flaxseed Drink for Sensitive Skin; Calcium-rich Smoothie; Apple Omega Drink; Creamy Salmon Mornay; Smoked Salmon and Eggs; Tuna and Avocado Wrap; Salmon Steaks with Peas and Mash; Rainbow Trout with Honey Roasted Vegetables and Marinated Whole Steamed Trout (avoid the sauce as it contains soy sauce/tamari). Cook with tiny amounts of butter or ghee (clarified butter) or plain, low salt butter – if you have dairy allergy avoid ghee and butter, and if you have severe salicylate sensitivity avoid olive oil.

Eat omega-3 rich fish two to three times a week. On the days you don't eat fish (or if you can't/don't eat fish at all), you can add 1–2 tablespoons of flaxseeds to your food or use flaxseed oil in salad dressings. You can also add flaxseeds (ground or whole) to the following recipes: Designer Muesli; Gluten-free Muesli; Vitamin E Muesli; Pear and Buckwheat Crepes. To get the most out of your high omega-3 diet it's necessary to *concurrently* reduce your intake of saturated fats. This helps to balance your 'hormone-like' substances/prostaglandins in your body. You can still have up to two servings of meat per week but it's necessary to avoid all dairy products during the Healthy Skin Diet.

Fresh oysters contain lots of zinc which is vital for healthy skin; biotin-rich egg yolk can help prevent dermatitis if you have biotin deficiency, so make Creamy Mayonnaise (homemade only as it cannot contain any raw egg white/whole egg). To get more antioxidants in your diet, eat Sweet Chicken Stir-fry; Roasted Sweet Potato Salad and Tasty Antioxidant Salad, however use Omega Salad Dressing instead of the ones recommended.

Enjoy dairy-free carob, decaffeinated coffee (no more than two cups a day), dandelion tea and chamomile tea (remembering the caution above). And are you drinking plenty of water? Water is vital for elimination of waste and it hydrates your skin. You will get all the information you need on water in Chapter 3. Other suitable drinks include Skin Juice for Sensitive skin No. 1 and No. 2; Skin Firming Drink; Green Water (from week 3); ACV Drink (from week 3) and Anti-ageing Broth.

Key points to remember

Step one: Identify triggers and irritants

- Limit chemical exposure, use natural cleaning products and wash fruits and veg.

- Eat less processed, chemical-laden products and eat more fresh food.

Step two: Identify allergies

- Identify allergies and avoid offending foods and environments.

Step three: Soothe your skin with topical treatments

- Moisturise your skin as often as needed (two to four times a day).

- Have a 'healing' bath once or twice a week.

Step four: Take anti-eczema supplements

- Have a therapeutic dose of glycine daily (look for a glycine supplement that also contains magnesium and vitamin B6).

- Take a probiotic supplement that is specific for eczema.

- Optional: If you have signs of biotin deficiency, take a supplement for eight weeks and if you present with chemical sensitivity, have a liver detoxification supplement for two weeks.

Step five: Eat moisturising foods

- Drink plenty of water – eight to ten glasses a day.

- Consume omega-3 every day.

- Adults with severe dry skin should also take an omega-3 supplement – read Chapter 4 for dosage and cautions.

Step six: Go on an elimination diet

- Limit saturated fat intake – avoid pork and dairy products and limit red meat intake (have one to two servings of meat a week, each serving smaller than the size and thickness of the palm of your hand).

- Avoid foods that are likely to cause flare-ups. Especially limit the types of fruit you eat. Favour pears, banana and papaya/papaw as they are salicylate-free, and have small amounts of apples and blueberries. Avoid all other fruits.

- Reduce omega-6 so avoid using margarine; safflower/sunflower/sesame/corn oil; nuts and seeds. You can use small amounts of ghee, butter or extra-virgin olive oil in cooking.

- Increase non-dairy sources of calcium (see Chapter 4). Use soya milk that is fortified with calcium carbonate. Butter and ghee are the only acceptable dairy products, unless you have a diagnosed dairy allergy.

Other important steps:

- Relax.
- Sweat for 15 minutes every day.
- In week 3 introduce Green Water and apple cider vinegar into your routine.

After your eczema has cleared up

- Celebrate!

- Gradually reintroduce dairy products into your diet. Have one serving only per day such as plain yogurt and see if it causes a flare-up. This step is necessary to identify if you should avoid or limit dairy for the long term.

- After you have tried dairy products and have experienced no reaction then add more foods back into your diet such as tomato, grapes and lemon. Introduce one new food every three days. If you get a flare-up then limit or avoid that food for another month then retest.

- Reduce supplement dosages gradually. Stop taking probiotic, biotin and liver cleansing supplement (if you haven't already).

- Important: Keep consuming omega-3 rich foods every day (fish, flaxseeds, etc.).

- Important: Continue having one bottle of Green Water (with added glycine and 2 teaspoons of chlorophyll) three to five times a week (or daily if desired).

Chapter 16

Children's Clear Skin Programme

The following programme is suitable for children with eczema, psoriasis, hives, rosacea and allergies. If a treatment is for a specific condition it will be mentioned by name.

If your child has an undesirable skin condition, you can begin by following the relevant advice in the eczema management plan for adults in the previous chapter – steps one to three. Here is a brief recap; for more information read pages 179–192.

Step one: Identify triggers and irritants

- Limit chemical exposure. You can do this by using natural cleaning products and washing fruit and vegetables in a bowl of water with a splash of vinegar (the vinegar helps with pesticide removal). You can also wash your child's clothes with sensitive-skin washing powder and avoid all bath products containing chemicals and artificial foaming agents.

- Feed your child fresh foods that don't contain artificial additives. Avoid food colourings, preservatives and flavour enhancers (see 'Additives to avoid' in Appendix 1).

Step two: Identify allergies

Have your child allergy tested if age appropriate. Talk to your doctor.

Step three: Soothe your child's skin with topical treatments

- Moisturise your child's skin as often as needed (two to four times a day).
- Apply creams in the same direction as the hair growth on your child's skin.

- Give your child 'healing' baths at least three times a week. If you bathe your child in a baby sized bath, see the 'Baby Bath Recipes' below, or if your child is old enough to bathe in an adult sized bath then follow the 'Big Bath Recipes'.

Baby Bath Recipes

1. For bacterial infections and healing of lesions: Add 1 tablespoon of apple cider vinegar to a lukewarm baby sized bath. Bathe your bub for approximately 5 minutes. Pat skin semi-dry (allowing some moisture to remain), then apply moisturiser or a thick barrier cream to affected areas.

> **CAUTION**
>
> Vinegar can increase itchiness, if this occurs, rinse skin with plain water or replace bath water and use bicarb of soda (described next).

2. For severely itchy skin: Add 2 table-spoons of bicarb of soda to a lukewarm bath. Bathe for 10 minutes. Afterwards, pat skin semi-dry and apply moisturiser or a thick barrier cream.

3. For dry, flaky, itchy skin: Add 1 capful (1 teaspoon) of oil/oil blend to a lukewarm bath. Suitable oils include coconut oil, emu oil, olive oil, jojoba oil and evening primrose oil. Bathe for 10 minutes. Pat skin semi-dry afterwards and apply a moisturiser or barrier cream to affected areas.

Big Bath Recipes

When children are older they can bathe in an adult sized bath, although keep the bath fairly shallow so less measured ingredients are needed:

1. For bacterial infections and healing of lesions: Add 120ml of apple cider vinegar to a lukewarm bath (white vinegar is the budget option). Bathe for 5 to 15 minutes. You may need to rinse the skin afterwards if your child suffers from itchiness. Pat skin semi-dry with a towel then apply moisturiser or a thick barrier cream to affected skin.

2. For severely itchy skin: Add 35g of bicarb of soda to a lukewarm bath. Bathe for 5 to 15 minutes. Afterwards, pat semi-dry and apply moisturiser or a thick barrier cream.

3. For dry, flaky, itchy skin: Add 1–2 capfuls (teaspoons) of natural oil/oil blend to a lukewarm bath. Suitable oils include coconut oil, emu oil, jojoba oil and evening primrose oil (olive oil may also be okay). Bathe for 5 to 15 minutes. Pat skin semi-dry afterwards and apply a barrier cream.

Never use bubble bath, antiseptics or soap as they will irritate the condition further. They also exacerbate vulvovaginitis (vagina inflammation, common in young girls). A vinegar bath (option 1, page 205) is most suitable for this condition.

CAUTION

Oils can make bath surfaces very slippery so use a non-slip mat in the bath and always clean the oil off your bath using a natural abrasive such as bicarb of soda. Vinegar and hot water is also an effective cleaning agent.

Topical evening primrose oil for babies and children with eczema

Pierce one capsule of evening primrose oil and mix it in with your child's usual skin cream then apply the mixture to unbroken skin (to test for reactions). If there is no swelling or redness you can then apply the emollient directly to the eczema-affected areas so your bub can absorb the beneficial oils through the skin.[1,2] Look out for moisturisers that contain evening primrose oil, blackcurrant seed oil or borage oil as these oils contain gamma-linolenic acid (GLA), which is beneficial for your child's skin.

After you have reviewed the first three steps, move on to step four.

Step four: Give your child suitable supplements

Supplements are necessary for children with inflammation for three main reasons. First, skin inflammation causes a high amount of nutrient loss in children – the body burns up vitamins and minerals in its bid to repair the damaged skin. The stress caused by having itchy or uncomfortable skin also depletes nutrients in the body. Second, a deficiency in B vitamins, glycine, magnesium and/or essential fatty acids can cause skin conditions because the liver needs these nutrients to safely remove chemicals, hormones and carcinogens (cancer-causing substances) from the body. Third, a deficiency of healthy bacteria in your child's gastrointestinal tract can

CAUTION

Please note that no supplements are to be given to a small child in a pill or capsule form as they may choke on them. If a supplement is packaged in a capsule, simply break open or pierce the capsule and add the contents to liquid or food as prescribed. Refer to the manufacturer's instructions for more information.

cause a proliferation of unhealthy microbes and this can hamper your child's digestion and absorption of foods. Poor digestion can prevent essential fatty acids, such as omega-3, from being absorbed properly and B vitamins cannot be manufactured by your child's body if friendly bacteria aren't present.

Suitable supplements for children

Please note that some supplements are essential only for certain skin conditions:

- glycine (essential for eczema, salicylate and chemical sensitivity, psoriasis, hives and may be beneficial for nut sensitivity)

- probiotic supplement (essential for all skin conditions, lowered immunity, allergies and sensitivities)

- liquid chlorophyll (essential for all skin conditions, allergies and sensitivities)

- children's omega-3 fish oil supplement (essential for psoriasis, rosacea and hyperactivity).

Glycine

As I mentioned in the Anti-eczema Programme in the previous chapter, glycine helps the liver to safely process salicylates and other chemicals. Glycine can help your child tolerate a wider variety of foods without getting an adverse skin reaction so it can help them to have a more normal diet! (read the information on glycine in Chapter 15). Glycine is available from most health food shops.

Dosage: For babies under one year: 100–200mg of glycine, added to formula or water. For children over the age of one: 600–800mg per day, added to liquid.[3] Glycine is sweet and pleasant tasting; you can also add it to Green Water in week 4 of the Healthy Skin Diet. Older children can have up to 1000mg (1g) per day; begin with a glycine dosage of 600–700mg per day in divided doses. After their skin has cleared up, give your child one to two maintenance doses a week to ensure there is always enough glycine stored in the liver for salicylate removal.

Tips for breastfeeding mothers

Salicylates end up in breast milk so babies with eczema and salicylate sensitivity may benefit if their breastfeeding mother takes a glycine supplement.[4] If you're breastfeeding, you can take glycine on its own or with magnesium and vitamin B6 (see the adult dosage in the previous chapter). You can also drink the Anti-ageing Broth twice a day as it's naturally rich in glycine.

Probiotic supplement

There is excellent scientific research showing that *certain strains* of probiotic bacteria can successfully reduce inflammation in many (but not all) people suffering from atopic and allergic conditions.[5]

Probiotic strains that have solid evidence of usefulness in infantile eczema and food allergies (however all children can benefit from taking a probiotic supplement) include:

- L. fermentum PCC (VRI-002)
- B. lactis Bb12 (now called Bifidobacterium animalis)
- L. rhamnosus GG, Lactobacillus GG (it must be the GG variety)
- L. paracasei shirota.[6]

Again, this information is confusing when presented on its own but when combined with brand information it becomes easy to find the right supplement for your child. As products and formulas can change at any time you can find up-to-date information at my website mentioned on page 371.

READER QUESTION

Q 'Are probiotics suitable for babies with eczema?'

A *Yes. Plain probiotic supplements are safe for babies. There are a couple of ways to administer probiotics if your baby is under the age of one. If you are still breast-feeding then you can take the probiotic yourself (as it may alter the flora in your breast milk) and you can also put a few grains of probiotic on your nipple before your baby breastfeeds (do this twice a day). If your baby is bottle fed then you can add a measured dose of probiotic to his or her bottle, twice a day.*

All babies should naturally develop healthy gut bacteria in their gastrointestinal tracts soon after birth. This helps them to have a healthy immune system and good digestion. However this flora proliferation doesn't always occur, especially if the baby was born by caesarean, prematurely or if the mother had a yeast/candida infection in the vaginal tract at the time of giving birth.

If babies don't have enough of the right gut bacteria then candida albicans (fungus/yeast) and other undesirable microbes attach to the gut lining. This increases your baby's chance of illness, allergies and skin conditions such as eczema (not forgetting that genetics also play a role). A suitable probiotic can help to improve a baby's gut health, reduce some allergic responses, and promote good digestion and proper immunity.

Dosage: From birth to seven months: 1 pinch (1/8 capsule) of probiotic grains sprinkled onto nipple or bottle nipple before suckling. Eight months to one year:

¼ capsule (⅛ teaspoon) added to a lukewarm bottle or room-temperature water. You can also sprinkle probiotic grains onto cooled baby rice cereal (never add probiotic to overly warm foods). Two to seven years old: ½ capsule (or less than ¼ teaspoon) added to liquid. Over the age of eight years: 1 full capsule opened (or ½ teaspoon) added to liquid. If you're unsure of the dosage, refer to the manufacturer's instructions for the appropriate measure for your child's age.

Give your child a suitable probiotic supplement twice a day, before breakfast and in the afternoon, preferably on an empty stomach (or about fifteen minutes before food). Add a measured dose of probiotic to rice/soya milk, water or diluted apple/pear juice, twice a day. If you're using apple or pear juice make sure it is preservative-free and diluted with water. Juices and rice milk generally aren't good for children's teeth so you should brush their teeth afterwards or before sleep.

Case study

A one-year-old boy had severe eczema on the back of his legs, on his back, chest and ears, and his arms and face were extremely dry. His dermatologist previously said the eczema wasn't food related and prescribed a medicated cream and the avoidance of dust mites. The child was later brought to me by his mother because his eczema still wasn't getting any better. Dietary changes were prescribed – no dairy/tomato/high salicylate fruits such as grapes/sultanas – and he was to take a probiotic and a children's supplement containing glycine. His eczema completely cleared up within two months of taking the supplements and making dietary changes. His mother happily reported that she threw away the medicated cream. After his eczema cleared up the mother reintroduced foods one-by-one so she could identify trigger foods which caused flare-ups (these were orange juice, tomato and dairy) and his diet was expanded to include healthy alternatives so he could continue to be eczema free.

Liquid chlorophyll

Liquid chlorophyll is ideal for children, especially if your child doesn't eat enough vegetables. Chlorophyll gives them an extra dose of 'green leafy vegetables', although children still need to eat four servings of vegetables a day for good health (two types of veggies with lunch and two with dinner). See Chapter 3, 'Guideline No. 1', for therapeutic information on chlorophyll.

You can give your child liquid chlorophyll via the Children's Green Water recipe overleaf. Buy a liquid chlorophyll supplement that is preservative free as preservatives can irritate the skin. Choose a supplement that is low strength – look on the ingredient panel for a chlorophyll concentration of around 200mg per 100ml.

Children's Green Water

¼ to ½ teaspoon of liquid chlorophyll (see dosages below)
1 small glass of water OR ½ water and ½ preservative-free apple or pear juice

> **Method:** Mix together and drink at leisure. Give your child Green Water once or twice a day. If your child doesn't drink much water, reduce water measurement to ½ or ¼ glass to ensure they drink it.

Dosage (four weeks after beginning the programme): Babies from eight months to one year: 5–10 drops of chlorophyll (with 1–2 tablespoons of pre-boiled, cooled water), once a day. One to four years: ¼ teaspoon of chlorophyll (with water, or apple or pear juice), once or twice a day. Five years and over: ½ teaspoon of chlorophyll (with water, or apple or pear juice), once or twice a day.

CAUTION

Chlorophyll is NOT suitable for babies under the age of six months. Liquid chlorophyll may initially cause a flare-up as it contains salicylates, so to reduce the chance of this occurring do not commence Green Water until your child is four weeks into the programme. Flare-ups should not occur if glycine is used concurrently.

Children's omega-3 fish oil supplement

Chewable omega-3 fish oil supplements are good for children over the age of one year who have psoriasis, rosacea or hyperactivity. Omega-3 from fish oil supplements and food sources can also enhance brain development according to recent scientific studies.[7] Omega-3 also helps to hydrate skin cells as omega-3 can literally draw fluids back into cells (where it should be).

Dosage: Age one year or above: 50–150mg of omega-3 marine triglycerides per day. Please refer to the packaging for the appropriate dosage for your child's age.

For other skin conditions: if your child eats deep sea fish at least twice a week then he or she may not need an omega-3 supplement. If your child has a fish allergy or if you are a vegetarian family then they can have flaxseed oil or ground flaxseeds (see step five).

CAUTION

Always supervise young children when taking chewable supplements and if your child has allergies, speak to your specialist before giving your child omega-3 fish oil.

Step five: Feed your child moisturising foods

When you have eczema your skin lacks the ability to hold adequate moisture. Even though this can occur genetically from enzyme insufficiency, specific foods can literally moisturise your child's skin from the inside out.

Omega-3 from food sources and supplements has a beneficial effect when consumed in high enough doses to exert a therapeutic effect. Omega-3 helps to produce the 'good' prostaglandins and it also suppresses the bad ones; but omega-3 will not work effectively if your child is consuming lots of saturated fats, fried foods (containing trans fats) and omega-6 rich vegetable oils, nuts and margarine. As I mentioned in the last chapter, a study found that margarine users were more likely to suffer with eczema than butter users, making butter a slightly better choice.[8]

All children with dry, irritated skin should have flaxseed oil or ground flaxseeds daily (unless they have an allergy to flax). Below is a formula that shows you how to use omega-3 rich products to decrease skin inflammation:

Reduce/avoid certain foods	**+**	Increase moisturising foods	**=**	Positive results
Limit saturated fats, nuts, vegetable oils, seeds, salicylates. Avoid dairy, margarine, fried foods, white bread and other high GI foods.		Omega-3, salmon, trout, sardines, flaxseed oil/ground flaxseeds, dark leafy green vegetables.		Fewer leukotrienes and more beneficial prostaglandins being produced in the body, for healthy, rash-free skin.

Dosage: For children over the age of one year: Give your child omega-3 rich fish three times a week (tinned sardines or salmon, or fresh, boneless salmon/trout) and

---

CAUTION

If your child has multiple allergies, especially seed allergies, then speak to an allergy specialist before giving your child flaxseed oil. Allergy is rare but possible. Fish oil and flaxseed oil naturally thin the blood so avoid supplemental omega-3 if your child has haemorrhaging problems or is undergoing surgery. If diarrhoea occurs from flaxseed oil then reduce the dosage and improve your child's digestion with a suitable probiotic.

flaxseed oil or a children's fish oil supplement on the days when fresh fish is not consumed. Flaxseed oil dosage: 1 teaspoon mixed into calcium-fortified rice milk, cooled breakfast cereal or vegetables (flaxseed is a pleasant tasting oil). See caution box on page 211.

Tip: Flaxseed oil goes rancid very easily. Only buy refrigerated flaxseed oil and chose one that's packaged in dark glass (not plastic). To keep it fresh always refrigerate the oil and use within five weeks. Flaxseed oil can be stored in the freezer to keep it fresh for longer. Heat damages flaxseed oil so never heat it or add to hot food.

Tips for breastfeeding mothers

- Improve the omega-3 content in your breast milk by regularly eating omega-3 rich foods including salmon, trout, sardines, herring, mackerel and freshly ground flaxseeds or flaxseed oil. Eat a variety of omega-3 rich foods, one serving daily.

- Avoid nuts, caffeine, chocolate, tomato, dried fruits, oranges and spicy foods.

- Avoid foods you are allergic to.

A note on baby formulas

If your baby is drinking formula then make sure it contains the amino acids taurine and glycine. Like glycine, taurine helps the liver detoxify chemicals, and taurine is also essential for brain development. When choosing a goat's milk or cow's milk formula make sure it contains added vitamins, minerals *and* omega-3, taurine and glycine. NEVER give standard milk to a baby under the age of one year because regular milks, on their own, are not nutritious enough to sustain a baby's health.

If your child has been diagnosed with a dairy allergy then speak to your allergy specialist or paediatrician about suitable dairy/lactose-free formulas. Otherwise, if your child has no dairy allergy it's best to use a dairy-based, lactose-free baby formula until the age of one year, then if your child still has a skin condition eliminate dairy products from their diet for one to two months. During this time, make sure your child is having 500–800mg of calcium daily to ensure proper bone and teeth development (age one to four years: 500mg of calcium per day; over the age of four: 800mg of calcium/day). Calcium sources include rice or soya milk that has added calcium. Other sources suitable for children over the age of one year include the Anti-ageing Broth and Calcium-rich Smoothie (give them 1 to 2 small cups per day, plus additional calcium-rich foods and drinks). Calcium can be found in many non-dairy sources: see Chapter 4, 'Guideline No. 2', under the heading 'Non-dairy calcium sources' for a list of non-dairy products.

Step six: Put your child on an elimination diet

This step can work on its own but it is enhanced when combined with the other steps. Your child's skin condition should completely disappear within eight weeks using dietary changes alone and much sooner if all six steps from this chapter are implemented. This is great news as it means your child won't have to suffer with eczema anymore.

Foods for babies with skin conditions

When your child is five or six months old, you can introduce 'solid' food (baby food that resembles mush). Begin with plain rice cereals mixed with cooled boiled water (it's necessary to pre-boil water to kill microbes). Every three days introduce a new food. Introducing new foods like this – separately – will help to identify any allergies as you go.

Baby's first foods (at five to six months old) should include 1 to 3 teaspoons of puréed food (begin with one and gradually increase) per day of the following:

- baby rice cereal (once a day for the first week, then twice a day in the second week)
- stewed, peeled pear (third week, cooked then pureed or mashed)
- very ripe banana, mashed with a fork (third week)
- mashed potato (fourth week, cooked then pureed or mashed)
- carrot (fourth week, cooked then pureed or mashed – contains salicylates*)

* If a vegetable contains salicylates, look for a reaction within 48 hours of consumption.

Baby rice cereal can be mixed with cooled boiled water, breast milk or formula. Continue to breastfeed or formula feed your baby.

At six to nine months old solid meals should be given to your baby *before* milk feeding, so they have a better appetite and favour their meals. You can now also give your baby:

- three 'mushy' meals and three to four milk feeds (breast milk and/or formula) per day
- dried peas (cooked and mashed)
- kidney beans, cooked and mashed

- steamed fish without bones^
- steamed free-range/organic chicken**
- cooked lamb**
- plain full-fat yogurt mixed with stewed fruit
- lentils (pre-soaked overnight, then cooked)**
- pumpkin, mashed (contains salicylates*)
- sweet potato, mashed (contains salicylates*)
- pawpaw/papaya, mashed

  * If a vegetable contains salicylates, look for a reaction within 48 hours of consumption.

  **These are iron-rich foods. Your baby needs to have at least one of the iron-rich foods daily to prevent anaemia. Make sure you remove the skin and fatty sections before puréeing or chopping finely (food can be a little bit lumpy as your child needs to get used to textured foods).

  ^ Avoid larger fish that contain high levels of mercury – see Chapter 5 for a list of suitable fish. Caution: fish allergy is possible in sensitive individuals.

At nine to 12 months old you can also give your baby:

- three solid meals including 'finger foods' and three milk feeds a day (approx. 600ml in total)
- mashed green peas (contains salicylates*)
- stewed peeled apple (contains salicylates*)
- brown rice (well cooked so it is very soft)
- tofu
- egg yolk (make Egg Soldiers and dip toast in)
- crusts of bread, fingers of toast
- steamed vegetables cut into slices
- pieces of banana
- macaroni pasta (no cheese or sauce)
- casseroles with meat/beans/veggies (see recipe section)
- Sweet Banana Porridge (see recipe section), omit honey

By this age each mealtime should include carbohydrates (cereal/bread/rice), plus fruit or vegetables, plus protein (fish/meat/lentils/tofu/beans/egg) to make it a balanced meal. Make sure breads are preservative free and wholemeal (get them used to eating brown bread). NEVER leave a child alone with any food as they may choke.[9]

After the age of one year

If your child has skin inflammation after the age of one, it's vital to stop giving them formula and switch to non-dairy milks (this is for two months only). You can continue to breastfeed if you wish but you may have to modify your own diet slightly (follow the adult guidelines in step six of the previous chapter, 'Eczema/dermatitis', for adults).

After the age of one, your child needs a wider variety of solid foods. Growth can be hampered if a child has too many bottles of milk (four or more per day) and not enough solid foods such as meats, fish, vegetables and carbohydrates. Give your child two bottles of calcium-fortified non-dairy milk per day. Your child also needs protein with every meal such as beans with grainy toast or tuna, egg or chicken sandwiches.

To help prevent skin inflammation (and for optimal health in all children) it's important to avoid giving your child artificial additives such as bread preservative (282), food colours and flavour enhancers (MSG, 635), found in products such as chicken salt, flavoured chips and biscuits. These additives offer no benefits to your child and according to the scientific research they can promote bad behaviour, poor concentration and learning, and skin inflammation.

Also avoid giving your child too many salicylate and MSG-rich foods ('flare-up foods') such as tomato, stone fruit, citrus, grapes, dried fruits, kiwi fruit, avocado, soy sauce/tamari, gravies, Vegemite and nut/chocolate spreads. For a full list, see 'Foods and drinks to AVOID' and 'Foods and drinks to LIMIT' for adults (also relevant for your child) on page 199.

READER QUESTION

Q 'My child loves sweets but she has eczema and rosacea and they seem to make her skin worse. Are there any treats that won't aggravate her condition?'

A *Coloured lollies are notorious for causing skin rashes because they contain artificial additives. Yellow food colourings are particularly bad for the skin: tartrazine (102) can cause allergic reactions, skin rashes, hyperactivity and headaches, and sunset yellow (110, FCF110) can cause skin rashes, sunlight allergy and upset stomach. Red, green and blue food colourings can also cause adverse reactions in children.[10] Flavoured chips, instant noodles, party pies and chicken salt often contain flavour enhancers such as monosodium glutamate (MSG, 621) and 635. These additives are not suitable for infants and small children as they can induce hyperactivity, skin rashes, stomach upsets, irritability, insomnia and asthma attacks in sensitive individuals.*

Luckily there are suitable alternatives. If your child is going to a party or if you want to give your child a treat, then favour products that are free from food colourings and artificial flavours. The best choices include plain lemonade ice lollies; white marshmallows; white jellybeans; plain potato crisps; plain corn chips; plain rice crackers; oat biscuits; and homemade cakes that don't contain food colouring. Always check the ingredient panel for suspect additives.

Case study

A four-year-old girl with a history of eczema and dust mite allergy had a severe flare-up when she ate coloured sweets and chocolate at her birthday party. Previously her eczema had been controlled by having a low salicylate diet, and by avoiding dairy, coloured sweets and preservatives but this diet ceased to work after the party and her eczema continued to get worse for the following two months. Glycine, chlorophyll and probiotics were prescribed, and ground flaxseeds were added to her breakfast cereal. Her eczema cleared up within five weeks and she could eat a more varied diet which included salicylate fruits such as mango, watermelon and lemon and other foods that previously caused flare-ups, and she could eat *small* amounts of dairy, tomato and party food without her eczema returning. Another positive was that after taking the supplements she no longer had reactions to dust mites and she could sleep with her fluffy toys for the first time in years.

Let's get practical

Meals and therapeutic drinks for children over the age of one (to teens):

Essential drinks: Pear Flaxseed Drink for Sensitive Skin; Anti-ageing Broth; Green Water; filtered water; calcium-fortified rice or soya milk twice a day in drinks such as Calcium-rich Smoothie.

Breakfasts: Gluten-free Muesli (no nuts); Pear and Buckwheat Crepes; Egg Soldiers; Sweet Banana Porridge; Kids Creamy Beans on Toast; Sardines and Lemon on Grainy Toast; Kids Scrambled Eggs; Delicious French Toast (modified).

Lunches and dinners rich in omega-3: Creamy Salmon Mornay; Salmon and Salad Sandwich; Salmon Steaks with Peas and Mash; and Rainbow Trout with Honey Roasted Vegetables; Marinated Whole Steamed Trout (avoid the marinade/sauce); Fish and Steamed Vegetables; Roasted Sweet Potato Salad; Kids Creamy Beans on Toast.

Other meals and snacks: Friendly Fruit Salad with Flaxseeds; Perfect Poached Eggs; Sweet Chicken Stir-fry; Therapeutic Veggie Soup; Salad Sandwich with Creamy Mayo; Lean Meat and Three Veg; Colourful Non-fried Rice (without the sauce: alternatively, flavour it with natural sea salt); Tasty Vegetable Casserole; Therapeutic Chicken Soup; Tuna and Salad Wrap (no avocado). And for special occasions: Banana Cake; Carrot Cake; Rhubarb Crumble (modified: use pear and juice instead of rhubarb and lemon); Stewed Pears with Vanilla Soya Custard; Sweet Banana and Carob Spread (makes delicious ice lollies, cake filling/icing or a light pudding).

Other steps to consider:

Baby massage: Gently massage your baby's or child's shoulders and scalp with natural oil such as calendula and coconut oil. Massaging your baby promotes relaxation: it calms an itchy, irritated child and increases bonding. Don't massage directly over the affected skin.

Extra hugs! Give your child lots of hugs – kids with skin inflammation need more cuddles and encouragement than usual as they're very sensitive. And a really warm and loving hug is basically 'touch therapy' which has been proven to trigger the release of endorphins. Endorphins help to reduce inflammation in the body so give 'hug therapy' a try. At least five minutes a day would be ideal.

Remain calm: Skin inflammation sufferers are particularly sensitive to stress so try not to shout at your child or argue in front of them as stress promotes the enzyme blockage that increases arachidonic acid and inflammation. (Of course you can calmly discipline your child if they're being naughty, as clearly set boundaries are also vital for a child's development.)

Key points to remember

Step one: Identify triggers and irritants

- Limit chemical exposure, use natural cleaning products and wash fruits and veg.

Step two: Identify allergies

- Get allergy testing if age appropriate.

Step three: Soothe your child's skin with topical treatments

- Moisturise your child's skin as often as needed (two to four times a day).

- Bathe your child three to four times a week and use therapeutic ingredients.

Step four: Give your child suitable supplements

- Glycine (for eczema, psoriasis, salicylate and chemical sensitivity and hives).

- Probiotic supplement (for all skin conditions and lowered immunity and digestive complaints).

- Liquid chlorophyll (for all skin conditions, and for allergy sufferers and reflux).

- Children's omega-3 supplement (for psoriasis, rosacea and hyperactivity).

Step five: Give your child moisturising foods

- Ensure your child has plenty of water to drink throughout the day.

- Give your child a daily omega-3 intake: fish two to three times a week (salmon, trout, sardines) and flaxseed oil or ground flaxseeds at least four times a week.

Step six: Put your child on an elimination diet

- Limit saturated fat intake – avoid pork and dairy products for two months.

- Avoid foods that are likely to cause flare-ups such as sauces containing dairy, tomato or soy sauce/tamari/oyster sauce. Also familiarise yourself – and your child if they're old enough – with the foods to avoid and the foods to limit (as for adults) on page 199, including additives and preservatives (see 'Additives to avoid' in Appendix 1).

- Reduce omega-6 so avoid giving your child margarine, safflower oil, sunflower oil, peanut oil, sesame oil and corn oil. Limit intake of nuts and seeds until eczema has disappeared. You can use *small* amounts of butter, ghee and extra-virgin olive oil in your cooking.

After your child's skin condition has cleared up

- Celebrate!

- Wait a couple of weeks then reintroduce dairy into your child's diet – do this gradually to avoid flare-ups. This step is necessary to identify if dairy should be avoided for the long term. If a flare-up occurs or if your child gets itchy skin (inflammation under the surface) then avoid dairy and wait for your child's skin to clear up before testing the next food item.

- After you have tested dairy (and your child's skin is clear of rashes) then test all of the other foods you've taken out of their diet (such as tomato, grapes and honey). Introduce one new food every three days. DO NOT test your child with allergy foods to which you know your child will have an anaphylactic reaction. This allergy may be permanent (and dangerous) so see an allergy specialist for guidance.

- Important: continue to avoid margarine, poor quality cooking oils, white bread, preservatives and artificial additives.

- Reduce supplement dosages gradually. Supplement with glycine and probiotics twice a week, on an ongoing basis if necessary.

- Important: continue giving your child Green Water on a daily basis to prevent eczema from returning. This drink will help your child's acid levels to remain within normal limits and can prevent minor food sensitivities from recurring.

- Important: keep giving your child omega-3 rich foods daily (fish or flaxseed).

- Use moisturiser if necessary.

Chapter 17

Psoriasis

Silvery scales were meant for fish not femme fatales. Psoriasis (pronounced sor-*rya*-sis) is an inflammatory skin disorder that can look silvery or red and it can occur on any part of the body. As mentioned previously, skin cells mature in approximately four weeks but with psoriasis they can mature in as little as three to four *days*, resulting in flaky build-up. It's as if the skin is desperate to expel something irritating from within so it prematurely forces skin cells to the surface. Psoriasis can be itchy and occasionally painful but it's not contagious.[1,2,3]

- Psoriasis affects 2–3 per cent of the population in the UK.[4]

- Psoriasis affects approximately one in 50 Australians and in 2001 there were approximately 335,000 Australians suffering with psoriasis.[5]

- Up to 7.5 million Americans have psoriasis according to the country's National Psoriasis Foundation.[6]

- Approximately 2 to 3 per cent of the world's population is affected by psoriasis (at the time this statistic was calculated it totalled approximately 125 million people!).[7]

- Psoriasis commonly develops between the ages of 15 and 40 but it can occur at any age. Seventy-five per cent of psoriasis cases occur before the age of 40.[8]

Psoriasis is more common in fair-skinned people and you're less likely to get psoriasis if you live somewhere tropical and sunny. It's a good excuse to move to the Bahamas.

Management plan

The management plan details how psoriasis can be managed, soothed and calmed. First let's look at what can trigger it:

People with psoriasis usually have an underlying genetic tendency that makes them susceptible to getting the condition. However, psoriasis can lie dormant for many years and may never appear unless it's awoken by some sort of 'trigger.' Psoriasis can be triggered by the following factors: high chemical exposure; injury; throat infection/poor health; drugs/medications; physical stress; emotional stress. If your psoriasis appeared during adulthood or in your later childhood years then it's a good idea to try to figure out what may have triggered it, with the following activity.

Activity

Think back to when your psoriasis first appeared – what was going on in your life at the time? For example, were you exposed to a new chemical or food? Did you move house? Did you renovate your house or put in new carpets? Was your home or office sprayed with pesticides or were the carpets chemically cleaned? Were you under great financial or personal pressure? Were you feeling rundown with a virus or throat infection? Were you prescribed a new drug or were you using pain-killers or another kind of medication? Were you self-medicating with alcohol or cigarettes?

It's important to work out what may have switched on your 'psoriasis' gene so you can see if you're still being exposed to the problem. For example, if you figure that stress triggered your psoriasis then you can make sure you include relaxation techniques in your healthy skin programme. If your trigger was a throat infection, then you can support your immune system with relaxation and supplements such as probiotics, zinc and foods such as garlic and the Anti-ageing Broth. If you suspect it may have been triggered by a prescribed drug (and you're still taking it) then speak to your GP about possible alternatives (DON'T stop taking the drug without speaking to your doctor first).

The following things aggravate psoriasis:

alcohol, heavy drinking	vitamin and mineral deficiencies
anxiety and worry	cold climates
chemical exposure	poor digestion, bowel toxemia
chemical cleaning products	impaired liver function
illness, serious throat infection	eating excess meats/saturated fats
medications/drugs	candida albicans
severe stress, trauma, inability to cope	cigarette smoke
trauma to the skin (scratch/surgery)	

Note: A cigarette may make you temporarily feel relaxed but don't light up thinking that it's doing your psoriasis any good. The fact is that smoking is shocking for psoriasis. A scientific study found that the more cigarettes you smoke and the longer the duration as a smoker, the more severe your psoriasis becomes.[9] Even being around smokers where you passively breathe in is doing your scaly skin harm.

Step one: Use water, oil and light therapy

READER QUESTION

Q 'I have psoriasis, it's extremely uncomfortable and I'm shedding skin every-where. What can I do to get some relief and reduce flaking?'

A *A common therapy for treating psoriasis is sunlight therapy and when you combine this treatment with water and oiled skin you can quickly reduce scales and get some relief. Water, oil and light therapy (I like to call it WOL therapy) is natural, it doesn't have the negative side effects that corticosteroids have, it's practically free (the price of a jar of oil) and it can be highly effective – it may even temporarily eliminate your psoriasis.[10] However, I recommend using WOL therapy in conjunction with the diet and supplement advice in the Anti-psoriasis Programme for long-term results.*

An eight-week study published in the International Journal of Hypothermia *found that warm bath treatments were also very effective in healing flaky lesions in psoriasis patients.[11] Seven people were asked to take very warm baths twice a week and three of them showed a rapid improvement in symptoms; the other four were told to increase bathing to every second day and three out of the four had improved symptoms. Only one person's lesions did not improve with bath therapy and coincidentally he was the only person in the study who was also using doctor-prescribed drug therapy. So WOL therapy may not work in conjunction with conventional psoriasis medications but please speak to your doctor first before discontinuing your prescribed drugs.*

Back to the 'warm bath' study ... Not only were psoriatic lesions completely healed in six out of seven of the people, swelling (oedema) was also markedly reduced and itching was relieved in all patients during the treatments, and this relief lasted for up to several months after treatment. An unexpected (and some would say positive) side effect was increased melanin content in the skin, which increased tanning ability in sun-exposed skin.[12]

Another study found that people with severe psoriasis have decreased blood levels of vitamin D, compared with clear-skinned people and people with mild psoriasis.[13] You can obtain a daily dose of vitamin D by simply going out in the sun, because UV rays from sunlight trigger vitamin D production in the skin. (Being cov-ered from head to toe with sunscreen can block vitamin D production so skip the heavy-duty sunscreen during WOL therapy – but use sunscreen if you are spending more than 15 minutes in the sun.) I don't recommend sunbaking for long periods of time. Keep sunshine therapy to a healthy minimum, which is about ten minutes a day.

WOL therapy step by step

- Begin by wetting your skin with warm water – either by having a very warm bath, a shower or by splashing yourself with water. Keep in mind that it's best to allow the water to soak into the skin for a few minutes. Bathing is also a safe and effective way to gently remove some of the excess skin.

- Pat your skin semi-dry, leaving some moisture on the skin, then rub in tiny (must be tiny!) amounts of olive oil, ointment or coconut oil. When applying the oint-ment or oil remember that *the less you use the better it works*. Gently rub in the ointment/oil until it's completely absorbed – according to psoriasis specialist Dr David Cohen the more you rub it in, the better this treatment should work.[14]

- Once you have applied a thin, well-rubbed-in layer of ointment or oil onto the affected areas, you may notice that these areas end up feeling dry again. IMMEDIATELY, while the skin is still partially moist, rub another smidgin of oint-ment over the same spots of scaly skin. Rub in thoroughly once again. Follow this procedure at least twice a day for best results. For severe psoriasis you can repeat this process up to five times a day for maximum relief. When symptoms markedly improve you can reduce this routine to once a day.

- For accelerated results, which may also put your psoriasis into remission, use natural sunlight therapy daily after one of your ointment applications: ten min-utes of sunshine daily, after wetting and moisturising the skin as described, is enough to encourage healing. After short sun exposure *don't* wash off the oil by having a shower. Instead, if it's necessary, you can gently blot any excess oil/ointment with a wet cloth (don't rub harshly).[15]

- *Don't* try to remove dry patches of skin unless they are first wetted with water.

- There is little or no benefit to putting a cream or oil onto the skin *unless* the skin is moist.[16]

Topical treatments

There are a number of beneficial topical treatments that can be used for WOL ther-apy, as listed below.

Extra-virgin olive oil. 'Extra-virgin' means it's less processed and has higher vita-min E content (antioxidant that's good for the skin) than regular olive oil. Apply a capful to bath water, suitable for WOL therapy. Use organic if possible. Cheap and effective.

Extra-virgin coconut oil. Contains capric acid which is anti-fungal, and also con-tains anti-microbial lauric acid which is naturally found in skin's sebum.[17] One of the most respected oils found in the British Pharmacopoeia. Protects the skin from microbes and dryness.[18] Suitable for WOL therapy.

Ointments. Ointments and balms are thick and greasy. Look for beneficial ingredients such as pawpaw, triglyceride wax, grapeseed oil, beeswax and vitamin E. Useful for scaly skin and extremely dry patches. May temporarily soothe itchy skin. Ointments can protect your skin from stinging when you go for a swim in the ocean or a chlorinated pool if a thick coat is applied beforehand. However, ointments can also stain your clothes if not used sparingly. Natural ointments are available from health food shops. May be suitable for WOL Therapy

Sweet almond oil/almond oil. These are antibacterial, and contain fatty acids and triglycerides to moisturise the skin. Moisturising, soothes irritation and dryness. May be suitable for WOL Therapy.

• Avoid psoriasis products that contain coal tar as this ingredient is a skin and eye irritant that has promoted cancer in animal studies (keeping in mind that this has not been proven in human studies).

The Anti-psoriasis Programme

You can use WOL therapy in conjunction with the Anti-psoriasis Programme. This programme is like an insurance policy that helps to prevent your psoriasis from returning.

Please note that this is an adult programme for anyone over the age of 15 years only. For a suitable children's programme see Chapter 16, 'Children's Clear Skin Programme'. Children with psoriasis should also use WOL therapy four days a week.

Step two: Improve liver health

As I've mentioned before, I've had a personal relationship with psoriasis so I realise how ostracised you can feel when you have this skin condition. As you may recall, my psoriasis was triggered when I flea-bombed the house with a strong chemical concoction bought from the supermarket. I've a family history of eczema, contact dermatitis, arthritis and heart disease (lots of inflammation in the family tree) so getting psoriasis was no big surprise. Psoriasis can also be triggered in people who have no family history of the condition and no genetic tendency, if they're exposed to a large dose of stress or chemicals. Stress is covered soon but let's first consider psoriasis that is caused by chemical exposure.

We were never meant to inhale or ingest large amounts of toxic substances. In fact, even low but regular exposure to chemicals puts a great burden on the liver (and immune system). Your liver is designed to deactivate chemicals, toxins, hormones and drugs, and safely remove them from your blood. To demonstrate this, picture your liver as a big sponge that filters the blood – chemicals go in and then they exit the other end of the sponge in a different form as they are now 'deactivated' so they can be removed from the body. This is called detoxification.

To deactivate chemicals, the liver needs little 'helpers' – tiny worker nutrients such as B vitamins, minerals, omega-3 and amino acids – to assist with the detoxification process. But what happens if you're not getting enough of these helpers in your diet? Your liver cannot work on its own and if it runs out of helpers – the essential nutrients – the liver will send chemicals back into the blood stream, without deactivating them, so they stay in the body.

Imagine what happens over time ... your body has more and more chemicals in the blood and to prevent damage they have to be stored in your body's tissues. What happens to this excess waste? Your body wants to remove unwanted materials any way it can and another way to do this is through the skin. Chemicals are expelled through the skin, which may explain the exceptionally fast skin-turnover process in psoriasis sufferers. The skin may shed quickly to help eliminate excess chemicals.

After my chemical exposure I ended up with a small circular patch of flaking skin on my neck and it didn't go away. It quickly spread over my chest, and my torso ended up completely covered within a month of the first patch appearing. I was embarrassed about my patchy red scales and going for a swim at the local pool became a test in confidence as I exposed my mottled skin. With the help of the Anti-psoriasis Programme and WOL therapy my psoriasis completely disappeared within four weeks. My psoriasis has never reappeared, not even a single patch.

To help your liver to recover from chemical exposure, drugs/medicines, alcohol, illness or a stressful period in your life, you need in your diet nutrients such as omega-3, selenium, vitamin E, zinc, magnesium, vitamin B6, glycine, taurine and vitamin C. If you're not getting these nutrients in your diet, your liver can't do its job properly. Exercise, adequate sleep and drinking plenty of water also help the liver to function at full speed.

The antioxidant enzyme glutathione peroxidase is abnormally low in many psoriatic patients and this can result from the excessive loss of skin cells, or other factors such as alcohol misuse and eating too much greasy fast food. Low glutathione is bad news for you because glutathione is vital to keep you looking young and gorgeous, and it's an antioxidant that is vital for liver detoxification of pesticides, alcohol and heavy metals. The antioxidant mineral selenium, when combined with vitamin E, can bring glutathione levels back up to normal levels.[19]

Take a liver detoxification supplement to improve liver health – this is the first line of defence or the first supplement to use when treating psoriasis. A good liver detox supplement (and one that is suitable for psoriasis) should contain selenium, vitamin E, vitamin A/beta-carotene, zinc, magnesium, vitamin B6, glycine, taurine, glutamine and vitamin C. Take a liver detox supplement for two to four weeks.

Step three: Improve your digestion and bowel health

Poor digestion of protein can contribute to psoriasis. If your digestive system does not break down and absorb protein correctly, high levels of amino acids and polypeptides are left in the bowel. You don't have to remember their names just know that they're converted by bowel bacteria into toxic substances, such as polyamines. Increased polyamine levels have been found in psoriasis sufferers, which may explain why psoriatic skin cells mature too quickly.[20]

- Psoriasis sufferers have incorrect cell division caused by not enough cyclic AMP and too much cyclic GMP (both are internal control compounds).

- Polyamines decrease production of cyclic AMP, which contributes to skin cells maturing too quickly (causing scaly, rough skin).[21]

Polyamines may sound a bit confusing but all you have to do is focus on the remedies for inhibiting these toxic substances – the main remedy being to improve your protein digestion as this is the true source of the problem.[22] This may involve relaxing more often, chewing your food better and having drinks, such as the Papaya Beauty Smoothie, to improve digestive juices. Read Chapter 3, 'Guideline No. 1', for more information.

You can also protect yourself against toxic polyamines by taking vitamin A and the herb goldenseal (hydrastis canadensis).[23]

People with psoriasis are often deficient in vitamin A and zinc – both of these nutrients are vital for healthy skin.[24] So when buying a liver detoxification/cleansing supplement make sure it contains vitamin A and/or beta-carotene, and zinc.

Bowel health questionnaire

Let's see if you have any signs of poor bowel health. Circle any signs or symptoms that you experience on a regular basis (weekly):

foul-smelling wind and/or stools

excessive gas

excessive burping

bloating

food allergies, food sensitivities

abdominal discomfort/pain

chronic fatigue

premature ageing

constipation and/or diarrhoea

nausea

unexplained back/shoulder/abdominal pain*

If you have circled more than three symptoms then you may have poor bowel health that could be caused by poor digestion, poor diet, not enough water/hydration, candida albicans (yeast infection), poor bowel flora or parasites. If you have any concerns see your doctor (*especially if you have pain). Also look at Chapter 3, 'Guideline No. 1', to see what you can do to keep your gut in good working order.

Hydration

Make sure you're drinking enough water and other hydrating liquids to keep your skin looking gorgeous and clear of psoriasis. Other hydrating liquids include herbal teas, fresh vegetable juices, mineral water, dandelion tea and any of the drinks listed in the recipe section.

Step four: Consume omega-3

According to an international study, psoriasis sufferers have decreased levels of omega-3 in their blood.[25] Omega-3 is an essential fatty acid (EFA) that is absolutely essential for gorgeous skin. Your cells need EFAs such as omega-3 (linoleic acid) to function properly because without adequate EFAs skin cells can become rigid. Skin cells may also leak fluids, which can irritate the surrounding tissues, causing redness and swelling. Omega-3 is anti-inflammatory so it can reduce the inflammation seen in psoriasis.[26]

Omega-3 needs to convert to EPA and DHA in the body before it can be used to prevent inflammation and dry flaking skin. If taking an omega-3 fish oil supplement it is important to get a therapeutic dose of EPA and DHA. Fish oil works better than flaxseed oil when treating psoriasis but you can also add this omega-3 rich seed oil to your diet. For correct dosages of omega-3 supplements, see Chapter 4.

Step five: Stress less and relax more

As mentioned earlier, psoriasis can be triggered by emotional stress and anxiety but don't get me wrong, stress isn't always a bad thing: short-term stress can give you a boost of energy and motivate you to excel. But chronic emotional stress and bouts of anxiety can cause all sorts of health problems. Stress and anxiety have the ability to drain your body of essential nutrients. For example, you are panicking about your high school end-of-year exams and you can't sleep. You worry about failing and by the time you have completed your tests, your body is so depleted of B vitamins and liver detoxifying minerals that your liver hasn't got enough 'helpers' to keep your blood clean, so you end up with psoriasis. Your skin bears the burden if your liver and immune system are overworked.

Stress affects the immune system as it increases your levels of adrenal gland hormones. These stress hormones include corticosteroids and adrenaline which can eventually suppress your immunity. One study has found that stress commonly triggers psoriasis, with the psoriasis appearing anywhere from two days to one month after significant stress was experienced.[27]

Dealing with your stress

So you've identified that you're prone to stress, but you can't possibly give up your busy life to go and meditate for a week in Nepal so what else can you do? There are plenty of alternatives to help you temporarily switch off your inner busyness and find some inner peace.

1. Have **a warm bath** at the end of your action-packed day. A bath is fantastic for psoriasis, as mentioned in the WOL therapy section, and it also helps your body switch to the 'rest and digest' part of your nervous system; so having a humble bath is truly good for you. Have a relaxing bath three to four times a week. You can combine this with WOL therapy.

Clear Skin Bath Recipe

Fill the bath with warm water and add the following: 1 cup Epsom salts, 1 tablespoon extra-virgin olive oil or coconut oil. Bathe for 10–20 minutes and do nothing but breathe in and out, and look at the water. For a moment forget your life and your worries – they *can* wait. Remember, bath time is your precious time out, not time to make a 'to do' list.

2. **Breathing exercises** are also fantastic for inducing relaxation. But I'm not talking about any old breathing in and out, I mean true diaphragmatic breathing that

'tricks' your body into thinking it's calm and happy, if only for a few moments. Mastering a few of these techniques can be useful for when you're at work and you have a panic attack or if you're feeling overwhelmed; you just sit at your desk and focus on very specific inhalations and exhalations and you'll soon feel better. These breathing exercises are covered in Chapter 19: 'Beauty breathing'.

3. **Exercise** is one of the best ways to reduce stress. See Chapter 7, 'Guideline No. 5', for more information.

4. **Getting adequate sleep** is a great way to counter stress. When you sleep your body heals itself. Your cells are like little doctors and nurses, working though the night, making you all better. However, when your sleep is disturbed by lights or sunlight (if you're a shift or night worker), noise or insomnia then your skin won't be able to rejuvenate itself properly. Wounds may not heal effectively and you end up ageing prematurely. Make sure you get to bed by 10.30 p.m. and have about eight hours of quality sleep.

If you are having trouble getting to sleep, see Chapter 6, 'Guideline No. 4', for more information.

Let's get practical

To get more vitamin A and beta-carotene in your diet: I recommend you simply eat more carrots, eggs and colourful vegetables rather than taking a supplement. After all, one carrot contains approximately 20,253 IUs (international units) of beta-carotene. Try recipes from the Healthy Skin Diet such as Roasted Sweet Potato Salad; A&C-rich Apricot Chicken; Sweet Raspberry, Avocado and Watercress Salad; ACE Smoothie; Spot-Free Skin Juice; Mango and Buckwheat Crepes; and Perfect Poached Eggs.

   To get more zinc in your diet: eat oysters and Lamb's Fry in Rich Tomato. Snack on a small handful of brazil nuts twice a week as they contain selenium.

   To increase omega-3 (EPA/DHA) in your diet: eat deep sea/oily fish at least twice a week. Recipes include Marinated Whole Steamed Trout; Salmon Steaks with Peas and Mash; Rainbow Trout with Honey Roasted Vegetables; Creamy Salmon Mornay; Smoked Salmon and Eggs; Tuna and Avocado Wrap. Essential: Add 1–2 tablespoons of flaxseeds to your food or use flaxseed oil in one of the following skin drinks: Flaxseed Lemon Drink; Pear Flaxseed Drink for Sensitive Skin; Berry Beauty Smoothie; Papaya Beauty Smoothie; Calcium-rich Smoothie; Apple Omega Drink.

CAUTION

Keep your vitamin A intake low if you're pregnant – don't eat too much liver. Natural (not synthetic) beta-carotene is a safer option for you. Pregnant women should also limit their nut intake, especially if you have a family history of allergies.

Key points to remember

Step one: Water, oil and light therapy

- Use WOL therapy approximately four times a week.

Step two: Improve liver health

- Follow the Healthy Skin Diet (either the standard eight-week programme or the structured menu).

- During the first two weeks take a liver detox/cleansing supplement. Look for one that contains selenium, vitamin E, vitamin A/beta-carotene, zinc, magnesium, vitamin B6 (and other B vitamins), glycine, taurine, glutamine and vitamin C.

Step three: Improve your digestion and bowel health

- Improve bowel health with a probiotic supplement (see Chapter 3).

- Drink plenty of water and other hydrating fluids.

Step four: Consume omega-3

- Take an omega-3 fish oil supplement containing EPA and DHA. Make sure you're having a therapeutic dose (read Chapter 4).

Step five: Stress less and relax more

- Have relaxing baths once or twice a week.

- Relax for at least ten minutes a day, do breathing exercises (found in Chapter 19).

- Sweat daily and exercise three to four times a week (see Chapter 7).

- Get adequate sleep (see Chapter 6).

Chapter 18

Rosacea

The rosacea sufferer is not only blushing like a beetroot, they're also suffering with an uncomfortable skin disorder that may eventually disfigure their face. Rosacea (pronounced rose-*ay*-sha) first appears as a mild redness of the skin that looks like sunburn but the redness doesn't disappear. Rosacea isn't contagious or infectious, the rosiness is actually caused by enlarged blood vessels under the skin and these blood vessels fail to function like normal ones. Rosacea sufferers may also develop spots and have dry, burning and gritty sensations in the eyes. A thickening of the skin, caused by enlarged sebaceous glands, can also lead to the nose becoming larger and disfigured (bulbous).[1,2]

- There are approximately 45 million rosacea sufferers worldwide.[3]
- Fair skinned adults are more likely to get rosacea than darker skinned folks.
- Rosacea can occur at any age, however it's more common in middle-aged women.

How to eliminate rosacea

In the rosacea management plan you'll find out how to look after your skin condition and minimise discomfort. The management plan details factors that can exacerbate rosacea as do the 'What to avoid' and 'Topical treatments' sections. I've listed heaps of information below but you don't have to follow every bit of advice; you should decide what's relevant to your condition and keep it simple, and as 'doable' as possible.

After the management plan comes the Anti-rosacea Programme. This programme shows you how to improve your health and clear up your skin condition from the inside out. Rosacea is said to be irreversible once it becomes chronic but I believe any stage of rosacea can be eliminated or at least minimised and controlled with the right health programme. This programme is divided into six steps.

The supplemental advice in the Anti-rosacea Programme is designed for adults. If you have a child with rosacea, you can read this section however you should follow the 'Children's Clear Skin Programme' (Chapter 16) and implement a daily exercise routine for your child.

Management plan

Facial skin contains hundreds of blood vessels of different shapes and sizes and with rosacea, where the facial skin becomes easily flushed, the underlying facial blood vessels don't behave as they should. So rosacea is primarily a disorder of the facial blood vessels.[4]

To understand rosacea better, it's important to look at the *functional* and *structural* changes that occur in the blood vessels of rosacea sufferers.

Normal blood vessels perform these important functions to keep the skin healthy:

- Facial blood vessels *deliver* essential nutrients and oxygen to the skin. Just like the postman delivers letters to your home each day, your blood vessels transport and deposit vitamins, minerals, fats and oxygen to your outer layer throughout the day (and night) so your skin can function properly.

- Facial blood vessels *remove* waste products that have been produced by facial skin cells. Just as you put out your household rubbish each week for collection by the local dustbin men, your facial skin cells also put out their rubbish daily and the bloodstream takes these waste products away for removal from the body.

- Facial blood vessels help to *regulate* internal body temperature. If your body's internal temperature gets too high it triggers the blood vessels to dilate. This expansion of the vessels allows an increase in blood flow, which releases large amounts of heat from the skin's surface. This helps the internal body temperature to normalise and afterwards, healthy blood vessels return to their regular size.[5]

The abnormal functioning of facial blood vessels in rosacea sufferers:

- Rosacea blood vessels expand (dilate) when exposed to ordinary substances that normal blood vessels do not respond to.
- Rosacea blood vessels can expand wider than normal blood vessels.
- Rosacea blood vessels can continue to dilate for abnormally long periods of time.

All three of these changes cause an abnormal increase in blood flow to facial skin and this results in facial flushing.[6] In rosacea, the *functional* changes occur first and if these functional changes are left untreated then more serious *structural* changes may eventually occur.

The normal structure of facial blood vessels:

- Blood vessels are hollow tubes which transport blood that is rich in nutrients and oxygen from the heart to the body's outermost organ – the skin.
- Facial blood vessels contain vascular smooth muscle cells and endothelial cells which work to control blood flow and change the blood vessel diameter.

Imagine that vascular smooth muscle cells and endothelial cells are like nightclub bouncers. A bouncer acts as a regulator, usually increasing the flow of people through the door when the club is empty but restricting the amount of patrons who come through the door when they get instructions from management to do so. In a similar way, normal blood vessels should dilate and constrict on cue, to meet the body's demands and maintain good health.[7]

The abnormal structural changes in the facial blood vessels of rosacea sufferers:

- Rosacea facial blood vessels may become permanently dilated from dysfunctional endothelial cells – like a balloon that has been blown up and let out so many times that it eventually fails to deflate back to its original size.
- Damage may occur to vascular smooth muscle.
- New blood vessels may branch out from existing blood vessels (angiogenesis) and more blood vessels near the surface of your skin will make your skin appear red.[8]

You don't have to fully understand the structural and functional changes in rosacea to be able to treat your condition; you just need to remember things that make your condition worse so you can limit your exposure to them. This is important because you can help to prevent your blood vessel functional changes from becoming *permanent* structural changes (FYI: structural changes are bad news so you want to treat this condition as early as possible).

Let's identify factors that can aggravate rosacea. This will vary from person to person. See if you can identify some of your facial flushing triggers from this list:

allergies (triggering histamine release)	extreme temperatures
alcohol	foods containing histamine
anxiety and worry	hot drinks
dairy products	illness
embarrassment	laughing, crying
exposure to sunlight	physical activity*

poor diet and lifestyle	spicy and hot foods
saunas or hot baths	skin-care products
sudden temperature changes	stress, inability to cope
sunshine	vitamin and mineral deficiencies
some medications (such as topical steroids)	windy weather

> * Although physical activity aggravates rosacea, exercise should not be avoided as it's an important part of recovery.

Step one: Limit histamine reactions

Because the redness of rosacea is created by enlarged blood vessels under the skin, we'll look very closely at histamine foods and their ability to enlarge blood vessels. Read and fill in the following questionnaire to identify whether you have a histamine/amine sensitivity.

Histamine/amine sensitivity questionnaire

	Always	Sometimes	Never
If you eat too much chocolate do you get a headache or migraine? OR do you suffer from frequent headaches or migraines but don't know the trigger?	10	5	0
Does alcohol, especially red wine and beer, cause increased flushing of the face, excess body heat, swelling of the tongue/throat/face, or is there any other sensitivity reaction?	10	5	0
Do you notice a reaction when you eat cheese, raw egg or citrus?	10	5	0
Do you notice a reaction when you eat fish, deli meats or sausages?	10	5	0
Do you notice a reaction when you eat preservatives (in breads, etc.)?	10	5	0
Do you react to perfumes, household cleaners or pesticides?	10	5	0

If you scored 20 or above then you may have an amine sensitivity. If you scored over 30 then you are highly likely to have amine sensitivity. However, even if you scored lower, I believe *all* people with rosacea should limit their intake of histamine-containing foods to prevent the progression of rosacea.

Histamine can trigger facial flushing in rosacea sufferers. There are two ways you can be exposed to histamine. First, histamine is released within the body when exposed to stress or an allergen (an allergen causes an allergic histamine reaction such as redness or swelling). Second, histamine is naturally found in many delicious foods and drinks such as wine, cheese and chocolate. Let's look at these two points in more detail.

Histamine release

When you have an allergic response, the substance you've come into contact with stimulates the release of antibodies, which then attach to your mast cells and cause histamine to be released.[9] For example, you might be allergic to the yellow food colouring tartrazine, found in the packaged dessert you just ate, so your body goes into panic mode and releases the antibodies that attach to mast cells. Then histamine is freed into your bloodstream, which causes your skin to itch and flush with redness.

Histamine/allergic symptoms include: itchy nose, sneezing and increased mucus production; watery or burning sensation in eyes; skin rashes or hives; congested sinuses; headache or migraine; wheeze in lungs or spasms; stomach cramps, diarrhoea; skin itchiness; skin flushing/redness.

Histamines are able to cause such havoc in your body because they are present in almost all body tissues, waiting for a trigger to release them into the bloodstream.

Histamine is stored in the skin, lungs, intestinal lining, mast cells and basophils.

- The release of histamine can be triggered by anything your body deems an allergen, such as drugs, chemicals, inhaled particles such as pollen, insect venom and some foods.

- Histamine release can also be triggered by stress – so if you're an anxious worrywart then you are probably flooding your body with havoc-wreaking histamines.

Histamines in foods and drinks

As mentioned earlier, histamine is naturally found in many foods and drinks, in varying amounts. Large amounts can be found in chocolate, cheese, wine, spicy food and beer which is why they're more likely to cause a reaction than other histamine-containing foods.

- Histamine has the ability to signal to your body to enlarge the blood vessels and allow maximum blood flow, which leads to a facial flush.

- Headaches can be caused by histamine-containing chocolate because histamine causes the blood vessels in the brain to dilate and this increases pressure in the head.

Histamine-rich foods and drinks include:

anchovies, sardines, tuna	jams and preserves
avocado	cooked meats, processed meats
beer, brandy, liqueur, port, rum, sherry	sour cream
canned foods	spinach
cheese	mushrooms, champignons
chocolate, cocoa powder/drinks	tomatoes, tomato juice and sauce
ciders, cider vinegar, vinegar	wines, especially red wine
cola soft drinks	yeast extract
aubergine	oranges, orange juice
fermented drinks	gherkins
fermented foods/yogurt/soy sauce	olives[10]
coloured fish (not white-fleshed fish)	

Histamine-releasing foods, which cause a histamine reaction in the body, include:

alcohol	milk/dairy products
bananas	papaya/pawpaw
certain nuts	pineapple
chocolate	shellfish
eggs	strawberries
fish	tomatoes[11]

It's not necessary to avoid all of these foods but you must limit them. Also take note of any negative reactions that occur after eating any of these foods. If hot flushes or heart palpitations happen after eating a particular food, then avoid that substance for the duration of the Healthy Skin Diet.

Amine-free foods – ENJOY! – include the following:

most vegetables	soya milk, tofu
lentils, beans	carob
peas	lemonade
pears	decaffeinated coffee
apples	coffee, tea
custard apples	peppermint tea
mangos	garlic
apricots	shallots
peaches	herbs
rhubarb	vanilla
berries	arrowroot
cherries	barley
currants	buckwheat
guava	cornflour
lychees	malt
nectarines	rice, rice flour
pomegranate	rolled oats
cantaloupe melon	rye
watermelon	wheat
freshly cooked beef*	polenta
skinless chicken*	honey
lamb, veal*	maple syrup
rabbit*	sunflower oil
fresh white fish*	cashews[12]

* Amine levels increase during storage of cooked meats, so avoid eating cooked leftovers that have been stored/refrigerated overnight.

If you want to drink alcohol for a special occasion your best choices would be gin, vodka or whisky as they don't contain amines (although they can still cause a histamine reaction). You can drink them with soda or mineral water (but *not* lemon squash, tonic water or any other mixer). However, you really should avoid alcohol until your condition improves.

Histamines may not be the initial cause of your rosacea but they usually play a role in exacerbating the problem. In a properly functioning body, the liver helps to safely remove histamines by a process called sulfation, and people with rosacea may have poor sulfation ability. When sulfation and other liver detoxification reactions are overburdened, histamine is not removed from the body fast enough and problems such as vasodilation may be the result.

What is sulfation?

Sulfation in the liver sounds a bit confusing but whenever I explain liver detoxification I liken it to a horse race around a race track. Histamine is the race horse that is travelling along the blood vessels and it needs to be sternly guided to the finish line for safe removal from the body. Now histamine 'race horses' can't find the finish line all by themselves – horses just aren't that disciplined on their own – they need 'jockeys' to steer them in the right direction. In your body, sulphur is the jockey that can ride histamine horses safely to the finish line. When sulphur is available in the body, histamine is quickly removed from the blood stream, so only the appropriate amount of blood vessel dilation can occur.

You can improve sulfation (and histamine removal from the bloodstream) by including sulphur-rich foods such as garlic, onion and cabbage in your diet. Sulphur-containing amino acids (methionine, cysteine and taurine) are found in protein-rich foods such as chicken. All of the other detoxification pathways need support to take the burden off the sulfation pathway in the liver, so also take the other liver 'jockeys' – omega-3, glycine, magnesium, B vitamins, selenium and vitamin C.

- Poor sulfation (not enough jockeys) in the liver detoxification (race track) can make you more susceptible to environmental illness, rheumatoid arthritis and nervous system problems such as Parkinson's disease and motor neuron disease.

Step two: Soothe your skin

You may need to soothe your skin with anti-inflammatory and moisturising topical treatments to minimise discomfort. When choosing a moisturising and cleansing product look for the following key ingredients:

omega-3 (linolenic acid)	rosehip oil
chamomile	sea buckthorn berry oil
calendula	hemp seed oil
vitamin E	gamma linolenic acid
blackcurrant seed oil	grapeseed extract/citrus seed
sweet almond oil	vitamin C
evening primrose oil	licorice

Read Chapter 8, 'Guideline No. 6', for further descriptions and information on what product ingredients to avoid.

READER QUESTION

Q   'I get awful facial flushing, especially in summer. What can I do to quickly relieve the flush?'

A   *People with severe rosacea produce a lot of body heat so they feel hot and uncomfortable much of the time. If you are having a facial flush or experiencing excessive heat, try the following:*

- *Suck on an ice cube.*
- *Wet your skin with cold water or fill a plastic bag with ice cubes and hold next to the skin.*
- *During a flush if you have no ice cubes or access to cold water, you can **visualise** bathing in a swimming pool filled with ice cubes. This works because studies have shown that the brain can't tell the difference between what is real and what is vividly imagined.[13] Picture bathing with ice cubes floating around you, even pretend to shiver and you will cool down in no time.*

READER QUESTION

Q   'I have rosacea and my skin gets itchy all the time. Is there anything I can do to get some relief?'

A   *If you're feeling itchy try the following:*

- *Fill a plastic bag with ice cubes and hold next to the skin.*
- *Add ¼ cup of bicarb of soda to a lukewarm bath and soak in it (refer to bath recipes on page 188).*
- *Immediately after bathing, before the skin is totally dry, gently dab sensitive skin moisturiser or ointment on the affected areas.*
- *Take a supplement containing quercetin and vitamin C (see step five).*

Anti-rosacea Programme

The Anti-rosacea Programme takes a deeper look at why rosacea may appear in the first place – it goes way beyond trying to soothe the hot flush and looks at possible causes so you can eliminate the root of your problem and improve your blood vessel function and structure.

Step three: Exercise!

Exercise is essential for eliminating rosacea. I found this out the hard way ...

My own personal experience is with mild rosacea. It wasn't so bad because luckily I found a way to get rid of it before it had a chance to get worse. The first signs of rosacea began to appear eight years ago; my chin was always red and I had to camouflage it with make-up, but my skin colour suddenly improved after I took dairy products out of my diet.

I had a skin prick test and blood test for allergies and intolerances and modified my diet slightly so I enjoyed having a clear complexion for a while. However a few years later, even without having dairy in my diet, I started getting facial flushing. If the gas heater was on in winter I would flush. I was also overly sensitive to the summer heat and I couldn't splash my face with warm water in the morning without my face being pink for the rest of the day.

I also got patchy, red flushing during and after exercise. This was embarrassing so I used to apply make-up *before* going to the gym, just so I wouldn't look like a blushing beetroot. Not that I ever exercised much! As I've mentioned before, I just never liked exercise; it always fatigued me and sometimes brought on cold and flu symptoms so I'd feel rotten for a whole week. However whenever I did stick to an exercise routine my rosacea would magically disappear. Then I would find another excuse to ditch the regime and my rosacea would soon return. So I did some extra research to see if this was a common reaction.

The Rosacea Support Group website states that 'Many rosaceans have noted that moderate (not strenuous) exercise seems to help alleviate their rosacea symptoms'.[14] Other specialists have also said that many sufferers find the same success with exercise, which could be due to increased sympathetic constrictor tone to the facial blood vessels.[15] Other scientific reasons why exercise can improve rosacea:

- Moderate exercise burns up the body's lipid stores, which potentially leaves less fat available for the inflammatory response. However, excessive exercise, such as running a marathon, does the opposite and promotes inflammation in the body.[16]

- Moderate exercise decreases blood levels of arachidonic acid (AA).[17] AA from meat and dairy can be used to make inflammation in the body so it's important to reduce AA levels by exercising and avoiding dairy if you suffer from rosacea.

- Exercise enhances the amount of anti-inflammatory endorphins in the bloodstream.

- Excess glucose in the blood can damage blood vessels and exercise reduces blood glucose levels.

Regular exercise also improves blood circulation and good circulation is vital for healthy skin. An efficiently pumping circulatory system is necessary to carry nutrients and oxygen to your skin. If you have poor circulation, your skin literally becomes *starved* of nutrients because you are giving it an inadequate supply of essential fatty acids, antioxidants and oxygen.

How does skin that is starved of nutrients survive?

Think about it … skin that lacks oxygen and nutrients will rot and die (as is the case with gangrene). So when your blood supply is sluggish or hampered in some way, the skin needs *extra* blood vessels to supply more nutrient-rich blood and it needs wider blood vessels to allow more flow with less effort.

Poor circulation also means there is an inefficient removal of bodily wastes such as industrial toxins, pollution, dead cells and chemicals. Increased waste and skin cell turnover can cause the facial oil glands to become blocked and enlarged. This can eventually lead to nose and skin disfigurement seen in chronic rosacea.

Some exercise tips

- Initially when you exercise, you will get flushing and feel uncomfortable but bear with it as this reaction will eventually disappear.

- If possible, exercise in air-conditioning or go swimming to avoid negative symptoms.

- Exercise and sweat for at least 15 minutes a day. However, keep your routines moderate and under one hour until your rosacea has cleared up. See Chapter 7, 'Guideline No. 5', for more information.

Step four: Promote good intestinal health

Rosacea may also be exacerbated by poor gastrointestinal tract health and intestinal permeability. Ideally, your intestines should only allow tiny particles (that have been extracted from properly digested foods) to enter the bloodstream. These microscopic amino acids, glucose, vitamins, minerals and fatty acids are small enough to pass through a healthy gut wall while the larger particles stay in the intestines then pass through to the colon for removal in the faeces.

But when the intestinal wall is unhealthy, it can develop *larger* than normal holes that allow the wrong-sized particles into your blood vessels. To get a clear idea of what I mean, picture that you're in a kitchen, you've cooked some rice and you're now using a strainer to drain the water from the rice. The rice ends up in the strainer and the liquid passes through. Imagine what would happen if the colander holes were too large: when you strained the rice, some of the grains would pass through – this is not ideal.

When your gut lining is permeable, foreign particles pass though, enter your bloodstream and cause an immune system response. This basically means your body panics at the invasion and a cascade of histamines is released from your cells. And as you know, histamines cause blood vessel dilation.

All rosacea sufferers should make sure they have good digestion and intestinal health. A probiotic supplement and chewing your food properly may help. See Chapter 3, 'Guideline No. 1', for more information.

Step five: Take supplements that promote healthy blood flow

These include natural antihistamine supplements, omega-3 fish oil and chlorophyll.

Natural antihistamine supplements

There are many nutrients that have an antihistamine effect; here are the top two: quercetin and vitamin C.

Quercetin

Quercetin is the most studied flavonoid because it's abundant in nature. Quercetin is found in high doses in red (Spanish) onions and it's an antioxidant that is more potent than vitamin E. Flavonoids – sometimes referred to in the media as 'bioflavonoids' – are fruit pigments; they give berries and other fruit and vegetables their colour. Flavonoids have antioxidant properties so they help to protect your cells from oxidation and cancer.

Quercetin is anti-inflammatory and a natural antihistamine, making it ideal for rosacea sufferers. Apart from onions, quercetin is found in apples, leafy vegetables such as spinach, green cabbage, cranberries, kale, grapes, pears, garlic and grape-fruit.

Dosage: Take 500mg of quercetin twice a day with foods, to reduce histamine build-up in the body and eat quercetin-rich foods. If you have a histamine reaction such as hay fever or facial flushing after eating an amine-rich food or beverage, you can have one extra dose of quercetin and vitamin C.

Vitamin C

Vitamin C also has an antihistamine effect and is a well-known antioxidant. The human body can't manufacture its own supply of vitamin C so we must consume it every day. Vitamin C is abundant in vegetables and fruit, fruit being the original sweet treat before lollies and cake were invented. Without vitamin C, your skin would come 'unglued' and you'd bleed (this is a deficiency disease called scurvy). So your desire for sweets may be an ancient life-preserving craving for fruits that contain vitamin C (and no, cake doesn't have vitamin C in it).

If you want to see vitamin C work its magic, just give 1000mg to an adult who is acutely suffering from hay fever and see how quickly the symptoms disappear (see caution box)!

Dosage: Take 1000mg of vitamin C three times a day during an acute rosacea attack. Reduce dosage to 500mg per day once rosacea begins to improve.

> **CAUTION**
>
> Vitamin C is an acid so don't buy chewable vitamin C tablets as they will wear away teeth enamel and leave your teeth feeling sensitive (this is painful!). Vitamin C thins the blood so don't take a vitamin C supplement if you are on blood thinning medications (heart medications, aspirin, etc.), if you're a haemophiliac or having surgery. If you have any medical condition requiring drugs, speak to your doctor before taking vitamin C. Also do not rely on natural antihistamine treatments if you have a life-threatening histamine reaction (swelling of the lips, tongue or throat). Please continue to strictly avoid anything that causes swelling and get advice from your doctor or allergy specialist.

It's more convenient to buy one supplement that contains both quercetin and vitamin C.

Omega-3

Omega-3 fish oil supplements can increase peripheral circulation as it thins the blood. Omega-3 also decreases skin inflammation as it alters inflammation-making hormone-like substances (prostaglandins) so it's very specific for rosacea. Omega-3 can also be obtained from non-fish sources such as flaxseeds, flaxseed oil, freshly shelled walnuts and tiny amounts are found in dark leafy vegetables.

Dosage: See Chapter 4, 'Guideline No. 2', for dosage and cautions.

Chlorophyll

Chlorophyll is the green pigment in plants and liquid chlorophyll supplements are useful for improving red blood cell health. Read Chapter 3, 'Guideline No. 1', for more information as chlorophyll is an essential treatment specific for rosacea.

Step six: Eat a healthy diet

Don't forget to do the eight-week programme, the Healthy Skin Diet. There are histamine-containing foods in the Healthy Skin Diet, but not as many as the average Western diet so you shouldn't have any problems enjoying the delicious recipes. I'm not giving you an amine-free diet as you want to be able to eat amine-containing foods *and* be rosacea free. Exercising on a daily basis and taking the essential supplements will help you to achieve this.

Let's get practical

You can get a fantastic dose of omega-3 (EPA and DHA) from oily fish such as salmon, trout, herring, sardines and mackerel. Eat fish twice a week but remember that fish contains histamines so don't overindulge and don't eat fish if you have a fish allergy. Omega-3 is also found in flaxseeds, flaxseed oil, walnuts and tiny amounts in dark green leafy vegetables. Eat one serving of these daily – one serving would be 1–2 tablespoons of flaxseed oil, 1–2 tablespoon of ground or whole flaxseeds, one small handful of freshly shelled walnuts a couple of times a week. **Eat two handfuls of dark green vegetables every day**. Recipes high in omega-3, EPA and DHA include Salmon Steaks with Peas and Mash; Rainbow Trout with Honey Roasted Vegetables; Creamy Salmon Mornay. Add 1–2 tablespoons of flaxseeds to your food or use flaxseed oil in one of the following skin drinks: Flaxseed Lemon Drink; Pear Flaxseed Drink for Sensitive Skin; Berry Beauty Smoothie; Calcium-rich Smoothie; Apple Omega Drink and drink plenty of filtered water.

To help your liver detoxify amines/histamines drink Green Water twice a day and eat sulphur-rich foods such as garlic, onion and cabbage. Recipes include Anti-ageing Broth; Therapeutic Veggie Soup; Herb and Garlic Chicken Casserole; Therapeutic Chicken Soup.

Add quercetin-rich produce to the shopping list such as Spanish onions, apples, grapefruit and cabbage. You can also snack on amine-free foods such as Amine-free Fruit Salad, lychees, watermelon, apples, pears, peas, mangos, berries, carob, rice and rolled oats (review the list 'Amine-free foods').

Key points to remember

Step one: Limit histamine reactions

- Avoid alcohol, chocolate, cheese, oranges, spicy food and allergy foods.

- Stress and anxiety also trigger histamine release so read Chapter 19, 'Beauty breathing', for effective relaxation techniques.

Step two: Soothe your skin

- Use a cleanser and moisturiser that contain anti-inflammatory ingredients.

Step three: Exercise!

- Improve your circulation. Exercise for at least 15 minutes every day, sweat and breathe deeply.

- Exercise is the most essential step to improving your rosacea; without it, all other steps will only offer minor benefit.

Step four: Promote good intestinal health

- Take a probiotic supplement if necessary; chew your food properly; drink water.

Step five: Take supplements that promote healthy blood flow

- Take a quercetin and vitamin C supplement; drink Green Water; and take an omega-3 supplement.

Step six: Eat a healthy diet

- Follow the Healthy Skin Diet for eight weeks.

- Improve liver function with garlic, onion, cabbage and omega-3 rich fish.

- Include flaxseed oil in your diet.

- Eat dark leafy green vegetables every day.

Part 4

Being beautiful and healthy

Chapter 19

Beauty breathing

The person with strong lungs has soft, lustrous skin and glossy hair. Skin that is dry, dull or rough is a sign of lung imbalance.

– Paul Pitchford, author of Healing with Whole Foods

Feeling stressed? If you know a couple of simple breathing techniques then you can make yourself feel relaxed in an instant. In fact, good quality breathing can enhance your health in many ways, which is why breathing exercises are an important part of the Healthy Skin Diet.

Breathing exercises are important for your skin's health. Correct breathing increases lymph and blood flow to the skin, giving you a fresher looking complexion. Correct breathing also enhances oxygen and nutrient flow to the skin so it facilitates wound healing and cell renewal. And it reduces stress and anxiety so it decreases the likelihood of skin rashes caused by stress-induced inflammation. Breathing exercises also teach you to breathe correctly during exercise, making it easier to do strenuous activities for longer (and remember, you must work up a sweat for gorgeous skin).

The skin is the last organ to receive nutrients (supplied by your meals). Better breathing can enhance digestion and absorption of nutrients, which means more essential fatty acids and antioxidants from the Healthy Skin Diet can get to your outermost organ – the skin.

The act of breathing in and out also directly affects your lymphatic system, which is one of the main body systems responsible for healthy skin as well as immunity and resistance to disease.[1]

The stress response

Stress triggers your 'fight or flight' nervous system to kick in. This is the hyped-up part of your nervous system but you don't want it to be switched on for too long. If you're chronically stressed or *always* shallow breathing then the stress hormone cortisol will be released. High or continual cortisol levels accelerate ageing and decrease the body's ability to fight bacteria and viruses.[2] Fight or flight stress responses can also prevent your body from making beauty-boosting prostaglandins (remember, prostaglandins were covered in Chapter 4, 'Guideline No. 2'). No wonder stress makes you look and feel older.

Breathing exercises are also a useful tool if you suffer from anxiety or depression. According to the principles of traditional Chinese medicine (and mounting evidence), clouded emotions and thoughts can be 'cleansed' by long, deep breathing and many doctors and psychiatrists are now prescribing breathing exercises to their patients as a part of their wellness programmes.[3]

READER QUESTION

Q 'My doctor said I am a shallow breather. What does this mean and what can I do about it?'

A *Weak or shallow breathing, where you predominantly breathe into your upper chest and only partially inflate the lungs, is becoming a common problem for many in our community. According to renowned breathing teacher Sophie Gabriel, author of* Breathe for Life, *poor breathing habits can be triggered by a variety of factors, such as an inability to cope with stress and anxiety, tense muscles, a sedentary lifestyle, illness, injury and smoking.[4] Even poor posture, where you slouch for long hours towards your computer (or this book) can decrease your breath quality and lead to chronic upper chest breathing.*

*To change your pattern of shallow breathing you need to first become aware of it. You can also check your posture and learn some simple breathing techniques (later in this chapter). Practise your breathing exercises daily to help retrain the breath. However, it must be said that simply breathing in deeply cannot make a lasting change to your health: it's the breathing **technique** or breath quality that makes all the difference.*

Case study

A 36-year-old woman presented with mild obesity, anxiety, pasty skin and a low tolerance to exercise. Her breathing was observed: her shoulders moved upwards on inhalation and she breathed into her upper chest in a shallow manner. She was given daily breathing exercises and was also advised to do them whenever she felt anxious. She reported the breathing exercises helped control her feelings of anxiety, enabling her to leave the house more often and exercise. After three weeks she felt less tired after exercise and she joined a netball team. After six weeks she had lost nearly 1½ stone (9 kilos), her complexion was a healthier colour and skin tone appeared more even.

Becoming familiar with the breath

I really feel strongly about sharing with you the breathing techniques that Sophie Gabriel has taught me as I have experienced amazing benefits from incorporating them into my life. When I first learnt the technique of Throat Breathing I was amazed at how it helped with my yoga practice. If I felt fatigued while doing leg work I would just consciously start Throat Breathing and this increased my stamina so I could keep going during the class.

I also used to be one of the worst at balancing in my class (and there's a lot of balancing poses in yoga). Even the 60-year-olds in my class could stand on one leg with the other leg pointing skyward like elegant statues. But not me. In the class I was always the one who wobbled and kept my (supposedly skyward) leg hovering so low it would occasionally touch the ground and save me from an embarrassing fall. Now when I use Throat Breathing my balance instantly improves – it's a godsend!

Gabriel says that your balance improves because Throat Breathing engages the diaphragm, which is one of the body's strongest muscles and it works hard to stabilise balance and enhance core strength (strength around your torso – back and stomach). Throat Breathing also allows you to take in more breath (and with less effort) so it quickly enhances your energy and stamina.

Before I read Sophie's book it was a different story. For years I had heard that breathing exercises were 'good for you' and breathing exercises 'helped you to relax' and so on. So I would try to breathe in deeply a few times and think 'big deal!' I got nothing from them or worse; sometimes breathing exercises would make me feel light headed and so I thought feeling *bad* after breathing deeply was normal.

Maybe you've tried basic deep breathing exercises in the past and you've not had any positive results so you've given up too. If so, I want you to know that when breathing exercises are done correctly, they can help you to feel fantastic. I'd be lying if I said that this didn't take practice but once you get the principles of breathing correctly, you really don't have to have much willpower. All you need to do is be more conscious of your breath quality as you walk to the bus stop or sit at your desk. Then if you notice you feel tense or tired, correct your posture and then do a couple of breathing exercises for 30 seconds or more. These exercises are such simple tools for gaining both energy and relaxation and I hope you enjoy the benefits as much as I have.

The diaphragm

There are many ways to improve your breathing quality and this chapter covers abdominal breathing which utilises the diaphragm. The diaphragm is a thin muscle that sits horizontally between the lungs and the abdomen, like an upside-down dinner plate. It's an important skeletal muscle as it's used to power lung expansion during breathing. However it can lose some of its flexibility if it's not utilised properly with good quality breathing.[5] A more rigid diaphragm makes it harder to take in a good quality breath and this can make exercising, singing or relaxing more of a challenge. Athletes and trained singers all have strong and toned diaphragms.[6]

Exercise 1: Observe yourself

Stand in front of a mirror and relax your shoulders. Now take a long, deep inhale followed by a long deep exhale. Do this a few times and observe the way your body moves when you breathe in and out.

- Do your shoulders rise up when you inhale? If so, a little, or a lot?
- Is your upper chest expanding upwards when you inhale? If so, a little, or a lot?
- Do your neck and shoulders look strained?
- Are you holding in your stomach and not allowing movement in the abdominal area?
- How does your posture look? (Go on, have another look in the mirror.)
- Take a really deep breath in through your nose: does it sound like you are *sniffing* in air?
- Take another deep breath in as you look in the mirror: do your nostrils close up slightly?

If you answered 'yes' to any of these questions then this could indicate that you are struggling to take a good quality deep breath and that your breathing may possibly be shallow.

According to Sophie Gabriel, your shoulders should remain relaxed and not move upwards when you breathe in.

Exercise 2: Listen to your nose

An exercise in 'what not to do' as described by Gabriel is to exaggerate the sound of *sniffing* in air. Pretend you're smelling a bunch of flowers; 'sniff' in the aroma as you take a deep breath in. Try to 'sniff' your out breath as well.[7] Observe how this feels. Does your nasal passage feel contracted?

When breathing in consists of subtly (or not so subtly) sniffing air into the upper chest, you create tension in the upper body. Less air is mobilised and less energy is created (so you may feel lethargic for no apparent reason). 'Sniffing in air is what you want to avoid doing at all times,' says Gabriel. 'There is never a need for it, unless you want to smell brewed coffee, a baked cake or flowers.'

Throat Breathing exercises

'Throat Breathing' is a non-technical term used by Gabriel to describe the next breathing exercise – the throat doesn't actually do the breathing but when breathing deeply, it's where the *sensations* are felt. It's important to understand Throat Breathing before learning any other type of breathing exercise, especially the ones that utilise the diaphragm, as it helps you to understand which throat muscles to engage when doing the breathing exercises.[8]

Throat breathing is also a fantastic tool to use during meditation and exercise. During exercise it allows more air to quickly enter the lungs, with less strain, so you have more energy available to you. Meditating with poor breathing habits can leave you feeling tense and frustrated, but using Throat Breathing (and good posture) during meditation helps to create a sense of relaxation in your body and this can make meditation more enjoyable.

The sensation of Throat Breathing automatically happens when good quality deep breathing occurs.[9]

Exercise 1: Prepare for Throat Breathing

Initially it's best to learn this exercise in a quiet environment, breathing in and out of your mouth. This breathing exercise will eventually be done with the mouth closed, breathing in and out of the nose but still achieving the same sound and sensation in the throat area.

Sit in a chair or lie down flat on your back and relax your shoulders. Take three slow, deep breaths and tell yourself to relax on each exhalation. Keep your chest lifted. Relax! Relax! Relax!

Now you're ready to practise Throat Breathing.

Throat Breathing

Exhalation exercise. When you do this exercise remember not to strain or create tension in your body, and as you exhale don't let your chest drop at all.

- Breathe in a nice, slow, deep breath.

- Then open your mouth wide and as you breathe out make a long 'HHH' sound: 'HHHHHHHHHH…'

Notice how your throat muscles respond – there should be a feeling of the throat passageway relaxing so the air passes with ease. Try this a few times and take note of how your throat feels (so you can eventually do this with your mouth closed, and so that the air is moving in and out of the nose only).

Practise this Throat Breathing exhalation exercise until you understand how it works.

Inhalation exercise. The inhalation exercise demonstrates the second part of Throat Breathing. According to Gabriel, everyone finds that the inhalation is harder to grasp than the exhalation, so you'll need a bit more patience with it. The easiest way to approach it is to simply remember what you did with the exhalation, but in reverse. You are still after the same sensation in the throat and the same sound. Voice coach James Hagan uses this inhalation exercise to teach people how to improve voice quality:

- Look in the mirror. Open your mouth wide and breathe in until the soft pallet (the uvula or 'dangly bit' at the back of your throat) retracts upwards.

This will sound a bit like Darth Vadar's breathing on a good day. See how it looks in the mirror – the throat is opened in a similar manner to the throat exhalation exercise and the tongue feels like its being pulled down (out of the way) by the throat muscles. If you cannot move your uvula upwards it doesn't matter as long as you are opening the throat and allowing air to pass in with ease. You'll know you are doing it correctly when you feel the sensation of air passing the roof of your mouth and you'll feel your throat relaxing.

Practise this in front of the mirror until you have memorised the feeling of what is happening in the throat. When you eventually do this exercise with your mouth closed and you are only breathing through your nose, there will be a more subtle relaxing of the throat. Initially exaggerating the movement helps you get a clear idea of what you are trying to achieve.

Sophie Gabriel claims that learning how to take a good quality throat breath is the most important part of breathing training. In fact, she does not continue training unless a person has grasped this properly. It's better to spend more time mastering Throat Breathing before moving on to the next breathing exercise. Remember this is for your own benefit. Wouldn't you like to have a great tool for boosting your energy when you feel tired and stressed? And having better balance may also be useful, especially if you play sports. Keeping this in mind, go over your Throat Breathing exercises for as long as necessary until you feel you have mastered it.

Test yourself. Now that you understand how Throat Breathing works, do both the inhalation and exhalation exercises *without looking in a mirror* and see if you can get the same relaxed-throat feeling. Can you feel the air on the back of the throat and sense the throat muscles working? Remember to be careful not to strain your throat. Relax your throat and take your time.

The next step is to practise Throat Breathing *without* opening your mouth:

Throat Breathing (closed mouth version)

- Close your mouth and breathe *in* through your nose (remembering to avoid 'sniffing' in air).
- Remember to relax your whole throat area so that the breath passes easily on the way down to your lungs.
- Breathe *out* through the nose, remembering to keep the throat relaxed so the breath passes out with ease.

Practise this for as long as necessary. Once you understand how the closed mouth version of Throat Breathing should feel, you can practise it any time: while you're walking down the street, when you're sitting in front of your computer or when relaxing by the pool.

- Throat Breathing is the opposite of 'sniffing' in air.

Tip: As you practise Throat Breathing, count the length of your inhalations and exhalations to see if they are equal in length and strength. If your inhalation is shorter and weaker than the exhalation, then work on increasing the inhalation so it becomes equal. When breathing, most people find that it's natural for the exhalation to be longer than the inhalation. However when doing breathing exercises, aim to keep the in and out breath equal in length and strength as this will improve the quality and depth of your inhalation and enhance your breathing in general. It's a big mistake to continue strengthening and lengthening the exhale if the inhale remains weaker and shorter.[10]

Abdominal Breathing

According to Sophie Gabriel, Abdominal Breathing is one of the best ways to relax the mind and body, as it triggers the 'rest and digest' part of your nervous system. Once you've mastered it you can use it anytime so you can call upon this tool to de-stress after a big day at work. You can even do Abdominal Breathing at work if you suddenly feel uptight or anxious. During Abdominal Breathing, you basically relax your abdomen and expand your belly as you inhale. It's a little like a small balloon being inflated behind your belly button. Don't worry, your workmates won't even notice you using this relaxation technique, especially if you're sitting behind your desk.

This exercise may be called Abdominal Breathing but your breath doesn't really end up in your abdomen; it's your diaphragm pushing downward that creates the expansion. However when you *imagine* breathing into the abdominal area, it helps you to grasp the exercise.

Gabriel suggests this exercise is initially practised lying down on your back and you can bring your knees up, with your feet flat on the floor, if it's more comfortable to do so.

- Place a small flat pillow or towel behind your head so your neck is comfortably lengthened and your chin moves slightly towards your chest.

- Place your hands on your belly with fingers resting towards your belly button.

- Remembering to throat breathe, take a deep and very slowly breath in through the nose and imagine this breath travelling to the abdomen as it expands.

- Be aware of the movement in your hands as you breathe. Are they moving outward or skyward as you inhale (they should be)? Keep breathing in and out gently, and expand your abdomen slowly. Your upper chest should not be moving. If it is and your belly is stationary then you need to make sure you're Throat Breathing (as this helps you to use the diaphragm correctly). Continue to visualise the breath inflating your belly and tell yourself to relax as you exhale.

Tip: To slow your breathing down during the exercises, imagine that you are slowly breathing in and out *through a straw*. (This is for when you are practising, *not* during high impact exercise.).

Practise this over and over again so you can master the exercise before you try it standing up or sitting down. And don't be alarmed if you experience difficulty in moving your belly on cue. If you're used to breathing in a shallow manner into your upper chest, your diaphragm may not have good tone and flexibility. But you can still do this exercise with some persistence and patience. Any small improvement is really a breakthrough so give yourself a bit of praise as you go. Also, you should not force your breathing and have a break if you begin to feel light-headed.

Now try the same exercise sitting up or standing in front of a mirror.

Tip: As you inhale and exhale, keep your hands placed on your belly and mentally visualise this area expanding and contracting like a balloon *slowly* filling up and *slowly* deflating. If you want to advance to the next stage you could also try expanding the front of your lower rib cage. Then you may want to try to expand the side and back ribs. (This is a whole new exercise so you may want to read Sophie's book for more information)

What you're aiming to achieve during the breathing exercises:

- relaxation;
- smooth air flow so breathing is regular;
- the ability to breathe more slowly, gently, longer and deeply as well as being able to breathe powerfully too;
- a relaxed throat while breathing;
- inhalation and exhalation similar in length and strength;
- a relaxed abdomen and freer movement in your *lower* rib cage as you breathe in and out. (If this is difficult then remember the tip, 'keep imagining a balloon slowly expanding and contracting in your abdominal area.')

Gabriel has observed that athletes use specific methods of breathing during their performance. She also compared athletes to unfit people during exercise and noticed the relevant differences, which included the following:

- Athletes maintain *good posture* when they exercise. They keep their chest and rib cage lifted and open as much as possible, without letting it drop when exhaling. This allows them to breathe with ease.
- Athletes regulate their breathing. They breathe appropriately according to what their sport demands; for example, they breathe deeper if they're doing high impact exercise such as sprinting. Athletes *do not* take in an unnecessarily large amount of air – this means they keep their oxygen and carbon dioxide levels in a constant healthy balance as they exercise.
- Athletes learn the correct way to do an exercise or sport – they consult with experts.
- Unfit people typically have erratic, inappropriate breathing when exercising. They may also have poor posture.

When exercising, Gabriel recommends the following:

- Maintain correct form and posture at all times – even if you're feeling fatigued.
- Breathe through your mouth using good quality Throat Breathing for both the inhalation and exhalation.

- Focus on breathing into the diaphragm and allow plenty of movement in the rib cage area (expand your rib cage, especially the lower part) – remember this tip as it's very useful.

- Breathe appropriately according to the level of exertion and movement – for example, if you're walking your breathing will be slower and if sprinting you'll need to breathe in and out faster and more deeply.

- Don't hold on to your breath (unless instructed by a qualified trainer).

- When aiming for endurance, don't exhale or inhale with too much force during exercise if not required, as this can upset your body's oxygen and carbon dioxide levels, which can tire you easily and affect stamina.

You know you're breathing in or out too forcefully and upsetting your oxygen and carbon dioxide balance if you experience numbness in the feet and/or hands, light headedness or feeling faint (however these may also be caused by other factors).

Let's get practical

Invest at least five minutes each morning in practising Throat Breathing and Abdominal Breathing. Schedule it into your diary or planner now.

Chapter 20

How to be beautiful

Do not be so rigid or self-righteous about your diet as to annoy anyone. A bad relationship is more poisonous than one of Grandma's sugar cookies.

–Paul Pitchford, author of Healing with Whole Foods

The definition of beauty is perfect skin, strong jaw line, symmetrical face, white teeth, blonde hair (or at least glossy and fashionable hair), olive skin, blue eyes and abs to die for. We should all look like Angelina Jolie, Brad Pitt or Halle Berry (take your pick) and feel bad about ourselves if we don't fit the beauty mould.

Please argue with me: it's ridiculous to think that beauty has a set formula. You can conform, rebel, pine for it or make judgements about who is (or isn't), but you can't define beauty for the masses.

In fact, beauty is a highly debatable topic. Have you ever said 'She is so beautiful' only to have a friend look at you as if you're crazy and retort with 'No she's not'? Some people think Kate Moss is gorgeous while others wonder what all the fuss is about. Geishas are considered the epitome of Japanese beauty, and in certain parts of Thailand hill-tribe women coil massive lengths of brass wire around their necks to make their necks appear giraffe-like. The coils are a decoration of beauty and wealth so that the women can attract a good husband. However a Western woman would only draw bewildered glances if her neck was elongated with brass coils or her face painted white. So what is beauty?

Beauty is subjective.

This is probably *not* what you want to hear as it creates a new problem: how do you make yourself appear more attractive if everyone has a different opinion of what beauty is? Do you go blonde or red? Do you get a spray tan or bleach your freckles? And are wrinkles finally in this season? What can you aspire to look like if beauty is so damn indefinable?

This chapter is broken down into four beauty 'insights' so you can get the edge without surgery, starvation, or orange-stained sheets from a fake tan.

Insight No. 1: Inner beauty is beautiful to everyone

As you know, external beauty is subjective. It can be difficult to obtain and too easy to lose because if you live long enough, you *will* get wrinkly no matter how much nipping and tucking you have. However, on the up side, inner beauty never grows old; in fact it gets firmer and stronger as time goes by and it's certainly easier to obtain than abs because no gym membership is required. And best of all, inner beauty is beyond subjectivity because it is adored by everyone.

I saw an example of this recently when I was standing in the checkout queue at my local supermarket. The woman working behind the counter caught my eye; I had seen her many times before and remembered her to be chatty and friendly (which often slowed down her queue). On this day she was undoing a lollipop wrapper for a little boy and chatting with his mum. As I watched her I became curious. She looked a little dishevelled, with frazzled red hair and scabby sores on her arms and I admit I was wondering if someone loved her. The mother and son left and the frazzled lady began scanning my items. She was chirpy and welcoming as usual. When the photo album I was buying wouldn't scan she happily said she would scan the refill pages that I was also purchasing and give the album to me for the same price, saving me time and money. She had an ease about her that made me feel relaxed and as she handed me my receipt it suddenly struck me: she had loads of inner beauty and of course she was loved. I told a close friend about the lovely lady from the supermarket and my friend said, 'I know exactly who you're talking about; she's amazing! She even remembers my son's name.'

As you check your reflection in the mirror each day, you may analyse your skin, fuss with your hair and curse your bone structure, but does your beautiful personality ever rate a mention? Other people probably appreciate your good qualities more than you do. Shame on you! When you fail to appreciate yourself, you miss out on feeling beautiful.

Here are some questions to help you identify beautiful attributes:

- Are you kind to your mother? Do you help her around the house and keep your room clean (even if you are an adult and just visiting)?

- Are you a great home entertainer? Do you cook for others?

- Are you a good friend? Do you make others laugh? Do you remember birthdays?

- Do you do your best to conserve water and recycle?

- Do you pick up your litter? Maybe you also pick up other people's litter because you care about the environment.

- Are you patient?

- Are you grateful?

- Have you ever performed a random act of kindness?

- Do you respect other people's property?

- Do you have kind thoughts towards others?

There are many ways to be beautiful.

Activity

Write down ten positive attributes you have. If you can't think of ten then you're probably not trying hard enough. Then add to your repertoire by doing something kind and thoughtful today. Write this in your diary or planner right now.

Insight No. 2: People detect inner beauty on an energetic level

You could spend all your time meticulously choosing the right foods to eat and exercising fanatically to get your external appearance looking good but you could *still* be unattractive. If you neglect your inner goodness, you may find yourself *exuding* the wrong type of energy, one that repels people despite your exterior good looks.

After I finished my shopping at the supermarket and said goodbye to the frazzle-haired lady with inner beauty I continued my shopping at a material and haberdashery shop. Once I was in the store, I found some material and asked an assistant how much I'd need for the pillowcase I was going to make for my daughter (well, I was buying the material and my mum would do the sewing). She advised me to look at the pillowcases in the linen section. I found a pillowcase and took it out of its plastic packaging to measure it. When I had finished, I folded it and realised the pillowcase would not fit back into the packaging so I put it back on the shelf unpacked (I admit this was due to a mixture of laziness and lack of coordination when it comes to folding and packing).

I sensed someone watching me. I looked up and thought I saw a well-groomed woman on the other side of the shop glare at me, but she was so far away I thought I was just being paranoid. However, the next thing I knew she was beside me with the unpacked pillowcase in hand (she must have run from the other side of the shop). She immediately launched into a lecture on how to put the pillowcase back into its packaging and she gave me an efficient demonstration. I apologised profusely and said I would be more thoughtful next time, however she continued to lecture me until I said, 'Excuse me, I have already apologised and you don't need to lecture me as if I'm stupid.' She calmed down and said sorry but I left the shop a bit shaken up at being attacked for such a minor offence. The funny thing was I felt her aggressive rather unattractive energy before she had even said a word.

READER QUESTION

Q '**How can we feel other people's energy?**'

A *This can be difficult to describe scientifically but there is evidence that different thoughts create varying frequencies in our brain, which can be demonstrated by electroencephalograph (EEG) testing. For example, delta waves are the lowest frequencies (vibrations) emitted from thoughts, recording only 0.1 to 3 Hz on an EEG. Delta waves occur when you are unmotivated, lethargic, inattentive or when you have attention deficit disorder (ADD) and try to focus. Delta waves are also recorded during sleep.*[1]

*Alpha waves create a little more energy, reading between 7.5 and 13 Hz. You can initiate alpha waves by sitting still and shutting your eyes or with deep breathing exercises and meditation. Alpha waves are associated with relaxation, inner awareness and healing. Alpha waves stop being produced when you engage in thinking, calculating and physical action. On the other hand, mid-range beta waves **increase** with alert mental activity (as long as you're not agitated). Mid-range frequencies range from 15 to 18 Hz.*[2] *If you were to be thinking agitated thoughts then your brain's energy frequencies would alter accordingly.*

*Of course in everyday life you can't **see** the energy you emit with each passing mood but that doesn't mean such energy doesn't exist. Just like electricity: you can't see it, you can't explain it, but it still has an effect. Flick on a switch and you create energy in the form of light.*

In humans, we instinctively sense strong and harmonious energy fields in people and we label it 'charisma'. These people have the ability to hold your attention without them having to say a word; they feel 'power-full' and we sense it when they walk into a room. On the other hand, the people who feel 'power-less' haven't learnt to harness their energy or they limit it with self-degradation, also known as negative self-talk. As a result they may feel sad for no reason and they can feel overlooked or invisible when in other people's company.

*The good news is **everyone** has the ability to raise their energy field so they feel more powerful, loved and appreciated. You just need to know how.*

However, I say 'Seeing is believing' so at the end of this chapter I've included three activities that can alter your energy field and increase your inner beauty. Do these activities for two weeks and see if people start responding differently to you.

Activity

Assess what type of energy you are emitting on a daily basis: you can tell this about yourself by the way people interact with you in everyday situations. Do people generally like you? Do you have good friends? Do you consider yourself lucky? Do you quickly recover from bad situations? If you answered yes to these questions, you may be giving off positive energy.

On the other hand, do you attract arguments? Are you unlucky in love or struggling financially? Are you accident-prone? Do you feel misunderstood? Do you feel anxious or depressed? If you answered yes to these questions you may be giving off inharmonious energy.

There are also shades of grey in between: you may be lucky sometimes, for example, and have great misfortune at other times. Your energy emissions can change as your thoughts and feelings shift. However, if you always seem to be misunderstood or mistreated then you may want to alter your energy emissions and see what happens.

Insight No. 3: As you see and appreciate beauty, you become more beautiful

Yes, inner beauty is important but you *are* allowed to improve your appearance while you work your inner beauty 'muscle' (after all, the Healthy Skin Diet is designed to help you achieve beautiful skin). So this insight goes beyond inner beauty and it helps you to literally programme yourself to *naturally* gravitate towards good habits that promote health and beauty, such as nutritious food and exercise. If you have ever sabotaged your health routine or lamented about your poor willpower then this is the secret that you have been waiting for!

Your subconscious mind helps you achieve this insight. It stores data for you including the actions you have performed over and over again. For example, practise driving a car every day and pretty soon it becomes automatic. If you do something 'without thinking' then you know your subconscious mind is at work.

The subconscious also stores repressed memories, painful things we don't want to deal with. For example, when I was four years old I was attacked by a dingo but I can only remember what happened before and after the attack. I was terrified before it occurred but I told myself to stop running as the puppy just wanted to play. The next thing I remember is thinking that my mother was hurt because she had blood all over her white T-shirt. However, after that event if a dog came near me my heart would race and I'd feel uncontrollable panic, and if the dog growled at me I would experience physical pain and cry even though I couldn't ever remember the attack itself.

Five years ago I made an effort to change my experiences with dogs. I did this by taking a friend's dog for a walk on a regular basis. It was fun and I assured myself over and over again, 'Most dogs are friendly'. In essence I reprogrammed my responses to dogs. My automatic reactions to dogs eventually changed and I stopped freaking out around them.

The subconscious mind records the events you have attached strong emotions to (both good and bad). You may reason you are being silly when you react inappropriately to a situation (like me and dogs) but your subconscious beliefs can override your logical, conscious mind. If this occurs you need to give your subconscious mind *new* data to draw from, just as I did when I created lots of *positive* experiences with dogs.

On the other hand, your subconscious mind generally will not record events to which you are indifferent. If you meet a person who interests you, you're likely to remember their face but when introduced to a person who does not grab your attention in any way, you're likely to forget the meeting ever occurred.

Your subconscious mind also affects how beautiful you *allow* yourself to be. When you appreciate beauty, your subconscious mind records that beauty is a positive attribute. You may think, 'Of course beauty is a positive attribute!' But you'd be surprised how many people programme into their subconscious mind the instructions, 'Beauty is bad and must be avoided!' If you acknowledge a beautiful sunset with a few emotionally charged wows then your subconscious records 'Beauty is good!' If you appreciate a beautiful face: 'Beauty is good!' If you genuinely compliment a woman with beautiful skin and feel happiness for her then 'Beauty is good!' Pretty soon your subconscious mind has formed a new belief: 'Beauty is good ... I've got to have it!'

Appreciation of beauty, in all its forms, helps you to have more beauty of your own. You can quite literally become more attractive. (Okay, don't take this out of context: your jaw line won't physically change but you *will* gravitate towards healthy living, which can promote good skin health and a better waistline.) This is because appreciation of beauty reduces the likelihood of self-sabotage.

Self-sabotage

Have you ever sabotaged your good looks with binge eating or laziness? Do you often have a *conscious* goal to enhance your skin health or lose some weight but then you always fail to stick with your fab new diet? This is called self-sabotage and it's awfully confusing when you're trying to make positive changes to your life.

Let's say you look in a glossy magazine and see a couple of female models with perfect skin. You may think (with lots of gusto) 'These models are only skinny because they don't eat and they're 15 years old so of course they have perfect skin!' This deduction makes you feel bad (because you have unfairly compared yourself to them). Or you may go to a bar and see a beautiful person enter the room and you subsequently feel bad about yourself, or you visit the beach and look at someone slimmer than you and you then feel bad. You go to a café and spot someone with better skin than you and you feel bad. And you do this over and over again until your subconscious mind registers that beauty makes you feel awful so therefore beauty is a negative attribute and one that must be avoided in order to avoid pain.

What's worse is now your subconscious mind has registered that beauty is only available to young people who starve themselves. Of course your subconscious mind doesn't want you to go hungry or feel bad so it reasons it must *protect* you from this detestable thing called beauty. Your subconscious mind subsequently employs self-sabotage or poor willpower to keep you from falling prey to beauty. Same too with other beliefs such as 'beautiful people are dumb', 'beautiful people get hassled and ogled', and 'beautiful people are fake'. And you wonder why you go on a diet, with good intentions to lose weight or clear up your skin and then sabotage yourself with binge eating, or you join a gym and never go. You think it's your 'lack of willpower' when in fact you have programmed yourself to fail because you've created a subconscious belief that beauty is a negative thing.

Willpower is your subconscious mind following through with *your instructions* about beauty. Positive observations about beauty = strong willpower when dieting and exercising.

What are your beliefs about beautiful people? Do you bitch or praise? Are you happy for other people who are beautiful or are you more than a teensy bit jealous? Your subconscious mind helps you achieve your goals such as getting fit and healthy; it enhances your willpower and prevents you from overeating. It promotes the satiety response so your body will tell you it's full sooner rather than later so you stay slim. You need willpower to change your diet and achieve your beauty goals but how do you programme 'Beauty is positive' into your subconscious mind so you get the drive you need, minus self-sabotage?

- To programme 'Beauty is positive' into your subconscious mind, you need to attach strong positive emotions to beauty, and you need to do this over and over again until you have formed a strong belief.

As you appreciate beauty and programme 'Beauty is positive', your subconscious mind helps you become more beautiful: it ensures you stick to the Healthy Skin Diet and it urges you to put on those running shoes!

Insight No. 4: People detect inner beauty by your actions and habits

Now, let's get back to the gorgeous topic of inner beauty ... Your actions and habits have a strong effect on the people around you, even more so than your words. Actions and habits can contradict a spoken lie and reveal the truth for everyone to see. Unfortunately your habits are largely driven by your subconscious mind so they are hard to consciously control. This means you cannot fake inner beauty because your subconsciously driven actions will eventually give you away. Your subconscious mind reveals the most when you are relaxed. Alcohol also has a reputation of bringing hidden or suppressed beliefs out in the open and you can ruin your reputation with one drunken rant.

Where do these subconscious 'truths' come from and how do we get rid of them? Your words and actions don't necessarily come from your daily life experiences; they come from how you *interpret* them. Say you had a bad experience with a Jewish kid at school. He teased you and took your lunch money. You could *interpret* this to mean 'all Jews are bad' or alternatively you may decide 'Jerry was mean to me, thank goodness not all people are like him' and you could go on to have healthy friendships with others.

Poor interpretations can shape your future and they can also ruin your life. Poor interpretations form unreasonable subconscious 'truths' (true in your subconscious mind but not reality) and they affect your actions in daily life so you can come across as defensive, angry or unlikeable *without you even realising it*.

For example, if you've decided that 'all men are bastards' because you've had your heart broken a few times, then you are likely to appear defensive when in the company of men. So on your next date, you may end up sounding arrogant or angry without meaning to. Your subconscious mind has worked against you (another case of self-sabotage) and you are unlikely to be asked out a second time because of your 'angry about men' habits. Guess what? This bad outcome once again backs up your belief that all men are bastards (when in reality most men just don't like defensive behaviour). *Poor* interpretations of your past relationships can lead you to sabotage your future relationships.

A remedy for negative interpretations is to *focus on beauty rather than faults*. For example, don't spend longer than a few moments thinking about a negative situation, instead turn your attention to the good things in your life such as your strengths and positive attributes. If intimate relationships are a problem then focus on your positive experiences with the opposite sex. If you don't have any good memories to draw from, then it's time to form some platonic friendships: have good clean fun *and* expect nothing from them in return, and you will create positive experiences that will condition your mind for healthy relationships in the future.

If you've had negative experiences with beautiful people then forge new friendships with people you consider attractive (who seem kind) so you can create new positive experiences with beauty.

People also experience your beauty via your words. When you genuinely care about other people, you make them feel good and who wouldn't want to be around someone who makes their life more enjoyable? When you say thank you (and mean it), when you show genuine gratitude, and when you offer help and then follow through on your offer you form strong bonds with people. These bonds cannot be broken easily: not by small arguments, not by distance and certainly not by you having a bad skin day. The recipients of your kindness will always remember your beauty (and if they don't, then they probably aren't worthy of your friendship).

A note on jealousy

What do you think your energy field is like when you're jealous or bitching about another? Do you think it gives you an attractive energy that others are drawn to?

Unfortunately it doesn't, as jealousy can temporarily block your inner beauty. Jealousy also makes you feel 'power-less' as it's a proclamation of inferiority. It is like holding up a sign saying 'I am not as good as the person over there'. Jealousy undermines your self-worth but it is a common feeling that can be hard to ignore, so what can you do when the green-eyed monster suddenly appears?

Be prepared!

Start to associate jealousy with weakness and all things bad. You can do this by considering the problems with jealousy:

Say to yourself (with great passion): 'Jealousy makes me weaker.'

'Jealousy is a sign I'm feeling inferior or inadequate.'

'Jealousy will not bring good fortune into my life.'

As mentioned before, your subconscious mind will stop you from striving for something you have perceived as bad. Jealousy is bad! It is a self-sabotaging emotion so limit it for your own good.

The famous Swiss psychoanalyst Carl Jung said that anything about which you feel strong emotions is a part of your shadow self, the suppressed or unacknowledged part of yourself. For example, when you feel strong *positive* emotions about another person's charisma then you should realise this quality can be yours too if you stop suppressing it (with negative self-talk) and then consciously cultivate it (with research and practice, practice, practice).

It also works the other way around: when you feel strong *negative* emotions about a person (such as jealousy of their beauty), your jealousy has nothing to do with the other person, but everything to do with your own negative feelings about yourself. It's fuelled by a suppressed part of yourself. If you are jealous of another person's good looks then you're really envious because you've either suppressed your own beauty or haven't acknowledged your own good features. Shame on you! Your beauty is being wasted by your own ignorance.

Do you despise fitness freaks? You may have sabotaged your own health and fitness for years so you don't like to see it in other people and this belief may come out in the form of jealousy or hate. However, when you allow yourself to be your best then you don't mind if others are also being their best.

I find that most people are hard on themselves and don't appreciate their good features so if this sounds like you then you're not alone. Instead, when you become jealous tell yourself: 'My jealousy is coming from a suppressed part of myself.'

If you see someone whom you consider beautiful, remember your shadow self and say to yourself: 'As I see the beauty in you, I allow the beauty in myself.' And remember you don't need to compete to be a contender. You will shine when you value your own worth – this simply means you should be happy to be you rather than wishing you were more like someone else.

A note on sisterhood

Just under 100 years ago, women were not allowed to vote. We have come a long way but today there are women who are still being treated like second-class citizens. And I'm sad to say that quite often it is other women who are the main offenders in treating them this way. We should not be putting other women down as many of them still feel 'power-less' and they need a boost not a kick.

I believe women should look after each other more and compete less. We are not in competition unless we are behind the starting line at the Olympic Games waiting for the starter gun to go off. We do not need to battle at bars, we are not contenders at clubs and we are not at war with good looking women, single or not.

We should also be looking out for one another. For example, there have been an alarming number of women who have been out socialising and had their drinks spiked with date-rape drugs. When this occurs they appear drunk and disorderly. If they have been separated from their friends they often have no one to care for them: instead onlookers may laugh at their behaviour and leave these women vulnerable to predators. It is up to us to make sure that this does not occur, first by making sure our own drinks are not left unattended and second by helping a woman find her friends if she appears drunk and disoriented, or consider calling an ambulance.

Don't snigger at someone else's poor judgement and don't compete on a beauty level. Inner beauty is created when you bond, help and care for another human being.

How to bump up your inner beauty in a flash

- Smile.

- Have integrity – be honest and authentic.

- Meditate or do breathing exercises – calm your mind.

- Value the present moment – observe your family, your children and the world around you and enjoy now.

- Enjoy being you – like yourself unconditionally.

- Treat yourself with respect – speak kindly of yourself and respect your body. This shows other people how you *expect* them to treat you.

- Find a charity and support it within your means. If you have time, give time; if you have a special skill, help out; if you have money, give donations.

- Be kind and generous, whether it is an anonymous random act of kindness or saying hello to an old person. Your kindness makes the world a better place.

- Appreciate beauty – expand your definition of beauty and choose to see it more often.

- Wish other people happiness.

- Be happy for other people's good fortune.

- When you glance at yourself in the mirror, look for beauty, not faults.

Here are three exercises to boost your inner beauty and enhance your energetic field or charisma:

Inner beauty exercise, level 1

This 'walking appreciation exercise' is a fantastic tool for expanding your definition of beauty so you can experience more beauty in your life.

Go for a brisk walk in a public place, preferably a popular nature walk, beach walk or park (anywhere will do just as long as you are walking past other people). Instead of focusing on yourself, focus your attention on the people you pass. Your task is to *look for the beauty in others*. Look for conventional and unconventional beauty: is there unconventional beauty in their eyes, their appearance or their smile? Look for inner beauty: strength, happiness, kindness, feminine/masculine power, wisdom, free spiritedness, loveliness. See the beauty in people of all shapes and sizes (including the overly skinny or overweight ones). It is your duty to break the 'size-barrier' that may exist in your mind – you cannot accuse the media of favouring the slim and beautiful if you yourself cannot see or appreciate beauty in all forms. The key is to look for beauty not faults.

If this activity brings up uneasiness in you, then a more subtle approach may be necessary. Try thinking 'Wouldn't it be nice if I could see the beauty in her (or him)?' If resistance occurs this is a sign you are suppressing your own beauty. If this is the case, when you see someone attractive say over and over again to yourself (with great passion/feeling): *'As I see the beauty in you, I see the beauty in myself'*.

As you walk and look for the beauty in others, don't be afraid of eye contact – just smile if a person catches you looking at them.

Do this walking appreciation exercise for at least ten minutes each day. After doing this for several days, you may notice that people seem friendlier and smile at you more often.

Seeing beauty in others is a great way to expand your definition of beauty and you also bond with your local community without having to utter a word!

Inner beauty exercise, level 2

Insight No. 2 taught us that people detect inner beauty on an energetic level and the following activity helps to alter your inner energy so you seem more attractive.

You can do this activity as soon as you wake up or when you go for a walk. For three to five minutes, list everything you are grateful for. You can either do this in your head or out loud but you must do this exercise with enthusiasm and passion (remember you need to use strong positive emotions to store new information in your subconscious mind). When your subconscious mind records how grateful you are, you will feel happier and emit a more powerful energy. This is the energy that attracts other people and makes you seem more alluring.

Begin by listing your positive attributes and strengths. For example, I'm so grateful I have two legs to walk with; I'm so thankful I'm good at table tennis; I really appreciate my green eyes and my perfect eyesight; I'm so grateful I can look after myself; I'm so grateful I'm fit and healthy (even if it's only wishful thinking). Then list what you appreciate about the people closest to you: I'm so grateful for my daughter, she is smart and kind and laughs at all my jokes; I'm so grateful for my partner, he pays the bills and loves me dearly; I'm so thankful for my mum, she is so generous and caring; I'm grateful for my dad, he loves me and supports all my decisions; I'm so lucky I have my sister, she is inspirational as she has overcome so many hurdles and this shows me that anything is possible, and I am so thankful that she calls me all the time to let me know she is okay (and so on).

You can also list the surroundings that you are grateful for: I'm so grateful for this beautiful beach; I'm so grateful for the warm sunshine; I'm so thankful for this lovely house; I'm so happy to be here today; I'm so lucky to be alive. You will find plenty of things to be grateful for if you start with the small stuff such as your hands, the food in your fridge or a pet.

Inner beauty exercise, level 3

This exercise is brilliant for changing your energy frequencies to be more like what you want. You can do this exercise while lying down or anywhere you can close your eyes and concentrate. The idea is to *imagine* what you would like to achieve as if you've already done it, and then say thanks. Do it with enthusiasm and you will feel great – you will feel the same happiness as if it were real *because the brain cannot tell the difference between what is actual and what is vividly imagined.*[3] So you may not already have a great life but you are able to emit the same energy frequencies as someone who is charismatic and rich, with beautiful skin, a great job and is happy. All you have to do is imagine having a good life and feel the associated good feelings.

Begin by closing your eyes and taking three deep breaths. Then spend five minutes daydreaming about what you would love to achieve. Since you are reading this book I assume you want better looking skin. If so, then imagine you already have beautiful skin. See people complimenting your gorgeous complexion and say thanks and smile because you're so grateful. Imagine looking at your reflection in a mirror and seeing your skin as smooth and fresh looking. Imagine you have beautiful skin every day during the eight-week programme.

It is the *positive feelings* you attach to these daydreams that will raise your energetic pull. So imagine you have beautiful skin and then get very excited about it. You can even cry happy tears and jump for joy in your daydreams (yes, look as silly as possible) so your subconscious mind will record that you love having beautiful skin. This is also a great confidence booster, which is another attractive quality to have.

What about reality checks?

Now, you may be able to imagine having perfect skin but what about reality? What can you do when you catch a glimpse of yourself in the mirror and see all your skin's faults, creases, canyons and moguls? For starters, you should avoid looking at your problem spots as much as possible, so limit using mirrors during the Healthy Skin Diet eight-week programme. This is a little tricky at first but fogging up the mirrors after a shower will definitely help. Don't worry, you can briefly use a mirror to apply make-up or check that you having nothing hanging out of your nose but do not judge yourself. Keep it brief and functional to make sure you are dressed properly and well groomed. Once you look good you can compliment yourself but you DO NOT want to comment on any imperfections. You can't feel good about yourself if you are constantly putting yourself down. *And you can't hate yourself into having better skin!*

Alternatively, each day look at a *good* patch of skin that is smooth and clear, such as the inside of your arms, and affirm 'I'm having a great skin day!' or 'I have gorgeous skin!' You need to love the skin you're in because it is a vital part of you. Loving all parts of you, no matter how imperfect they seem to be, is imperative for your inner beauty and it is the key to true self-confidence, which is one of the most attractive qualities you can possess.

Do all three inner beauty exercises, levels 1 to 3, daily and try to keep the happy feelings they create with you throughout the day. If at any time you begin to feel stressed then counteract this negative feeling by listing the things you are grateful for. Within a few weeks you just may see a shift in the way people respond to you.

Key points to remember

- Inner beauty is beautiful to everyone.
- People detect inner beauty on an energetic level.
- As you see and appreciate beauty, you become more beautiful.
- People detect inner beauty by your actions and habits.
- Jealousy makes you feel powerless as it's a proclamation of inferiority.
- Smile and laugh more.
- Be kind and thoughtful, and look after each other.
- Inner beauty exercise level 1: As you walk past people, look for beauty not faults.
- Inner beauty exercise level 2: For three to five minutes each day, list everything you're grateful for.
- Inner beauty exercise level 3: Spend five minutes daydreaming about having

beautiful skin. Imagine you already have it and say thanks.

- Avoid critiquing yourself in the mirror. Don't affirm what you hate about yourself as it will ruin your self-confidence. You can't hate yourself into having better skin.

- Look at a good patch of skin and compliment yourself on having a gorgeous complexion. This will raise your energy field to an attractive level.

It is easy to be beautiful. All you have to do is expand your definition of what beauty is, appreciate beauty and emulate it. Cultivate a good-looking aura with daily inner beauty exercises and remember as you glimpse in the mirror, *look for beauty not faults.*

Chapter 21

The Healthy Skin Diet

As I've mentioned elsewhere in this book, there are many reasons why the Healthy Skin Diet works so well to improve skin health and overall vitality. But what are the *specific* foods and liquids that make this diet exceptional? Let's take a quick look at the top 12 ingredients in the Healthy Skin Diet.

The Top 12 healthy ingredients

1. Apple cider vinegar (ACV)

ACV has an alkalising effect in the body. This may explain apple cider vinegar's reputation for reducing pain and inflammatory conditions such as arthritis and eczema. It's also anti-fungal, anti-viral, anti-bacterial, promotes healthy red blood cells and can help improve digestion if you have low stomach acids. Only use good quality apple cider vinegar that contains the 'mother', the dark cloudy substance that looks like strands linked together, settled at the bottom of the bottle (shake the bottle before use). This indicates that minimal processing has occurred and valuable enzymes and minerals are present. You can eat the mother as it's the most nutritious part.

CAUTION

Although apple cider vinegar is alkalising once digested, keep in mind that it's an *acid before* digestion and acids can aggravate ulcers and slowly strip enamel off teeth (other acids include orange juice, citrus fruits, vitamin C tablets and other types of vinegar). If discomfort occurs then have Green Water as an alternative. If you have sensitive teeth, you can also rinse your mouth with a bit of bicarb mixed with water or brush your teeth after having ACV.

Prescription

For adults with poor digestion: 2 teaspoons daily in a glass of water (in divided doses); use before meals to increase digestion. For a more pleasant drink have ACV in 125ml (4fl oz) of preservative-free apple juice and 125ml (4fl oz) water. Use ACV in salad recipes such as Tasty Antioxidant Salad.

2. Avocado

Avocado is a nutrient-dense fruit which is high in monounsaturated fatty acids (omega-9 and some omega-6). Avocado can be used as a nutritious spread, and it's a healthy alternative to butter and margarine. It contains vitamins B6, B3 and C, beta-carotene, folic acid, copper, magnesium, iron, potassium, amino acids and antioxidants. Avocado improves digestive health, is moisturising for the skin, is gluten free, low GI and highly alkalising.

> **CAUTION**
>
> Avocado is very high in salicylates and amines so temporarily avoid avocado if you have eczema.

Prescription

Use avocado as a nutritious spread instead of butter or margarine. Have ¼ to ½ avocado per day, twice a week.

3. Buckwheat

Buckwheat contains the antioxidant quercetin, which has anti-inflammatory properties. It is high in vitamin B3, folic acid, calcium, magnesium, potassium, zinc and antioxidants, is anti-inflammatory, and low GI (the flour has a higher GI than the grains). Buckwheat isn't technically a grain but resembles grain and is a gluten-free alternative to wheat.

Prescription

Incorporate buckwheat into your weekly diet to increase your intake of anti-inflammatory antioxidants. Buckwheat crêpes make a great breakfast or dessert. Buckwheat grains cook like rice and can be served with curries, fish or meat.

4. Chlorophyll

Chlorophyll is the green pigment in plants; the drink called chlorophyll is a combination of green plant pigment and spearmint oil (some brands also contain alfalfa extract). Chlorophyll supplies magnesium needed for cardiovascular and respiratory health, and also contains potassium and iron. It prevents anaemia, is highly alkalising and is both blood purifying and blood thinning. Chlorophyll increases oxygen-carrying capacity in the blood (so it can increase your energy and stamina); it promotes friendly bacteria in the bowel (so it can reduce harmful bowel microbes); promotes healthy digestion; and prevents bad breath and body odour.

> **CAUTION**
>
> The super strength chlorophyll supplements are darkly pigmented (dark green/black) and may stain teeth if used in high doses. Use low dose chlorophyll (containing approximately 200mg of chlorophyll per 100ml).

Prescription

Adult dosage for *normal/low strength* liquid chlorophyll (see caution box): 1–2 teaspoons diluted in water once or twice a day, beginning on a low dosage. Drink Green Water daily. If you have hypoglycaemia or blood sugar level problems (energy crashes/irritability in between meals) mix 2 teaspoons of liquid chlorophyll in a 1.5 litre bottle of water and sip throughout the day.

5. Dandelion root

Dandelion root, also known as taraxacum officinale radix, contains bitter compounds called inulin and taraxacin, which rapidly improve digestion in people with poor bile secretion. Dandelion root also makes a great morning cuppa. Contains mineral salts and vitamins; activates phase II liver detoxification; prevents constipation; good for liver and gallbladder.

> **CAUTION**
>
> Dandelion root can increase appetite and overstimulate digestion; do not use if you have ulcers, reflux or excess digestive acids in stomach.

Prescription

Enjoy a cup of Soy Dandé' from the recipe section up to three times a day (before meals). But be aware that too many cups can overstimulate digestion; if this occurs, reduce dosage and strength.

6. Dark leafy green vegetables

This group includes Chinese greens, kale, dandelion greens, silverbeet, spinach, chicory, beet greens, mustard greens, rocket, watercress and baby spinach. Such vegetables are highly alkalising to the blood; they deliver *more nutrients for fewer calories*; and the calcium in kale and watercress is easy for the body to absorb. They contain antioxidants, folic acid, magnesium, calcium, vitamins A and C, B vitamins, potassium, fibre and cancer-protective phytonutrients; they're gluten free and low GI.

> **CAUTION**
>
> These vegetables are high in salicylates; spinach is also high in amines and natural MSG so eat with caution if you have severe eczema (parsley and iceberg lettuce are low in natural plant chemicals so they are the better green choices for eczema sufferers).

Prescription

Adults: Have two handfuls of dark leafy greens every day. That's EVERY SINGLE DAY OF YOUR LIFE. **Children:** Have one child-sized handful a day.

7. Fish

Oily or deep sea fish contains therapeutic amounts of omega-3 (EPA and DHA) and is a potent anti-inflammatory food. Studies have shown that two to three servings of fish a week are good for elevating mood and increasing health of the brain, skin and heart. A good source of protein, vitamin D and iodine; metabolism-boosting; low GI; gluten free.

Good sources of EPA and DHA include salmon, trout, mackerel, sardines, herring, eel, and salmon and tuna oil supplements. Other minor sources of EPA and DHA include low-fat fish such as carp, pike and haddock, and oysters, clams, scallops and squid.

Salmon and trout are commonly farmed and it has been suggested that these fish contain less omega-3, and less vitamin A and C, than fish fresh from the ocean – but any amount of omega-3 is better than none.

Prescription

Both adults and children should eat oily fish two to three times a week.

8. Flaxseeds (also known as linseeds) and flaxseed oil

Flaxseeds are anti-inflammatory because they contain a whopping 50 per cent omega-3 essential fatty acids; they also contain omega-6, phyto-chemicals, silica, mucilage, oleic acid, protein, vitamin E and fibre, and are a potent bowel cleanser. Flaxseeds aid with weight loss; treat constipation; may improve cardiovascular health; may improve female reproductive health; are liver protective; stabilise blood sugar levels; are soothing to the digestive tract; alkalising; may inhibit tumour formation. Flaxseed oil and ground flaxseeds should be refrigerated at all times. **Note:** Think of flaxseed oil as a healthy ingredient not as a supplement: I don't recommend buying flaxseed oil in capsule form as I don't want you popping pills all day and it is more beneficial as a food, incorporated into salad dressings and smoothies to increase their nutritional value.

> **CAUTION**
>
> A bottle of flaxseed oil needs to be consumed within five weeks of opening to ensure freshness. Keep oil refrigerated and grind flaxseeds fresh monthly. Flaxseed oil can also be stored in the freezer to increase shelf life. Drink *plenty* of water when having whole or ground flaxseeds as the fibre absorbs a lot of water (about five times the seeds' weight!).

Prescription

Adults: Have 1–2 tablespoons of ground flaxseeds or flaxseed oil per day – not necessary on the days you eat oily fish. Use flaxseed oil in the Flaxseed Lemon Drink, Skin Firming Drink and in homemade salad dressings. Add whole flaxseeds to Designer Muesli or grind them in a coffee grinder for use on breakfast cereal or fruit salad.

9. Lecithin granules

Lecithin is naturally found in soyabeans (edamame), eggs, beef and liver and can also be bought in the form of soya lecithin granules, which kind of look like tiny yellow beads. Lecithin is a special type of lipid that helps break down fats in the body much the same way detergent does when washing greasy dishes; it contains choline for healthy brain neurotransmitters and inositol for healthy cell membranes. Lecithin breaks up cholesterol; helps with weight loss and removal of fats from the body; aids removal of chemicals and cholesterol from the body; is low GI, is brain food and is gluten free; it enhances phase II liver detoxification; improves digestion; and due to inositol it may decrease the risk of eczema, hair loss, cellulite and eye problems.

Prescription

Adults: 1 tablespoon of lecithin granules per day. **Children** aged one to six years: ½ teaspoon per day; children over seven years 1 teaspoon per day. Add lecithin to Papaya Beauty Smoothie, Flaxseed Lemon Drink and muesli/cereals.

10. Lemons and limes

Lemons and limes contain vitamin C, folic acid, calcium and potassium; they enhance phase II liver detoxification and have a strong alkalising effect. The pectin from the citrus pulp (white part of the fruit) contains valuable flavonoids, and both these fruits aid removal of toxins from the bowel.

Prescription

Adults: Have a squeeze of lemon/lime with the ACV Drink, Tangy Papaya Cups or Green Water. Drink the Flaxseed Lemon Drink at least once a week; this recipe uses all parts of the lemon, including the skin and pulp. Use lemon/lime in salad dressings, and squeeze lemon/lime onto fish before serving.

> **CAUTION**
>
> Lemons and limes are high in salicylates and amines so may initially cause flare-ups in some individuals with eczema. Although alkalising once digested, they are acidic pre-digestion and may aggravate sensitive teeth; if this occurs brush your teeth after contact.

11. Seaweed

Seaweed such as kelp and kombu contains a good dose of metabolism-boosting iodine and is a weight-loss aid; it is helpful in combating fatigue caused by slow thyroid activity; and it helps prevent skin irritations. Seaweed is a good source of iodine, beta-carotene, B vitamins, vitamin A, D, E and K, folic acid, calcium, magnesium, potassium, iron, selenium and zinc; it is skin cleansing and is good for constipation and arthritis. Seaweed has anti-cancer properties, is anti-bacterial and anti-viral.

> **CAUTION**
>
> If you have hyperthyroidism (or a speedy metabolism) avoid seaweed as it may speed up your metabolism further.

Prescriptions

Add a sprinkling of kelp or a soaked strip of kombu to meals such as soups and stir-fried vegetables. It adds a mild salty flavour. Add kombu seaweed when cooking beans and pulses to make them easier to digest (this helps prevent gas).

12. Turmeric

Turmeric is a spice that contains curcumin, a flavonoid that has an anti-cancer and anti-alzheimer effect. Contains calcium, magnesium, potassium and antioxidants, and is anti-inflammatory; low GI; gluten free; promotes phase II detoxification; lowers blood sugar levels; helps prevent blood clotting; alkalising.

> **CAUTION**
>
> Turmeric is high in salicylates so it may initially aggravate eczema.

Prescription

Adults: Have 2 teaspoons a day in a small amount of water or fresh vegetable juice. Best used in meals such as curries or dahl. Add ground black pepper to enhance the absorption of curcumin.

Now it's time to get practical. The Healthy Skin Diet is divided into two stages; the first is the Three Day Alkalising Cleanse and the second is the Healthy Skin Diet itself. You'll find all of the recipes mentioned in Appendix 2, starting on page 304.

READER QUESTION

Q 'Why do I need to cleanse for three days?'

A *If you were to plant a vegetable garden, ideally you would first prepare the soil and pull up the weeds so the veggies didn't have to compete for vital nutrients. It's the same with your body: preferably you should make your gastrointestinal tract undesirable for worms and candida albicans (fungus), and prime for good digestion and* absorption so you get the most out of your new diet. The Three Day Alkalising Cleanse does this for you.

As I mentioned in Guideline No. 1, parasites such as candida albicans are found in varying amounts in all humans and in healthy individuals such microbes aren't a problem as they're only present in minute amounts. However in an **acidic** internal environment, caused by the typical Western diet and lifestyle, these pests thrive and eventually cause all sorts of health problems including undesirable skin conditions. The Three Day Alkalising Cleanse changes the acid–alkaline balance in your body, making the body more alkaline so parasites die off during the first week of the programme.

This cleanse programme is different to traditional detox programmes as it contains solid food so you won't feel too hungry or lethargic (maybe just a little). This three-day programme also has specially designed alkaline-forming foods and beauty-boosting nutrients such as omega-3, selenium, vitamin C, vitamin E and chlorophyll to help neutralise the heavy load of free radicals during detoxification. This means that the Three Day Alkalising Cleanse shouldn't make you feel ill like a traditional detox might.

The Three Day Alkalising Cleanse is especially good for reducing spots, eczema, hives, premature ageing and cellulite when combined with the eight-week programme. However if you have eczema/dermatitis and a salicylate sensitivity you may initially have a worsening of symptoms. Don't worry: this is only a temporary salicylate reaction (possibly from the Green Water). Your body will stop being sensitive to salicylates as your acid levels reduce during the eight-week programme.

There are two versions of the Three Day Alkalising Cleanse to choose from: one for cold or winter-like weather and the other for warmer conditions (see pages 278–281). It's important to do a cleanse that is appropriate for the season. A salad-based cleanse is ideal in warmer weather as it is cooling in nature. On the other hand, in cold weather you need warm, soupy foods to cleanse effectively – such as root vegetable casseroles and broths. **Please note that children under the age of 15 years should not follow any detox programme, including this one.**

READER QUESTION

Q **'Do I need to take supplements during the Three Day Alkalising Cleanse?'**

A No, supplements aren't essential; however if you have any digestive problems, skin rashes, parasitic infestation or lowered immunity it's advisable to take a suitable probiotic supplement. Review Chapter 3, 'Guideline No. 1', for probiotic information. Probiotics are suitable for all ages but please use the correct dosage. If you're unsure of the dosage then contact the manufacturer for more details.

*If you suffer from chemical sensitivity, acne or psoriasis then I highly recommend you take a liver detoxification supplement for the first two weeks of the programme. Liver detoxification supplements help to decrease the chemical load in your body. Good liver detox supplements should include the following nutrients: glycine, magnesium, vitamin B6, selenium, cysteine, glutamine, taurine, vitamin B2, vitamin B12, folic acid, vitamin C, zinc and the herb St Mary's thistle (otherwise known as milk thistle or silybum marianum). However, if your skin is in reasonable condition you can simply drink **dandelion tea** every day as it stimulates digestion and promotes healthy liver function.*

If you're on a special regime such as the Anti-eczema Programme or the Anti-cellulite Programme then you can use whatever supplements are specifically recommended for your condition, although I suggest you take fewer than three types of supplements at a time as you don't want to be popping pills all day!

As I mentioned before, it's important to do a cleanse that is suited to the weather. Choose which version of the Three Day Alkalising Cleanse is most appropriate and then plan which day you'd like to begin. If you don't work on the weekends you might want to start the programme on a Saturday so you have time to rest during the cleanse. However, if you want to socialise on the weekend and you work during the week I'd recommend beginning the programme on a Monday, after the weekend, so you have no temptations during your cleanse programme.

Note: *During the first three days you should not do any vigorous exercise. This is a time to eat alkalising foods, master the 'Beauty Breathing' exercises and take relaxing baths. It is important to get plenty of rest because your body is restoring health during this time. It's also necessary to avoid caffeine and alcohol during this period as they are highly acidic and may negate some of the healing effects during the Three Day Alkalising Cleanse. Please gradually cut down on both of these substances **before** you begin the programme so you don't suffer withdrawal symptoms.*

The Three Day Alkalising Cleanse – Warm Weather Version

Drink options

Essential: 2 litres of water, sipped throughout the day; 3 glasses of Flaxseed Lemon Drink (make fresh daily and enough for 3 glasses); Green Water (if you have eczema or salicylate sensitivity also add glycine to this drink to prevent salicylate reaction). **Optional:** pau d'arco tea; dandelion tea (however be aware that it may stimulate your digestion which can make you feel hungry); vegetable juices containing cabbage, celery, parsley, carrot and ginger. As most fruit is acidic, fruit is not permitted during the Three Day Alkalising Cleanse, unless it's lemon, lime, avocado or green papaya. Raspberries are also permitted in one of the recipes.

Days 1 to 3

Before breakfast

As soon as you wake up, drink 1 small glass of Green Water, initially making it up with a low dosage of 1 teaspoon. Also make a bottle of Green Water (1 teaspoon of chlorophyll to 1.5 litres of water) and sip throughout the day (if you have eczema, also add glycine – refer to 'Eczema/dermatitis' chapter for dosage). Have your first dosage of probiotics 15 to 30 minutes before breakfast.

Breakfast

Eat a small handful of fresh, raw almonds.

Drink 1 glass of Flaxseed Lemon Drink – this drink is fabulous for your immune system and it's completely alkaline (if you are taking the liver detox supplement Thermo Phase Detox by Metagenics then have this mixed with a big glass of chilled water now).

If you have any signs of parasites also eat 35g (1¼oz) of pumpkin seeds. This can be a combination of white and green pumpkin seeds. However, the white ones are usually highly salted. You can wash off most of the salt or just have the green pumpkin seeds on their own. Eating pumpkin seeds during the three-day programme helps loosen compacted faeces in the bowel so any hidden parasites can be flushed out.

Lunch

Drink 1 glass of Flaxseed Lemon Drink then choose from one of the following:

Spicy Green Papaya Salad (anti-parasitic recipe)

Sweet Raspberry, Avocado and Watercress Salad

Tasty Antioxidant Salad

Tabbouli (can be used in conjunction with another salad)

Rich Mineral Salad with Papaya, Dill and Baby Spinach

Avocado Dip with Dipping Sticks

Roasted Corn and Cauliflower Soup

Optional 3 p.m. snack

If you are hungry you can have any of the following alkalising snacks: fresh, raw almonds and brazil nuts (no more than 1 small handful); ½ avocado flavoured with fresh lemon juice and a pinch of natural sea salt (NOT table salt as it is acid-forming); carrot, celery and capsicum sticks; Green Water.

Dinner

15 to 30 minutes before dinner, take your probiotic supplement and finish your bottle of Green Water (if you haven't already). Dinner consists of a light salad with salad dressing containing flaxseed oil, lemon, garlic and apple cider vinegar (refer to recipes in Appendix 2). Drink the remainder of the Flaxseed Lemon Drink just before dinner; the oil in this drink helps to trigger the satiety response and is wonderful for digestion.

Choose one of the following dinners:

Spicy Green Papaya Salad

Roasted Sweet Potato Salad

Sweet Raspberry, Avocado and
    Watercress Salad

Tasty Antioxidant Salad

Tabbouli (in combo with another salad)

Rich Mineral Salad with Papaya, Dill and
    Baby Spinach

Roasted Corn and Cauliflower Soup

If you are still hungry after dinner, then have a glass of Skin Juice for Sensitive Skin No. 1 or 2, Spot-free Skin Juice or Anti-ageing Broth. You can also have a second serving of salad and 1 small handful of raw almonds or brazil nuts.

The Three Day Alkalising Cleanse – Cold Weather Version

Drink options

Essential: 2 litres of filtered or spring water, sipped throughout the day; Anti-ageing Broth 1 to 3 cups per day; Green Water (if you have eczema or salicylate sensitivity also add glycine to this drink to prevent salicylate reaction). **Optional:** pau d'arco tea; dandelion tea (however be aware that it may stimulate your digestion which can make you feel hungry); vegetable juices containing cabbage, celery, parsley, carrot and ginger (NO fruit during the Three Day Alkalising Cleanse).

Days 1 to 3

Before breakfast

One glass of Green Water and have your first dosage of probiotics 15 to 30 minutes before breakfast.

Breakfast

Eat one small handful of fresh, raw almonds

Two cups of Anti-ageing Broth (if you are taking the liver detox supplement Thermo Phase Detox by Metagenics then have this mixed with big glass of chilled water now).

If you have any signs of parasites also eat 35g (1¼oz) of pumpkin seeds. This can be a combination of white and green pumpkin seeds. However, the white ones are usually highly salted. You can wash off most of the salt or just have the green pumpkin seeds on their own. Eating pumpkin seeds during the three-day programme helps loosen compacted faeces in the bowel so any hidden parasites can be flushed out.

Lunch

Choose from one of the following:

Roasted Corn and Cauliflower Soup (omit the toast)

Roasted Sweet Potato Salad

Multi-vitamin Dahl (Detox Dahl)

Therapeutic Veggie Soup (omit the toast)

Dinner

15 to 30 minutes before dinner, take your probiotic supplement and finish your bottle of Green Water (if you haven't already). Choose from one of the following dinners:

Roasted Corn and Cauliflower Soup (omit the toast)

Roasted Sweet Potato Salad

Multi-vitamin Dahl (Detox Dahl)

Therapeutic Veggie Soup (omit the toast)

If you are still hungry after dinner, then have a glass of Skin Juice for Sensitive Skin No. 1 or 2, Spot-free Skin Juice or Anti-ageing Broth. You can also have a second serving of soup and 1 small handful of raw almonds or brazil nuts.

Key points to remember (days 1 to 3)

- Drink two bottles of Green Water throughout the day, ideally before breakfast and in between meals.

- If your rash temporarily worsens during or after the Three Day Alkalising Cleanse then it's a sign you may be salicylate sensitive. If so, add glycine to your bottle of Green Water and reduce the amount of chlorophyll and lemon/lime used for the first two weeks. Read Chapter 15, 'Eczema/dermatitis', for glycine dosage.

- During the first three days you should not do any vigorous exercise as this will drain your energy. During the cleanse you are eating less food so you need to rest and relax to promote healing and restoration of vitality.

- Master the 'Beauty breathing' exercises in Chapter 19.

- Have at least one relaxing warm bath.

- Get plenty of rest, approximately eight hours of sleep at night.

- It's also necessary to avoid caffeine, cigarettes and alcohol during this period as they are highly acidic and may negate some of the healing effects during the Three Day Alkalising Cleanse. Please gradually cut down on these substances at least a week *before* you begin the programme so you don't suffer withdrawal symptoms.

- Relax while you eat and chew your food thoroughly.

- Do the exercises from Chapter 20, 'How to be beautiful'.

The Healthy Skin Diet eight-week programme

Step 1: Plan your diet

A new diet takes planning so if you don't have a personal assistant to say 'Now it's time to eat/relax/go for a walk', or a chef to prepare your tucker, then you'll need a diary or planner. A bit of organisation will help you achieve fabulous-looking skin.

Write your daily activities in your planner so you keep on track. Of course you'll then need to work out what day you're going to begin your healthy skin routine. Will it be Saturday, so you can relax on the weekend and quietly cleanse? Or will Monday be the first day you start the Healthy Skin Diet – a day when you'll be in work mode and far from the influences of your party pals? Once you have picked 'Diet' day then you can calculate the finishing date, exactly eight weeks after commencement.

Step 2: Prepare for your diet

- Gradually cut down on cigarettes, coffee, tea and cola (caffeine), and reduce your alcohol intake. If you're a big coffee/caffeine drinker or a-pack-a-day smoker then you may get withdrawals if you suddenly stop having them so it's best to begin cutting down at least one week before starting the Healthy Skin Diet.

- Choose the recipes you are going to have for the first week and shop for ingredients.

- Freeze some fresh fruit (such as diced mango, peeled whole banana) for the Skin Firming Drink or desserts such as Mango Ice (½ mango per container).

- Put filtered water and mineral water in the refrigerator.

- Pre-make the Anti-ageing Broth.

- Grind up 1 cup of fresh whole flaxseeds, place in a jar and store in the refrigerator.

What utensils do you need?

When cooking for the Healthy Skin Diet you'll need the following:

- A large non-stick frying pan (and a small pan would also be good for making crêpes).

- A large steamer (this could be a large pot with a strainer on top, plus a lid – make sure the pot/steamer is big enough to steam a small rainbow trout). If you are vegetarian, a medium-sized steamer would be suitable for steaming vegetables.

- Storage containers (empty jars for seed mix and small containers for frozen mango, etc.).

- A strainer (for straining rice, etc.).

- A juicing machine (this is optional as you can also buy fresh vegetable juices or simply eat plenty of fruit and vegetables).

- Tea strainer (an enclosed, ball-shaped one – for making dandelion or herbal tea).

- Coffee/seed grinder (this is essential for grinding up fresh flaxseeds and it's also handy for making breadcrumbs). Remember: don't buy pre-ground flaxseeds, they must be fresh.

Step 3: Do the Three Day Alkalising Cleanse

If you haven't already done this, see page 278 for details.

Step 4: Complete the Healthy Skin Diet

There are eight basic rules that will guarantee your success, outlined below. You may notice that some of these rules are the same as the Eight Guidelines for Healthy Skin.

Rule 1: Begin and end each day with an alkalising drink

Essential: One glass of Green Drink, twice a day (morning and evening) or 1 to 2 ACV Drinks per day. **Optional:** Anti-ageing Broth; Flaxseed Lemon Drink; freshly made vegetable juice; herbal teas.

Drinks to sip throughout the day (optional):

Flaxseed Lemon Drink	any fresh vegetable juice
Pear Flaxseed Drink for Sensitive Skin	Soya Dandé or Dandelion Tea (improves digestion)
Skin Juice for Sensitive Skin No. 1 and No. 2	herbal teas, e.g. rosehip tea
Spot-free Skin Juice	filtered water, natural mineral water
Apple Omega Drink	Anti-ageing Broth
ACE Smoothie	Skin Firming Drink

Rule 2: Eat breakfast every day

It is essential to eat breakfast every day. If you don't you may find you overeat later in the day. If you have no appetite in the morning, then have one of the recommended healthy drinks. If you have a good appetite then you can also have one of the drinks plus a moderate sized breakfast, approximately one plateful (minus 30 per cent). Make sure you get some protein with each meal and choose wholegrains over processed white flour products. If you're on a specific diet from the 'Specialised programmes' section or have nutritional deficiencies then you may need to take a supplement or two during breakfast. Take your specific probiotic 15–30 minutes before breakfast.

Choose from one of the following breakfasts:

Berry Beauty Smoothie	Tasty Omelette
Berry Beauty Porridge	Designer Muesli
Sweet Banana Porridge	Gluten-free Muesli
Delicious French Toast with Berries and Almonds	Vitamin E Muesli
Avocado on Toast	B Muesli
Smoked Salmon and Avocado on Toast	Mango and Buckwheat Crêpes
Sardines and Lemon on Grainy Toast	Pear and Buckwheat Crêpes
Whole Fruit Jam on Toast	Boiled Eggs, Vegetables and Rice
Friendly Fruit Salad with Flaxseeds	Fish and Steamed Vegetables
Amine-free Fruit Salad	Anti-ageing Broth with Grainy Toast
Perfect Poached Eggs	Vegetable Hand Rolls and Miso Soup
Smoked Salmon and Eggs	Beans on Toast
Egg Soldiers	Kids Scrambled Eggs
	Kids Creamy Beans on Toast

If you have a skin condition such as eczema or rosacea see the individual recipe descriptions as many of them have modification tips for you.

Breakfast café/take-away options

- Freshly squeezed juice (containing more vegetable than fruit) plus a handful of fresh, raw almonds or brazil nuts.

- Fresh fruit (as long as it hasn't been treated with preservatives).

- Muesli with soya milk and fresh fruit, no added sugar.

- Poached or boiled eggs (1–2) on grainy toast or sourdough, with *a side of spinach*.

- Salmon and avocado on sourdough or wholegrain toast.

Note: There is no snack between breakfast and lunch unless you're pregnant or unable to concentrate, or suffer from hypoglycaemia. If you get hypoglycaemia, you can also add 1–2 teaspoons of chlorophyll to a bottle of water and sip throughout the day to keep blood sugar levels steady. Also consider taking a chromium supplement (see Chapter 5).

Rule 3: Eat lunch every day

Have lunch between 12 p.m. and 2 p.m. (approximately five hours after breakfast). Lunch must be finished before 2 p.m. (unless you do shift work). If you do shift work then have your first meal after you wake up and eat 'lunch' five or six hours later.

Choose from one of the following lunches:

Spicy Green Papaya Salad

Omega Nicoise Salad

Colourful Non-fried Rice

Annie's Decadent Veggie Bake

Roasted Corn and Cauliflower Soup

Therapeutic Chicken Soup

Roasted Sweet Potato Salad served with protein

Rich Mineral Salad with Papaya, Dill and Baby Spinach, served with protein

Sweet Raspberry, Avocado and Watercress Salad, with protein (such as Cajun Chicken Breast)

Multi-vitamin Dahl

Tuna and Avocado Wrap

Chickpea Beauty Salad

Chicken and Salad Wrap

Chicken and Salad Sandwich

Tasty Antioxidant Salad, with protein

Vegetable Hand Rolls

Salad Sandwich with Creamy Mayo

Salmon and Salad Sandwich

Beef Barley Soup

Falafel Wrap

Rich Mediterranean Pasta with a side salad

Steak Sandwich

Healthy Hamburger

Boiled Eggs, Vegetables and Rice

Therapeutic Veggie Soup

Also see 'Choose from the following dinners' for more meal options.

Take-away options (lunch)

tuna, avocado and salad wrap

turkey, cranberry and salad wrap or wholegrain sandwich (sourdough is also okay)

chicken and tabbouli wrap (free-range or
organic chicken only)

sushi rolls, ohitashi spinach, edamame,
miso soup and green tea (Avoid raw
fish during the eight-week programme
as it may contain microbes.)

falafel in a Lebanese wrap/kebab with
tabbouli, onion, tomato and hummus (don't even think about getting
the meat variety!)

tuna and salad sandwich with avocado
instead of butter (on wholegrain or
sourdough bread). Turkey meat, tofu
or vegetarian patties are alternatives if you don't eat fish.

Note: Depending on your appetite at lunchtime either go for something light and colourful like an antioxidant-rich salad with a serving of protein, or pick something hearty and satisfying (but as always, the meat serving should be no bigger than the size of your palm – yes, a big palm means you can have a bit more).

Rule 4: Have a mid-afternoon snack

Many people feel tired at around 3 p.m. so this is a good time to have a snack that contains some protein and/or slow-release carbs. A 3 p.m. snack also helps to combat overeating at dinner time.

Choose from the following snacks (you can have one to two servings/snacks):

Avocado Dip with Dipping Sticks (equiv.
½ avocado each per day)

Avocado Beauty Snack

fresh fruit (1–2 servings per day)

pumpkin seeds (a small handful)

fresh vegetables (unlimited)

steamed soyabeans , or 'edamame'
(available from Japanese/sushi
restaurants)

fresh raw oysters (up to 6 per day, once
or twice a week)

Oysters with Dipping Sauce

low GI wholegrain crackers (no more
than 6 per day) with avocado and
tomato or lemon

fresh, raw almonds or brazil nuts
daily (up to 12 nuts per day
or 1 handful)

½ avocado with fresh lemon juice, diced
fresh tomato and sea salt

Vegetable Hand Rolls (raw spring rolls)
with Sweet Chilli Sauce

Rule 5: Eat dinner every evening

Take a probiotic supplement 15 minutes before dinner. Eat dinner at least two hours before bed so you have time to digest your food. You can also have one of the healthy desserts if you choose. If you tend to overeat then have 12 fresh, raw almonds or one of the drinks containing flaxseed oil about 20 minutes before dinner. The beneficial fats switch on the 'satiety response' (this takes approximately 30 minutes to kick in) so you are less likely to overeat when your main meal arrives.

Choose from the following dinners:

Roasted Corn and Cauliflower Soup

Sweet Raspberry, Avocado and Watercress Salad, with protein (such as Cajun Chicken Breast)

Seafood Hotpot

Beef Barley Soup

Kids Creamy Beans on Toast (or served with pasta)

Omega Nicoise Salad

Therapeutic Veggie Soup

Therapeutic Chicken Soup

Marinated Whole Steamed Trout

Multi-vitamin Dahl

Chickpea Beauty Salad

Colourful Non-fried Rice

Lamb's Fry in Rich Tomato

Creamy Chickpea Curry

A&C-rich Apricot Chicken

Creamy Tuna and Mushroom Mornay

Creamy Salmon Mornay

Slow Roasted Lamb with Steamed Greens

Rich Mediterranean Pasta with Garden Salad

Salmon Steaks with Peas and Mash

Rainbow Trout with Honey Roasted Vegetables

Herb and Garlic Chicken Casserole

Tasty Vegetable Casserole

Annie's Decadent Veggie Bake with Garden Salad

Prawn and Sweet Chilli Vegetable Stir-fry

Lean Meat and Three Veg

Roasted Sweet Potato Salad with Sweet Chutney

Thai Baked Fish with Sweet Corn

Lamb Stir-fry

Sweet Chicken Stir-fry

Healthy Hamburger

Chicken and Three Veg

Tropical Vegetarian Stir-fry

If not specified, meals can be served with brown rice, basmati rice (occasionally), buckwheat or quinoa.

Restaurant options

When eating out *avoid sauces* because you don't know how much sugar, fat, additives or dairy is in them.

Choose from the following:

- any salad (except Caesar salad). Ask for the dressing on the side and if it's dairy-free and homemade then you can use a small amount of it (olive oil and lemon is ideal);
- steamed or grilled fish (preferably salmon or trout, not high-mercury fish – refer to page 82) with no sauces;
- stir-fried vegetables with fish, tofu, beans or skinless chicken;
- steamed vegetables with fish, tofu, beans or skinless chicken;
- fresh oysters (snack);
- uncooked spring rolls (snack);
- (skinless) chicken and vegetables;
- any vegetarian dish that's not deep fried or overly processed, *no sauces*;
- side serving of vegetables with a protein food (fish, chicken, tofu or beans);
- vegetable soups as long as they're dairy free;
- lean meat (no bigger than the palm of your hand) and vegetables.

Desserts

If you crave something sweet, you can choose from a range of dessert recipes in this book. However, please follow these rules:

- Have no more than three desserts per week.
- If you have a heavy meal, such as Creamy Tuna and Mushroom Mornay, choose a light fruit dessert such as Mango Ice.
- If you have a light meal such as a salad then you can have a heavier dessert such as Rhubarb Crumble or Carrot Cake.

Other activities to schedule into your diary

- Sweat and exercise three to five times a week for 15 to 30 minutes. Your aim is to sweat for at least 15 minutes each day. This includes doing conventional exercise and having warm baths or saunas once or twice a week (see Chapter 7 for instructions). If you are exercising outdoors remember to wear sunscreen and a hat.

- Relax and make peace with your body. Do breathing exercises for at least five minutes a day (See Chapter 19, 'Beauty breathing').

- Do the inner beauty exercises from Chapter 20, 'How to be beautiful'.

- Get plenty of rest. Good quality sleep is essential to looking good and feeling fabulous. Go to bed by 10.30 p.m. and aim for eight hours' sleep a night.

- Exfoliate your body once or twice a week (see Chapter 8 to find out how).

- Call a friend or family member for a chat and a laugh (at least once a week).

- Smile and laugh (and make someone else laugh, at least once a day).

Read the next chapter 'The Healthy Skin Menu' to see how to implement these activities into your daily routine.

Chapter 22

The Healthy Skin Menu – structured plan

The Healthy Skin Menu is for anyone who wants a more structured meal plan. This menu is similar to a rotation diet as each day will either be a poultry, fish, vegetarian or red meat day. However you do not have to strictly follow this regime, it is just a guide to help you to monitor how much fish and red meat you're eating as it's important to balance your prostaglandins. Once or twice a week is a gluten-free day but all other foods are freely mixed so it is not strictly a rotation diet.

Of course, if you know you're allergic to something such as fish or any other ingredient then substitute the suggested recipe for a suitable alternative. If you have eczema or rosacea then you can choose the recipe that is most suitable for you. Read the recipe description with each recipe to see if it's suitable or modifiable.

Tips for success:

- Remember to have something green *every day*. Cup your hands together as if you are about to splash your face with water: this is the amount of greens you should be eating daily. The lunch and dinner recipes can help you achieve this.

- Have omega-3 rich foods every day: either salmon, sardines or trout, or 1–2 tablespoons of flaxseed oil, ground flaxseeds or whole flaxseeds. The drink and breakfast recipes can help you reach your daily omega-3 intake.

I hope you enjoy your new-found vitality and clear skin!

The Healthy Skin Menu

Days 1–3: The Three Day Alkalising Cleanse

Choose from the warm or cold weather versions (see pages 278–281). You may need supplements during this time.

Activities for days 1–3

Day 1

- Have a warm bath and exfoliate your skin (see Chapter 8).

- Practise breathing exercises for at least five minutes. Master the Throat Breathing exercises (see Chapter 19).

Day 2

- Continue your breathing exercises. Master the Throat Breathing exercises.

- Go for a walk and practise Inner Beauty Exercise Level 1 (see Chapter 20).

- Optional: enjoy a sauna.

Day 3

- Practise your breathing exercises for at least five minutes.

- Practise Inner Beauty Exercise Levels 2 and 3.

- Prepare the Anti-ageing Broth for the Therapeutic Chicken Soup on day 4 (there is also a non-soup option).

Day 4: Poultry day

During day 4 you are easing your way back into having heavier meals:

Breakfast

- Have one glass of Green Water on rising (at least 15 minutes before breakfast). Make one bottle of Green Water and sip it throughout the day.

- Tasty Omelette or muesli recipe of choice.

- Optional: Skin Juice for Sensitive Skin No. 1 *or* Anti-ageing Broth.

Lunch

Therapeutic Chicken Soup (one bowl) with one to two slices of plain grainy toast (or drizzled with olive oil, no butter/margarine) *or* Chicken and Salad Sandwich on grainy bread.

Optional 3 p.m. snack

Ten almonds; one pear *or* Skin Juice for Sensitive Skin No. 1 (as above).

Dinner

- One glass of ACV Drink 15 to 30 minutes before dinner.

- Therapeutic Chicken Soup (one large bowl) with one or two slices grainy toast (freeze any leftover soup).

Activities for day 4

- Exercise – your aim is to sweat for at least 15 minutes.

- Practise breathing exercises for at least five minutes.

- Grab a piece of paper and a pen right now. List your strengths and positive attributes. Acknowledge your good points on a daily basis to build self-confidence and decrease self-sabotage.

Day 5: Fish and gluten-free day

Even if you're not sensitive to gluten it's important to occasionally have a gluten-free day as it not only gives your digestive system a break from processing gluten, it also educates you on how to vary your diet.

Breakfast

- Have one glass of Green Water on rising. Make one bottle of Green Water and sip it throughout the day.

- If you have poor digestion you may also want to have one cup of Soya Dandé before breakfast as it stimulates digestive juices. Use 'malt-free' soya milk (barley malt is a sweetener that contains gluten).

- Friendly Fruit Salad with Flaxseeds (if you have eczema) but omit the rolled oats to make it gluten free *or* Amine-free Fruit Salad (especially suitable for rosacea), plus one glass of Calcium-rich Smoothie (with malt-free soya milk).

Lunch

Omega Nicoise Salad *or* Tasty Antioxidant Salad topped with one small tin of tuna (use Omega Salad Dressing as it's gluten free).

Optional 3 p.m. snack

Choose from the following:

- one small handful of pumpkin seeds or brazil nuts

- fresh vegetable sticks (carrot and celery) with Tuna Dip

- Soya Dandé
- one apple.

Dinner

- Drink the last of your Green Water bottle 15 to 30 minutes before dinner (if not already finished).
- One serving of Marinated Whole Steamed Trout. **Tip:** Don't drink cold liquids with meals as they dilute digestive acids.

Activities for day 5

- Exercise – sweat for 15 minutes.
- Do five minutes of breathing exercises (a great time for this is after work and before cooking dinner as it relaxes you and helps to restore energy).
- Drink 1–2 litres of water/Green Water in between meals.

Day 6: Vegetarian day

Breakfast

- Have one glass of Green Water on rising. Make one bottle of Green Water and sip it throughout the day.
- Avocado on Toast *or* Beans on Toast.

Lunch

One serving Chickpea Beauty Salad.

Optional 3 p.m. snack

Avocado Beauty Snack *and/or* Soya Dandé.

Dinner

- Drink the last of your Green Water bottle 15 to 30 minutes before dinner (if not already finished).
- Tasty Vegetable Casserole *or* Creamy Chickpea Curry.

Activities for day 6

- Rest day, no heavy exercise. Have a warm bath (or sauna).
- Practise Abdominal Breathing for five to ten minutes.

294 | The Healthy Skin Diet

- Have you been grateful today? (review Chapter 20).

Day 7: Red meat day

Breakfast

- Have one glass of Green Water on rising. Make one bottle of Green Water and sip it throughout the day.
- Muesli of choice from recipe section or buy an untoasted oat-based muesli and add ground flaxseeds and homemade Almond Milk.

Lunch

Healthy Hamburger *or* Salad Sandwich with Creamy Mayo.

Optional 3 p.m. snack

Choose from the following:

- four brazil nuts
- one piece of fruit (pear, banana and papaya are *low in salicylates*)
- Spot-free Skin Juice
- Soya Dandé.

Dinner

- One ACV Drink 15 to 30 minutes before dinner or drink the last of your Green Water bottle 15 to 30 minutes before dinner (if not already finished).
- Lean Meat and Three Veg; Lamb Stir-fry *or* soup recipe of choice. Only have one red meat meal on any given day (and only two per week in total).

Activities for day 7

- Exercise – sweat for 15 minutes.
- Practise Abdominal Breathing exercises for five minutes.
- Calculate how many glasses (or litres) of water you're consuming. Is it enough? (refer to Chapter 3).

Day 8: Poultry and gluten-free day

Breakfast

- Have one glass of Green Water on rising. Make one bottle of Green Water and sip it throughout the day.

- Boiled Eggs, Vegetables and Rice; Gluten-free Muesli or Mango and Buckwheat Crêpes (or Pear and Buckwheat Crêpes if you have eczema).

Lunch

Cajun Chicken breast fillet served with Sweet Raspberry, Avocado and Watercress Salad

Optional 3 p.m. snack

Choose from the following:

- Ten almonds and drink recipe of choice
- Soya Dandé (with malt-free soya milk) and vegetable sticks with Hummus Dip (see recipe section).

Dinner

- Drink the last of your Green Water bottle 15 to 30 minutes before dinner (if not already finished).
- A&C-rich Apricot Chicken with brown rice or buckwheat or Multi-vitamin Dahl.

Activities for day 8

- Exercise – sweat for 15 minutes.
- Practise breathing exercises for at least five minutes.
- Count how many times you check your reflection in mirrors. You may need to do your make-up or look to see if your outfit is on properly but if you glance or gaze at your reflection more than three times a day and criticise your looks/skin/weight then you need to restrict mirror use (see Chapter 20).

Day 9: Fish day

Breakfast

- Have one glass of Green Water on rising. Make one bottle of Green Water and sip it throughout the day.
- Sardines and Lemon on Grainy Toast and Papaya Beauty Smoothie or fruit salad recipe or porridge recipe of choice. Optional: Soya Dandé.

Lunch

Tuna and Avocado Wrap or Falafel Wrap.

Optional 3 p.m. snack

Choose from the following:

- 2–6 fresh oysters
- six tinned oysters on three to four whole wheat/grain crackers
- smoothie recipe of choice.

Dinner

- Drink the last of your Green Water bottle 15 to 30 minutes before dinner (if not already finished).
- Entrée option: 2–6 fresh oysters (if you didn't have them earlier).
- Prawn and Sweet Chilli Vegetable Stir-fry *or* Thai Baked Fish with Sweet Corn *or* Roasted Sweet Potato Salad, served with Sweet Chutney.

Activities for day 9

- Sweat *without* doing high impact exercise: sauna, warm bath or go for a walk on a hot day (avoiding the sun between the hours of 10 a.m. and 3 p.m.).
- Have you been wearing your hat when outdoors? You may have a cap for exercise/casual attire but do you need to buy another hat to suit dressier occasions/outfits? (see Chapter 9)
- List your strengths and positive attributes.

Day 10: Vegetarian day

Breakfast

- Have one glass of Green Water on rising. Make one bottle of Green Water and sip it throughout the day.
- Muesli of choice with Almond Milk or soya milk (containing calcium and 'whole' soyabean, *not* soya 'isolate').
- Optional: Skin Firming Drink

Lunch

Rich Mediterranean Pasta *or* Salad Sandwich with Creamy Mayo (if you don't eat egg, substitute Creamy Mayonnaise with Sweet Chutney in this recipe).

Optional 3 p.m. snack

Choose from the following:

- B-rich Avocado Salsa (optional: serve with 4 whole wheat/grain crackers)
- fruit
- one cup of alfalfa tea (add a squeeze of lemon and two slices of fresh ginger) *or* fresh vegetable juice of choice.

Dinner

- Drink the last of your Green Water bottle 15 to 30 minutes before dinner (if not already finished).
- Creamy Chickpea Curry.

Activities for day 10

- Exercise – sweat for 15 minutes.
- In the afternoon or before dinner, lie down and do your breathing exercises for five minutes.

Day 11: Red meat day

Breakfast

- Have one glass of Green Water on rising. Make one bottle of Green Water and sip it throughout the day.
- Berry Beauty Porridge served with Almond Milk or soya milk (with added calcium) *or* fruit salad recipe of choice with smoothie recipe of choice.

Lunch

Salad Sandwich with Creamy Mayo – if you're at a café skip the mayo and have avocado instead) *or* Falafel Wrap *or* Vegetable Hand Rolls.

Optional 3 p.m. snack

Choose from the following:

- a handful of raw almonds and brazil nuts (for selenium) and a handful of blueberries
- one cup Soya Dandé and vegetable sticks with Hummus Dip.

Dinner

- One ACV Drink to help with digestion *or* drink the last of your Green Water bottle 15 to 30 minutes before dinner (if not already finished).

- Slow Roasted Lamb with Steamed Greens *or* Beef Barley Soup.

Activities for day 11

- Exercise – sweat for 15 minutes.

- Practise Throat Breathing exercises for five minutes.

Day 12: Poultry day

Breakfast

- Have one glass of Green Water on rising. Make one bottle of Green Water and sip it throughout the day.

- Perfect Poached Eggs *or* Egg Soldiers.

Lunch

Chicken and Salad Wrap *or* chicken and salad of choice (e.g. Roasted Sweet Potato Salad)

Optional 3 p.m. snack

Choose from the following:

- carrot and celery sticks with Hummus Dip

- Soya Dandé

- Hummus Dip and 4 wholewheat/grain crackers.

Dinner

- Drink the last of your Green Water bottle 15 to 30 minutes before dinner.

- Sweet Chicken Stir-fry *or* Chicken and Three Veg.

Activities for day 12

- Go for a relaxing walk or stretch for 20 minutes.

- Practise breathing exercises for five to ten minutes.

- Have a shower/bath and lightly exfoliate your skin (face and body), then moisturise (see Chapter 8).

Day 13: Fish and gluten-free day

Breakfast

- Have one glass of Green Water on rising. Make one bottle of Green Water and sip it throughout the day.

- Mango and Buckwheat Crêpes. If you have eczema, have Pear and Buckwheat Crêpes or Gluten-free Muesli instead.

Lunch

Omega Nicoise Salad *or* gluten-free Japanese: nori rolls with real wasabi (very hot and green horseradish paste that can kill microbes in raw fish) and salmon/tuna/avocado/cucumber or other vegetables; green soya beans (edamame); pickled ginger; some miso soups (ones without soy sauce, barley or noodles). Soy sauce contains gluten so BYO tamari sauce, which tastes the same but is gluten free.

Japanese food that may contain gluten includes: products containing soy sauce; miso soup (if they have added soy sauce/barley/wheat noodles); tempura; fried and crumbed chicken; imitation crab (sushi with crab); green tea that contains barley; eel (as it's cooked in sauce); ramen; gyoza; panko; curry rice mix; dashi; salad dressing; tamago (omelette); flavoured roe; fish cakes; imitation wasabi (this is uncommon, however if you're a coeliac it's best to ask if the wasabi contains wheat starch or gluten).

Optional 3 p.m. snack

Choose from the following:

- one piece of fruit *and/or* a small handful of raw almonds and brazil nuts
- fresh vegetable juice *or* Flaxseed Lemon Drink
- steamed soyabeans (edamame).

Dinner

- Drink the last of your Green Water bottle 15 to 30 minutes before dinner.
- Seafood Hotpot *or* Salmon Steaks with Peas and Mash.

Activities for day 13

- Exercise – sweat for 15 minutes.
- Practise your deep breathing exercises.
- Have a relaxing bath before bed.
- Have an early night and get eight hours of quality sleep.

Day 14: Vegetarian day

Breakfast

- Have one glass of Green Water on rising. Make one bottle of Green Water and sip it throughout the day.

- Muesli of choice *or* Sweet Banana Porridge with Almond Milk or soya milk (with added calcium and 'whole' soyabean).

Lunch

Falafel Wrap.

Optional 3 p.m. snack

Choose from the following:

- Avocado Dip with Dipping Sticks
- one cup of Soya Dandé
- ¼ avocado with four whole wheat/grain crackers.

Dinner

- Drink the last of your Green Water bottle 15 to 30 minutes before dinner.
- Rich Mediterranean Pasta with Garden Salad *or* Colourful Non-fried Rice.

Activities for day 14

- Exercise – sweat for 15 minutes.
- Do 15 minutes of breathing exercises.
- Do an Inner Beauty Exercise of your choice from Chapter 20.

Continue with day 15 and if desired, follow the same pattern: poultry, fish, vegetarian and red meat. For example, day 15 would be a red meat day.

Life after the Healthy Skin Diet

You may have overcome an undesirable skin condition such as acne or eczema during the eight-week programme and you might now be wondering *are these results sustainable?* The answer could be yes or no.

Yes, because you have strengthened your health immensely during the eight weeks and you've also put into place new habits, many of which you'll now automatically follow. For example, you may have found a fab new hat and a good sunscreen so you continue with your sun-care programme; you might habitually add something green to your lunches and dinners and as you peek in the mirror you might look for beauty more often than faults. But I'll give you a tip: if you continue to be *kind* to yourself and speak highly of your strengths and positive attributes it will be much easier for you to continue to be healthy because your subconscious mind will work with, not against you.

However, I also say no because certain conditions are caused by *genetics* and although you may have 'switched off' your eczema, psoriasis or allergic reactions such as hives, they can reappear if triggered. Triggers include repeated stress, high chemical exposure, illness, a virus or poor diet and lifestyle habits. However there are ways to minimise the risk of relapse. Below I have listed the top four things you can do to keep your skin looking good beyond the Healthy Skin Diet. The Four Habits to Keep for a Lifetime can be followed by anyone who wants to maintain healthy skin, vitality and wellbeing.

1. Think green

Continue to alkalise your body with green drinks and green foods. Eat two handfuls of dark leafy greens every day. You can have a salad or a side of baby spinach leaves, steamed broccoli, silverbeet and Chinese greens. You should also continue to have a bottle of Green Water daily so you can cleanse your blood and keep track of how much water you consume. Think green for a healthy body and beautiful skin.

- If you drink alcohol or coffee (caffeine) then have one glass of Green Water afterwards to reduce acids in the body.

2. Moisturise your skin from the inside out

- Eat fish, especially oily deep sea fish, twice a week.
- Have ground flaxseeds or flaxseed oil twice a week.
- Drink plenty of water.

- Add lecithen granules to cereals/porridge/smoothies to promote healthy lipid (fat) digestion and hydrated cells.

3. Be a hat person

The easiest way to slow down the ageing process is to simply wear a hat and apply sunscreen when you go out in the sun.

4. Think beautiful thoughts to reduce your stress levels

Stress simply ruins your skin so you want to reduce its damaging effects as often as possible. The most effective way to cope with daily stress is to spend some time focusing on your good attributes, your strengths and your beauty.

Enjoy your beautiful skin!

Additives to avoid

The following food additives may cause adverse skin reactions:

Flavour enhancers	E620–E635	Especially **E635** and **E621** monosodium gluta-mate (**MSG**). Used in flavoured noodles, chicken salted chips, flavoured crackers, sauces, fast foods, traditional Chinese cooking
Artificial colours	E102	Tartrazine (yellow)
	E107, E110	Yellow
	E122–E129	Red
	E133, E142	Blue, green
	E151	Black
	E155	Brown
Natural colour	E160b	Annatto yellow (in some yogurts)
Preservatives	E200–E203	Sorbates (used in some processed fruits and veg, and wines)
	E210–E213	Benzoates (in most soft drinks, diet drinks, cordials, juices)
	E220–E228	Sulphites (wine, beer, processed meats, sausages, dried fruit)
	E249–E252	Nitrates, nitrites (processed meats – ham, salami, etc.)
	E280–E283	Propionates, especially **E282** calcium propionate in breads
	E310-E321	Antioxidants – not the natural kind (in oils, margarines, chips, fried snack foods, fast foods)
Artificial sweetener	E951	Aspartame (NutraSweet; Equal; diet and 'sugar-free' products)
	E954	Saccharin (in many diet and 'sugar-free' products)[1,2]

Recipes

Drink recipes

Green Water

SERVES 1, PREPARATION TIME 1 MINUTE

This mild-tasting drink is alkalising, gluten free, rich in magnesium and may help prevent some food intolerances, allergies and acid conditions such as skin rashes. Drink 1–2 glasses daily. Use low-strength chlorophyll and begin with 1 teaspoon and work up to having 2–3 teaspoons daily.

1–3 teaspoons liquid chlorophyll (or 1–3 capfuls)
1 glass chilled water (optional: chilled mineral water)

Method: Mix together and drink. To add more flavour and alkalinity you can add 1 teaspoon of fresh lemon juice.

If you suffer from blood sugar problems such as hypoglycaemia, you could also get a large bottle of filtered water (1–1.5 litres) and add 2 teaspoons of liquid chlorophyll and sip it throughout the day (don't add lemon juice as it's no good for the teeth if you're sipping it all day). If you have eczema or psoriasis also add a measured dose of glycine to this drink.

ACV Drink

SERVES 1, PREPARATION TIME 1 MINUTE

This alkalising drink has a mild apple cider taste. It's gluten free and stimulates digestion so ideally have it 15 minutes before breakfast or dinner. Drink 1–2 glasses daily as an occasional alternative to Green Water.

250–500ml (8–16fl oz) chilled water or mineral water
1 teaspoon apple cider vinegar

Method: Mix ingredients and drink slowly. Alternatively you can use 125ml (4fl oz) apple juice (sugar and preservative free), 240ml (8fl oz) water and 1–2 teaspoons of ACV for a sweeter-tasting drink.

Soya Dandé

SERVES 1, HAVE 1 TO 3 CUPS DAILY, PREPARATION TIME 2 MINUTES

This tasty, hot drink is a good coffee substitute as it is liver cleansing and caffeine free, and it stimulates digestive acids for improved digestion. May over-stimulate digestion; if this occurs reduce dosage. Use calcium-fortified soya milk that contains 'whole' soyabean (not isolate). Favour the ground dandelion root if available (it is the one that needs to be put into an enclosed tea strainer) as it is better than the instant dandelion root.

125ml (4fl oz) preheated soya milk
125ml (4fl oz) boiled water
1 teaspoon ground dandelion root (begin with ½ teaspoon)
1 teaspoon honey (optional) (*low GI*)

Method: Heat soya milk in a microwave for 30 seconds, then add boiling water (pre-heating the soya milk prevents it from curdling). Place the measured amount of ground dandelion root into a tea strainer and then dunk it into the hot liquid for about 5 to 10 seconds (it should darken the milk quickly). Remove the strainer and discard the contents. Add honey if desired. Also see Dandelion Tea.

Dandelion Tea

SERVES 1, PREPARATION TIME 2 MINUTES

½ teaspoon ground dandelion root
250ml (8fl oz) boiled water
1 teaspoon honey

Method: Place the dandelion root into an enclosed tea strainer. Dunk the tea strainer into boiled water and steep for about 5 seconds, until water is dark brown. Make it weak to begin with, as it can be quite strong in flavour. Add honey if desired.

Flaxseed Lemon Drink

SERVES 3, OR 1 DAY'S SUPPLY FOR ONE PERSON, PREPARATION TIME 5 MINUTES

This special therapeutic drink reduces body acidity and may balance weight, improve immune function and alleviate dry skin if consumed on a regular basis. The pectin and oils from lemon skin provide antioxidants, chelate toxins from the bowel and stimulate liver detoxification enzymes (cytochrome P450). The lecithin aids fat digestion and helps the body utilise the anti-inflammatory omega-3 oils. If you have eczema, have the Pear Flaxseed Drink instead. Gluten free. Omit the ginger and add honey if you're making this recipe for children.

400ml (14fl oz) water
½ organic lemon, washed, scrubbed and chopped into small chunks (including skin)
2 tablespoons lecithin granules (GMO-free soya)
2 tablespoons organic flaxseed oil
1 small knob ginger root, peeled and finely chopped
1 teaspoon vitamin C powder supplement (optional: for rosacea or hives only)

Method: Combine water, lemon, lecithin, oil and ginger in a blender and blend for 30 seconds on high. Strain mixture through a fine sieve to remove the pulp (mash the pulp to strain as much liquid as possible). Stir in the vitamin C powder if necessary. Drink 200ml (7fl oz) before breakfast and 100ml (3½fl oz) before lunch and dinner, preferably sipping slowly. Consume within 12 hours. (This recipe was adapted from the Whole Lemon Drink, author unknown.)

Pear Flaxseed Drink for Sensitive Skin

SERVES 3, OR 1 DAY'S SUPPLY FOR ONE PERSON, PREPARATION TIME 3 MINUTES

Specially designed for people with eczema, this drink is rich in omega-3 anti-inflammatory oils, ginger is anti-inflammatory and lecithin helps your body utilise the omega-3 oils. This recipe is also fibre-rich if using ground flaxseeds. If you have rosacea or hives you can add vitamin C powder to this recipe. Omit the ginger if you are making this recipe for children. Gluten free.

250ml (8fl oz) chilled water
140g (5oz) tinned pear slices plus natural juice, or freshly juiced pear
1 tablespoon lecithin granules (GMO-free soya)
2 tablespoons organic ground flaxseeds or flaxseed oil
1 knob ginger root, peeled and finely chopped
1 teaspoon vitamin C powder supplement (optional: for rosacea or hives only)

Method: Combine water, pear and natural juice, lecithin, oil and ginger root in a blender. Blend for 30 seconds on high. Stir in the vitamin C powder if necessary. Drink 100ml (3½fl oz) in between or before each meal. Consume within 12 hours.

Strawberry Rehydration Water

SERVES 1, PREPARATION TIME 2 MINUTES

This makes a refreshing drink to have after exercising as it replenishes electrolytes. Drink within 10 hours of making.

600ml (1 pint) water
2 fresh strawberries, rinsed and finely diced
1 pinch natural sea salt

Method: Combine water, strawberries and salt in a 600ml water bottle and shake.

Berry Beauty Smoothie

SERVES 1, PREPARATION TIME 3 MINUTES

This tasty drink is rich in antioxidants from berries, omega-3 from flaxseeds, protein and calcium from almonds and coconut oil is anti-fungal. Gluten free.

250ml (8fl oz) chilled Almond Milk (see p. 310) or water
1 tablespoon organic flaxseed oil or ground flaxseeds
1 tablespoon lecithin granules (GMO-free soya)
60g (2oz) frozen berries (raspberries or mixed)
2 tablespoons coconut milk

Method: Place all ingredients in a blender and blend on high until smooth. Consume within 2 hours.

Papaya Beauty Smoothie

SERVES 1 (LARGE SERVING) OR 2 (SMALL), PREPARATION TIME 5 MINUTES

This thick, tropical smoothie is a delicious and refreshing drink. It contains vitamin C-rich papaya, which enhances protein digestion; bananas are a great source of fibre and potassium, and banana, ginger and lime are alkalising. The only thing missing from this recipe is protein, which is vital for firm skin, so ideally you should use this shake as a digestion-enhancing appetiser and have it 15–30 minutes before a protein-rich meal. If had before dinner, it may also aid weight loss because flaxseed oil triggers the satiety response. Gluten free.

125ml (4fl oz) pure apple juice (preservative free, sugar free)
125ml (4fl oz) water
140g (5oz) chopped papaya (optional: pre-freeze chunks)
1 frozen banana (peel and chop before freezing)
2 tablespoons ground flaxseeds or flaxseed oil
2 tablespoons soya lecithin granules
½ lime, juiced (approx. 1 tablespoon)
¼ teaspoon grated ginger (optional)

Method: Place apple juice, water, fruit, lime juice and ginger into a blender and blend on high until smooth. Then add flaxseed oil and lecithin and blend for a further 20 seconds. Serve and drink immediately. For a thinner mixture add extra water.

Skin Firming Drink

SERVES 1, PREPARATION TIME 3 MINUTES

This fibre-rich drink helps to promote proper collagen formation and firm skin as it contains protein, glucosamine, copper, zinc and vitamin C*. Lecithin and omega-3 are essential for cell membrane health.

1 frozen banana (peel and chop before freezing)
250ml (8fl oz) chilled Almond Milk (see p. 310) or calcium-fortified soya milk
10 blueberries (or frozen raspberries)
Glucosamine complex supplement*
1 tablespoon ground flaxseeds or flaxseed oil
1–2 tablespoons lecithin granules (GMO-free soya)
2 dashes ground cinnamon

Method: Place all ingredients into a blender and blend until mixture is smooth.
Drink immediately.

*Choose a glucosamine supplement that also contains copper, zinc and vitamin C and follow dosage recommended by manufacturer. See Chapter 12 'Cellulite' for more information.

Calcium-rich Smoothie

SERVES 2, OR 1 DAY'S SUPPLY FOR ONE PERSON (SUPPLYING AT LEAST 600MG OF CALCIUM), PREPARATION TIME 3 MINUTES

This drink is a good calcium substitute when having a dairy-free diet. Choose quality soya milk that contains at least 300mg of calcium per 100ml. Flaxseed oil has been shown to increase calcium absorption. This drink is also ideal for eczema sufferers as it is low in salicylates. Banana and papaya contain amines so use other fruits if you have rosacea or hives. To make this recipe gluten free use malt free soya milk.

500ml (16fl oz) calcium-fortified soya milk
1 cup papaya or 1 banana, pre-frozen and diced
2 tablespoons flaxseed oil (or ground flaxseeds)
1 tablespoon soya lecithin granules (GMO-free soya)
1 teaspoon real maple syrup (optional)

Method: Place all ingredients in a blender and blend on high until smooth.
Consume within 8 hours.

Skin Juice for Sensitive Skin No. 1

SERVES 3 OR 1 DAY'S SUPPLY FOR ONE PERSON, PREPARATION TIME 5 MINUTES

A perfect juice, especially if you have chemical sensitivity or eczema as it is low in salicylates and rich in anti-inflammatory ingredients.

4 ripe pears
40g (1¾oz) cabbage
3 stalks celery
60ml (2fl oz) water
1 tablespoon apple cider vinegar
½ bunch parsley (including stalks)
1 knob ginger
1 tablespoon lecithin granules

1 teaspoon vitamin C powder (optional: only for rosacea and hives)

> **Method:** Wash and scrub all vegetables in water and apple cider vinegar. With a juicing machine, juice pears, cabbage, celery, parsley and ginger. At the end run 60ml (2fl oz) water through machine to flush though remaining juice and dilute drink slightly. Transfer juice to a blender and add lecithin and vitamin C powder. Blend for 10 seconds on medium speed. Drink 1 glass immediately and consume the rest within 8 hours.

Skin Juice for Sensitive Skin No. 2

3 SERVES OR 1 DAY'S SUPPLY FOR ONE PERSON, PREPARATION TIME 5 MINUTES

> A great drink, especially if you have chemical sensitivity or eczema as it is low in salicylates.

60g (2oz) green beans
4 ripe pears
40g (1¾oz) cabbage
½ bunch parsley (including stalks)
3 stalks celery

> **Method:** Wash and scrub all vegetables in a bowl of water with 1 tablespoon of apple cider vinegar. With a juicing machine, juice all ingredients. Mix and have one glass immediately. Drink the rest within 8 hours.

Spot-free Skin Juice

SERVES 2, OR 1 DAY'S SUPPLY FOR ONE PERSON, PREPARATION TIME 5 MINUTES

> This drink is ideal for anyone who wants clear skin.

1 pear (leave skin on)
2 apples (leave skin on)
60g (2oz) fresh beetroot
4 medium carrots
40g (1¾oz) cabbage
squeeze of fresh lemon

> **Method:** In a juicing machine, juice pear, apples, beetroot, carrots and cabbage. Add lemon before serving. Consume within 8 hours.

Apple Omega Drink

SERVES 2, PREPARATION TIME 2 MINUTES (PLUS OVERNIGHT SOAKING)

> This sweet drink is rich in omega-3 and fibre; low GI; gluten free; anti-inflammatory and promotes proper fat digestion. Use sugar-free and preservative-free apple juice or juice your own apples. Flaxseeds make the drink rich in fibre and a bit lumpy but it tastes surprisingly delicious.

2 tablespoons flaxseeds
100ml (3½fl oz) water
250ml (8fl oz) apple juice
1 small knob ginger, peeled and finely grated
1 tablespoon lecithin granules

Method: Soak the flaxseeds overnight in the water. The next morning put seeds and their water in a blender. Add other ingredients and blend on high for 30 seconds. Pour into glasses and serve immediately.

ACE Smoothie

SERVES 2, PREPARATION TIME 5 MINUTES

This tasty drink is rich in vitamins and minerals. It contains vitamins A and C from the fruits; vitamin E, B complex and chromium from wheat germ, and the egg yolk supplies B vitamins such as biotin. Don't use raw egg whites as they can cause dermatitis. Wheat germ contains gluten so to make it gluten-free use rice bran instead. Use antibiotic-free eggs.

2 tablespoons wheat germ
1 tablespoon ground flaxseeds or flaxseed oil
½ mango (70g (2½oz) diced mango), pre-frozen
70g (2½oz) papaya/papaw, peeled, sliced and pre-frozen
1 free-range egg yolk
500ml (1 pint) chilled plain mineral water

Method: Combine all ingredients in a blender and blend on high until smooth. Serve immediately.

Almond Milk

SERVES 4, PREPARATION TIME 2 MINUTES (PLUS OVERNIGHT SOAKING)

You can use Almond Milk in smoothies, on porridge or cereal instead of milk. It contains calcium and protein.

135g (4¾oz) whole raw almonds
750ml (1¼ pints) water
½ teaspoon vanilla essence
1 teaspoon honey or real maple syrup (optional)
dash of cinnamon or nutmeg (optional)

Method: Soak the almonds in the water overnight (highly recommended but not essential). Then put all ingredients into a blender and blend on high for 30 seconds. Strain the liquid. The leftover meal can be used on porridge or cereal. Consume within 3 days.

Breakfast recipes

Ground flaxseeds

MAKES 140G OF GROUND FLAXSEEDS, PREPARATION TIME 2 MINUTES

Flaxseeds are also known as linseeds and are available from health food shops and some supermarkets. Add ground flaxseeds to breakfast cereals, smoothies and porridge to increase the fibre, calcium and omega-3 content.

140g (5oz) whole flaxseeds
1 coffee bean or nut grinder

Method: Grind flaxseeds in a coffee grinder until they are a fine meal. Store in an air-tight jar in the fridge for up to 4 weeks.

Berry Beauty Porridge

SERVES 4, PREPARATION TIME 3 MINUTES, COOKING TIME 5 MINUTES

This hearty and warm breakfast is rich in antioxidants, fibre and omega-3, and it's low GI. If you have eczema, have the Sweet Banana Porridge instead. Oats contain gluten.

200g (7oz) rolled oats
1 litre (1¾ pints) water
4 teaspoons honey or sugar-free jam (optional)
2 tablespoons ground flaxseeds
240ml (8fl oz) calcium-fortified soya milk
120g (4oz) raspberries, fresh or frozen and thawed

Method: If possible, soak the oats overnight in the water to germinate the grain, making it more digestible and the nutrients more available. Place oats and their water in a small saucepan. Bring to the boil and simmer for 5 minutes, stirring regularly. Serve with honey or jam if extra sweetness is required then add flaxseeds, soya milk and berries. Other enzyme-rich options are blueberries, papaya, peach, grated apple or strawberries so you have a 'living' breakfast fit for a (beauty) queen.

Sweet Banana Porridge

SERVES 4, PREPARATION TIME 3 MINUTES, COOKING TIME 5 MINUTES

This hearty warm breakfast is low in salicylates so it's suitable for eczema sufferers and children love it too. It's also rich in fibre and potassium, flaxseeds supply omega-3 and whole rolled oats are low GI (instant oats are high GI and not suitable). Oats contain gluten.

200g (7oz) rolled oats
1 litre (1¾ pints) water
4 teaspoons real maple syrup
2 tablespoons ground flaxseeds
240ml (8fl oz) calcium-fortified soya milk
1 ripe banana, thinly sliced

Method: If possible, soak the oats overnight in the water to germinate the grain, making it more digestible and the nutrients more available. Place oats and their water in a small saucepan. Bring to the boil and simmer for approximately 5 minutes, stirring regularly, until cooked. Serve with maple syrup, flaxseeds, soya milk and banana.

Delicious French Toast with Berries and Almonds

SERVES 4, PREPARATION TIME 5 MINUTES, COOKING TIME 10 MINUTES

Full of skin-loving antioxidants, protein and fibre, low GI, gluten free if using gluten-free bread; vanilla extract and cinnamon help to keep blood sugar levels steady; use sugar-free berry jam that has been naturally sweetened with grape juice; you can also use strawberries or frozen raspberries (thawed) if desired. If you have eczema, avoid strawberries, cinnamon and jam and use blueberries or banana, and substitute jam with real maple syrup.

3 large eggs
180ml (6fl oz) calcium-fortified soya milk
dash of cinnamon (optional)
8 slices grainy bread (preferably low GI)
1 teaspoon vanilla extract
Extra-virgin olive oil
4 teaspoons sugar-free berry jam
1 punnet blueberries or raspberries (thawed if frozen)
40g (1¼oz) raw almonds, toasted and chopped
1 tablespoon ground flaxseeds

Method: In a shallow bowl, whisk together eggs, soya milk, cinnamon and vanilla extract. Dip bread slices into liquid mix, turning to coat. Grease a large frying pan with a small amount of olive oil and set on medium heat. Using a spatula, remove bread slices and let excess egg mixture drain off. Cook two slices at a time for approximately 2 minutes each side, until slightly golden. Sparingly spread jam onto French toast and top with berries and almonds, then sprinkle with ground flaxseeds. Serve immediately.

Avocado on Toast

SERVES 2, PREPARATION TIME 4 MINUTES

This breakfast is super quick and rich in vitamins and minerals. Not suitable if you have eczema or gluten intolerance.

4 slices grainy bread (soya and flaxseed)
½ avocado
1 banana, thinly sliced (optional)

Method: Toast bread and add the desired amount of avocado. Top with banana and serve immediately. If not using banana, you can add a squeeze of lemon to the avocado and sparingly add quality sea salt and pepper.

Smoked Salmon and Avocado on Toast

SERVES 2, PREPARATION TIME 4 MINUTES

This breakfast is rich in omega-3, vitamins and minerals. If you have eczema then omit the avocado and use hummus instead. If you have gluten intolerance, choose gluten-free bread.

4 slices grainy bread (soya and flaxseed)
½ avocado
100g (3½oz) smoked salmon
a squeeze of fresh lemon
15g (½oz) baby spinach
ground black pepper (optional)

Method: Toast bread and add the desired amount of avocado. Top with smoked salmon, lemon juice (use sparingly) and pepper, and add a side of spinach. Serve immediately.

Sardines and Lemon on Grainy Toast

SERVES 2, PREPARATION TIME 4 MINUTES

This breakfast is quick to prepare and rich in omega-3. Low GI and contains gluten if using wheat bread. If you have eczema use sardines in spring water (not oil) and a tablespoon of flat-leaf parsley instead of the greens.

4 slices grainy bread (soya and flaxseed)
1 small tin sardines in olive oil or spring water
a squeeze of fresh lemon
60g (2oz) dark leafy greens (rocket/spinach/lettuce)
ground black pepper (optional)

Method: Toast bread and spread the desired amount of sardines onto the toast. Top with lemon and pepper and add a side of greens (finely chopped parsley could also go on top). Serve immediately.

Whole Fruit Jam on Toast

SERVES 2, PREPARATION TIME 4 MINUTES

This breakfast is super quick to make, rich in antioxidants, naturally sweet and suitable as an occasional breakfast. Use sugar-free jam that is full of fruit and sweetened with grape juice (NOT artificial sweetener). Low GI, contains gluten and not suitable if you have eczema or gluten intolerance. **Note:** gluten-free bread is not a good alternative as it's high GI and low in nutrition so use sparingly.

4 slices grainy bread (soya and flaxseed)
2 tablespoons sugar-free jam
1 banana, sliced thinly (optional)

Method: Toast bread and add the desired amount of jam. Top with banana and serve immediately.

Friendly Fruit Salad with Flaxseeds

SERVES 2, PREPARATION TIME 5 MINUTES

This fruit salad is low in salicylates and is suitable for people with eczema. It contains amines so people with rosacea or hives should choose the Amine-free Fruit Salad. If you have gluten intolerance or are having a gluten-free day, use rice bran instead of oats.

1 pear, peeled and diced
1 ripe banana, chopped
210g (7½oz) papaya, diced
1 tablespoon ground flaxseeds
1 tablespoon rolled oats (or rice bran)

Method: Combine all ingredients and serve immediately.

Amine-free Fruit Salad

SERVES 4, PREPARATION TIME 6 MINUTES, COOKING TIME 4 MINUTES

This fruit salad is suitable for most people including those with rosacea or hives. People with eczema should have the Friendly Fruit Salad with Flaxseeds instead.

30g (1oz) raw almonds
1 red apple, diced
½ mango, diced

150g (5½oz) strawberries
125g (4½oz) blueberries
140g (5oz) cantaloupe, diced
1–2 tablespoons ground flaxseeds

Method: Toast the almonds on medium heat for approximately 4 minutes, being careful not to burn them. Remove from heat and set aside to cool. Then carefully chop the toasted almonds into smaller pieces. Combine fruits and sprinkle with flaxseeds and almonds.

Perfect Poached Eggs

SERVES 2, PREPARATION TIME 4 MINUTES, COOKING TIME 4 MINUTES

There is an art to cooking perfect poached eggs so it may take you a couple of attempts to master this one (but these tips will turn you into a pro in no time!). This recipe is a healthy way to cook eggs as there is no frying involved. Rich in B vitamins (approximately 64mcg biotin), protein, fibre and antioxidants, and it's low GI and contains gluten if using wheat bread. Use antibiotic-free eggs.

2–4 large free-range eggs
1 tablespoon white vinegar
2–4 slices wholegrain or sourdough bread
½ avocado
2 tablespoons parsley, finely chopped
natural sea salt and ground black pepper (optional)

Method: Fill a medium-sized saucepan with enough water to cover the eggs. Bring to the boil and add vinegar (the vinegar keeps the egg whites together while cooking). Keep the eggs whole in their shells for the first part of preparation: wash eggs if necessary and then, using a spoon, put the eggs into the boiling water for 10 seconds only. Remove eggs and set aside. Remove boiling water from heat so the water ceases movement then carefully crack the eggs into the water (initially only cook two eggs at a time to ensure correct cooking times). Return saucepan to heat and reduce to a simmer and set timer immediately. A 59g egg should take approximately 4 minutes to cook for a soft yolk. Toast the bread and spread with avocado. After 4 minutes, carefully and swiftly remove eggs with a spatula/slotted spoon and if desired, rinse vinegar from eggs using slow-running hot water. Drain water off eggs then place eggs on toast and top with parsley, and salt and pepper if desired. Serve immediately.

Smoked Salmon and Eggs

SERVES 2, PREPARATION TIME 4 MINUTES, COOKING TIME 4 MINUTES

Salmon is rich in omega-3 and eggs supply a good range of B vitamins and protein. If you have eczema, avoid using avocado and use salt-free butter sparingly instead.

2–4 large free-range eggs
1 tablespoon white vinegar
2–4 slices wholegrain or sourdough bread
½ avocado
2 tablespoons parsley, chopped finely
50g (2oz) smoked salmon
ground black pepper

Method: Follow the Perfect Poached Eggs recipe and add smoked salmon. If desired sprinkle pepper and a small amount of lemon juice on the fish. Serve immediately.

Egg Soldiers

SERVES 2, PREPARATION TIME 2 MINUTES, COOKING TIME 5 MINUTES

This meal is fun for children and grown-ups alike as it is served in egg cups with toast dipping sticks. It's a healthy way to cook eggs as no frying is involved. Parsley is alkalising and supplies antioxidants and chlorophyll. Use antibiotic-free eggs. The vinegar and salt help to prevent the egg shells from cracking during cooking. If you have eczema, omit the olive oil and chutney and use salt-free butter sparingly.

1 tablespoon white vinegar
pinch of salt
2–4 slices grainy bread
2–4 free-range eggs
2 teaspoons parsley, finely chopped
extra-virgin olive oil or Sweet Chutney/mango chutney (optional)

Method: Fill a small to medium-sized pan with enough water to cover eggs. Bring to the boil then add vinegar and salt. Gently spoon the eggs into the water and boil for 5 minutes (for a 59g egg), turning eggs occasionally to promote even cooking. Toast the bread and cut into strips and, if desired, top with a splash of olive oil or mango chutney. Remove eggs from water. **Tip:** If the egg shell dries immediately the egg is hard boiled, if it dries slowly then the egg is soft boiled. Place eggs in egg cups and cut off the top third. If some of the top egg white is uncooked, scoop the runny whites out or return the top third back onto the egg for 2 minutes to allow the whites to set. Sprinkle with parsley and serve with toast 'dipping sticks' and a teaspoon (to eat the cooked whites).

Tasty Omelette

SERVES 2, PREPARATION TIME 3 MINUTES, COOKING TIME 8–10 MINUTES

This omelette is bursting with antioxidants and flavour. When choosing a sweet chilli sauce look for one free from artificial flavour enhancers (MSG, E621 and E635).

4 free-range eggs
1 tablespoon water
½ teaspoon tamari sauce (or soy sauce)
1 teaspoon sweet chilli sauce
½ red onion, diced
1 tablespoon extra-virgin olive oil
30g (1oz) baby spinach or Swiss chard, chopped
1 fresh tomato, diced
ground black pepper (optional)

Method: Preheat grill on high. Lightly beat the eggs together, then add water, tamari and sweet chilli sauce to the eggs and mix. In a small frying pan on medium heat, sauté the onion with olive oil for 1 minute then add spinach and sauté for a further minute or two. Add the tomato and mix, then divide vegetables into two and remove half from the pan as you want to cook one omelette at a time. Spread vegetables evenly across the pan before adding half the egg mix. Cover saucepan with a lid and cook for 4 minutes on low heat, being careful not to burn omelette. If egg is still uncooked on top, transfer the pan to the grill and grill the omelette (keeping the pan's handle away from heat) for 1 minute or until egg has cooked through. Remove omelette from the pan and repeat the process for the second omelette. Add pepper if desired and serve immediately.

Designer Muesli

SERVES 4 (60G = 1 SERVING), PREPARATION TIME 3 MINUTES, COOKING TIME 8 MINUTES

This is a tasty treat at breakfast time. Full of fibre, low GI and rich in protein. Use quality soya milk containing added calcium and 'whole' soyabean (not 'isolate').

300g (10½oz) rolled oats (not instant)
2 tablespoons honey
70g (2½oz) almonds
70g (2½oz) pumpkin seeds
70g (2½oz) whole flaxseeds
35g (1¼oz) lecithin granules
30g (1oz) rice bran
Raspberries (fresh or frozen and thawed)
Almond Milk (see p. 310) or quality soya milk

Method: Preheat the oven to 200°C/400°F/gas 6. Combine oats and honey, mixing well. Spread evenly on a large baking tray. Toast in oven for 6 minutes, checking regularly to avoid burning, then stir and add almonds and pumpkin seeds. Cook for another 2 minutes (until mixture slightly browns). Allow to cool. Then add flaxseeds, bran and lecithin granules. Leftovers can be stored in an air-tight container in the cupboard for two weeks. Serve with a small handful of raspberries and Almond Milk or soya milk.

Gluten-free Muesli

SERVES 3 (60G = 1 SERVING), PREPARATION TIME 3 MINUTES, COOKING TIME 4 MINUTES

This muesli is medium to high GI as gluten-free grains are generally high GI. If you have eczema, favour soya milk instead of Almond Milk. If you have rosacea, have berries instead of banana. If using soya milk please note that barley malt contains gluten so use gluten-free or malt-free soya milk.

30g (1oz) almonds
30g (1oz) puffed brown rice
30g (1oz) puffed amaranth
60g (2oz) rice bran
35g (1oz) pumpkin seeds
70g (2½oz) whole flaxseeds
40g (1¼oz) of soya lecithin granules
honey (optional)
chilled malt-free soya milk or Almond Milk (p. 310)
1 banana

Method: Preheat oven to 200°C/400°F/gas 6 and toast the almonds for 4 minutes (do not burn them). Remove from heat and allow to cool. Mix puffed rice, puffed amaranth and rice bran with the almonds, pumpkin seeds, flaxseeds and lecithin granules. Store in an air-tight container. Serve 60g (2oz) per person and add chilled malt-free soya or Almond Milk, honey and banana.

Vitamin E Muesli

SERVES 1, PREPARATION TIME 3 MINUTES, (PLUS OVERNIGHT SOAKING)

If you have eczema, leave out the sunflower seeds and replace with 1 teaspoon flaxseeds and use soya milk instead of Almond Milk. Quality soya milk contains calcium and 'whole' soyabean (not soya 'isolate').

50g (1½oz) rolled oats
1 tablespoon sunflower seeds
250ml (8fl oz) water
1 tablespoon wheatgerm
1 teaspoon apple cider vinegar
250ml (8fl oz) Almond Milk (see p. 310)
1 teaspoon honey or real maple syrup
Fruit (raspberries/blueberries/banana)

Method: Combine oats, sunflower seeds, water, wheatgerm and apple cider vinegar in a breakfast bowl and soak overnight. Serve with Almond Milk, fruit and honey.

B Muesli

SERVES 4, PREPARATION TIME 5 MINUTES (PLUS OVERNIGHT SOAKING)

This sweet bircher muesli recipe is rich in B vitamins thanks to the rice bran, fruit and raisins. Soak the grains and seeds overnight to make the nutrients more available. Oats are great for the nerves and skin. Use mango if it's summer or pears if it's winter or if you have eczema. Omit the raisins if you have eczema.

150g (5oz) rolled oats
30g (1oz) rice bran (or wheatgerm)
1 tablespoon whole flaxseeds
45g (1½oz) raisins or sultanas
500ml (16fl oz) apple juice (cloudy and preservative free)
1 mango, sliced (or pears or prunes)
1 banana, sliced
30g (1oz) raw almonds, chopped (optional)

Method: Place oats, bran, flaxseeds, raisins and apple juice in a large bowl and soak overnight. The next morning, divide into bowls, add extra apple juice if necessary and top with fresh fruit and almonds.

Mango and Buckwheat Crêpes

SERVES 1, PREPARATION TIME 4 MINUTES, COOKING TIME 4 MINUTES

This tasty crêpe recipe is gluten free and rich in flavonoids from buckwheat flour and mango.

2 free-range eggs
2 tablespoons buckwheat flour
60ml (2fl oz) water
1 teaspoon ghee, coconut oil or olive oil
1–2 teaspoons of honey (optional)
1 tablespoon ground flaxseeds
½ fresh mango, sliced

Method: Beat eggs in a large bowl, and then mix in buckwheat flour until free of lumps. Add water and mix well. The mixture should be runny so you can make thin crêpes. Grease a medium-sized non-stick frying pan with oil or ghee and pour in enough mixture to make a thin crêpe. Use a spatula to turn over the crêpe once it is lightly cooked. Do not brown the crêpe. Repeat the process until all of the mixture is used. Top the crêpes with honey, ground flaxseeds and mango.

Pear and Buckwheat Crêpes

SERVES 1, PREPARATION TIME 4 MINUTES, COOKING TIME 4 MINUTES

This tasty crêpe recipe is low in salicylates so it's suitable for people with eczema. It's also gluten free and rich in flavonoids. You can also use banana instead of pear.

2 free-range eggs
2 tablespoons buckwheat flour
60ml (2fl oz) water
1 teaspoon ghee or unsalted butter
1–2 teaspoons of real maple syrup (optional)
1 tablespoon ground flaxseeds
1 ripe pear, peeled and chopped

Method: Beat the eggs in a large bowl, and then mix in the buckwheat flour until free of lumps. Add water and mix until smooth. The mixture should be runny so you can make thin crêpes. Grease a small frying pan with ghee or butter and pour in enough mixture to make a thin crêpe. Use a spatula to turn over the crêpe once it is lightly cooked. Do not brown the crêpe. Repeat the process until all the mixture is used. Top the crêpes with pear, maple syrup, ground flaxseeds and serve immediately.

Boiled Eggs, Vegetables and Rice

SERVES 2, PREPARATION TIME 10 MINUTES, COOKING TIME 20 MINUTES

200g (7oz) brown rice
1 tablespoon white vinegar
2–4 eggs (1–2 per person)
1 tablespoon extra-virgin olive oil
½ red or brown onion, sliced
100g (3½oz) mushrooms (6 medium)
100g (3½oz) courgettes, sliced thinly on the diagonal

Method: Boil the rice in plenty of water for 15–20 minutes, then drain. In a small saucepan, add enough water to cover eggs and add the vinegar to stop eggs from cracking. Bring water to the boil and add the eggs, cooking on high for 5 minutes for soft boiled or 7 minutes for a hard-boiled yolk. Heat the oil in a saucepan and sauté the onion and mushrooms on high heat for 2 minutes, stirring often. Then add courgette and sauté for a further 1–2 minutes, mixing constantly. The courgette should not be overcooked; it should be crisp and slightly browned. Peel the eggs, halve them and place the eggs and rice on a plate. Serve vegetables on top of the rice.

Fish and Steamed Vegetables

SERVES 2, PREPARATION TIME 5 MINUTES, COOKING TIME 6 MINUTES

This meal makes a healthy breakfast, lunch or light dinner. Favour using omega-3 rich salmon or trout.

2 pieces fish of choice (375g/13oz in total)
90g (3oz) broccoli, cut into chunks
45g (1½oz) spinach or Swiss chard, chopped
1 large carrot, thinly sliced
juice of ½ fresh lemon
ground black pepper

Method: Place some water in a saucepan that has a steamer attached and bring to the boil. In a large frying pan, cook fish for 2 minutes on each side or until cooked through. Place vegetables in the steamer and cook for 2 minutes (maximum of 3 minutes) on high. Garnish fish and vegetables with lemon juice and pepper if desired. Serve immediately.

Beans on Toast

SERVES 2, PREPARATION TIME 5 MINUTES, COOKING TIME 10 MINUTES

This simple and tasty vegetarian breakfast is rich in fibre, B vitamins, vitamin C and copper. If you have eczema, omit the tomato and olive oil, and instead use 1 tablespoon butter and season with sea salt if necessary.

1 teaspoon extra-virgin olive oil
½ onion, finely chopped
½ teaspoon paprika
85g (3oz) tinned kidney beans, drained and rinsed
85g (3oz) tinned butter beans (or other white beans), drained and rinsed
85g (3oz) tinned tomato, diced
1 tablespoon parsley, finely chopped
1 teaspoon oregano, chopped
4 slices wholegrain bread, toasted
ground black pepper

Method: Heat the oil in a large saucepan on medium heat. Cook the onion and paprika for 3 minutes until onion becomes translucent. Then add the beans and tomato and simmer for 6–8 minutes, stirring occasionally until sauce thickens. Mix in parsley and oregano and serve on toast. Season if necessary.

Kids Scrambled Eggs

SERVES 4 CHILDREN, PREPARATION TIME 4 MINUTES, COOKING TIME 4 MINUTES

Children love fun food and depending on your child's preferences you can either make normal scrambled eggs or Dr Seuss ones. Make eggs fun for fussy kids and tell them it's 'Green Eggs' or 'Shrek' Eggs – just add chlorophyll to the mix to make the eggs a pleasant green.

2 eggs, lightly beaten
1 tablespoon calcium-fortified soya milk
iodine-enriched sea salt
1 teaspoon parsley, finely chopped
½ teaspoon low-strength chlorophyll (optional)
½ teaspoon butter or ghee
4 slices wholegrain bread, toasted

Method: In a bowl, mix eggs, soya milk, salt, parsley and chlorophyll. Melt the butter in a non-stick pan on medium heat, and add egg mixture. Stir continuously for 2–4 minutes, until egg is just cooked. Do not burn or brown eggs. Serve with grainy toast.

Kids Creamy Beans on Toast

SERVES 2 TO 4 CHILDREN, DEPENDING ON THEIR AGE, PREPARATION TIME 5 MINUTES, COOKING TIME 5–10 MINUTES

This recipe is suitable for children over the age of one, especially those with eczema and other skin problems. The bean mix can also be puréed for children as young as eight months old (but leave out the salt and syrup). Make this recipe even more fun for children by colouring it with green chlorophyll and telling them it's 'Shrek Beans on Toast'. However, don't use 'high-strength' chlorophyll as it's likely to be black in colour. You need liquid chlorophyll that has approximately 200mg per 100ml. Chlorophyll shouldn't change the flavour of the beans. The maple syrup is added to this meal for fussy children who don't generally like beans. For all other kids, omit the maple syrup as this meal is also nice when savoury. Make sure the bread used is preservative free (no calcium propionate/282). White haricot beans or cannellini beans are best for this meal.

60–120ml (2–4fl oz) calcium-fortified soya milk
1 teaspoon plain wholemeal flour
170–340g (6–12oz) tinned beans (haricot, cannellini or kidney)
dash of sea salt
½–1 teaspoon real maple syrup (optional)
1 teaspoon fresh parsley, finely chopped
½–1½ teaspoons liquid chlorophyll (optional)
2 slices wholegrain bread, toasted and crusts removed

Method: In a small saucepan, mix soya milk and flour until lump-free, then heat, stirring as it simmers. Add beans, sea salt, maple syrup and parsley, stirring often. Cook until thickened and beans are soft. Remove from heat and stir in the liquid chlorophyll, half a teaspoon at a time until desired colour has been achieved. Serve warm, on top of grainy toast. Plain butter can be sparingly used on toast. Note that children generally prefer a bright green colour over a pale insipid green (the first time I cooked this, my daughter complained that the Shrek Beans weren't green enough). So when determining the colour of the mix, it's a case of 'more is more'.

Sauces, dips and salad dressings

Creamy Mayonnaise

MAKES 230G (8oz), PREPARATION TIME 10 MINUTES

This tasty mayonnaise is unique as it's made with omega-3 rich flaxseed oil and is a good source of B vitamins. It's also free of raw egg white so it won't cause a biotin deficiency. The apple cider vinegar is not only alkalising but it also works as a natural preservative. The leftover egg whites can be used in an egg-white omelette: see Tasty Omelette recipe on p. 316 (substitute two of the eggs for three egg whites). If you have eczema, omit the curry powder and mustard.

3 free-range egg yolks
1 tablespoon apple cider vinegar
1 tablespoon lemon juice
pinch of fine sea salt
60ml (2fl oz) extra-virgin olive oil
125ml (4fl oz) flaxseed oil
dash of finely ground pepper
dash of curry powder (optional)
dash of Dijon mustard (optional)

Method: Using a wooden spoon, whisk or a small food processor, beat together the egg yolks, vinegar, lemon juice and salt for a minute until smooth. Then gradually add olive oil one tablespoon at a time, and beat very well after each. Then add the flaxseed oil one tablespoon at a time and beat until thick and creamy. Adjust the taste to your liking: you can add another tablespoon of lemon juice or a dash of curry powder or Dijon mustard, and salt and pepper. Store in a sterilised jar and keep refrigerated (see Sterilisation Tips on p. 326). Will keep for 1 week, possibly longer if the jar has been sterilised correctly.

Tartare Sauce

MAKES 230G (8oz), PREPARATION TIME 10 MINUTES

This healthy and tasty tartare sauce is a great addition to steamed or pan-fried fish.

1 teaspoon capers, finely chopped
1 teaspoon parsley, finely chopped
1 teaspoon shallots or onion, minced

Method: Make Creamy Mayonnaise as described on p. 323 then add the ingredients and mix.

Aioli

MAKES 230G (8oz), PREPARATION TIME 10 MINUTES

Aioli is a delicious garlic dipping sauce suitable for fish and vegetable sticks such as carrots and green beans.

2 cloves garlic, minced
1 teaspoon parsley, finely chopped

Method: Make Creamy Mayonnaise as described on p. 323 then add the ingredients and mix.

Tuna Dip

MAKES 500G (16oz), PREPARATION TIME 15 MINUTES (INCLUDING THE TIME IT TAKES TO MAKE THE MAYONNAISE)

This delicious dip is perfect for serving guests and goes well with plain crackers, sourdough bread and chopped vegetable sticks. Only use chunky-style quality tuna in spring water or olive oil (not sandwich tuna). If you can't find a large can of quality tuna then use smaller cans: 2 x 185g and 1 x 95g.

425g tinned chunky-style tuna (quality tuna), drained well
¼ cup finely chopped shallots (green parts)
1 tablespoon lemon juice
1 large clove garlic, minced

Method: Make Creamy Mayonnaise as described on p. 323. Then mash the tuna in a separate bowl and add 230g of Creamy Mayonnaise (there should be no dry or chunky bits of tuna). Mix in the remaining ingredients and add sea salt and ground black pepper if desired. For presentation, top with a sprig of parsley or a few chopped shallots.

Hummus Dip

SERVES 8, PREPARATION TIME 15 MINUTES

This dip is rich in vegetarian protein and calcium, and contains alkalising lemon and garlic. Gluten free. If you have eczema, omit the olive oil and use flaxseed oil instead. Use flaxseed oil instead of olive oil if you want this dip to contain omega-3.

1 x 400g tinned chickpeas
3 cloves garlic, minced
5 tablespoons tahini (sesame seed paste)
2 lemons, juiced (8 tablespoons juice)
3 tablespoons extra-virgin olive oil (or flaxseed oil)
sea salt and pepper to taste
paprika and chopped parsley for garnish

Method: Drain and rinse the chickpeas and discard any discoloured ones, then place in a food processor. Add the remaining ingredients (except the garnish) and blend on high speed for up to 5 minutes, until puréed. Add extra lemon juice if the dip is too thick. Taste the mixture and season with extra salt and pepper if necessary. Garnish with paprika and fresh herbs and serve with carrot, celery and pepper sticks. If refrigerated, hummus will stay fresh for up to a week.

Sweet Chutney

MAKES JUST UNDER 1KG (2–3 JARS), PREPARATION TIME 15 MINUTES, COOKING TIME 1 HOUR

This sweet mango chutney has a slight Indian flavour and it's so much better than any chutney you can buy at the supermarket. It also contains less than half the sugar of store-bought chutneys but tastes just as sweet. This chutney goes superbly with chicken or tuna in sandwiches and wraps, and can even be served on curries, Annie's Decadent Veggie Bake, mixed in with the Roasted Sweet Potato Salad recipe and it's also wonderful for marinating fish. Not suitable for children with eczema. Gluten free.

1 tablespoon extra-virgin olive oil
2 teaspoons cumin seeds
1 teaspoon mustard seeds
4 cloves garlic, finely diced or minced
1 large onion, chopped
2 teaspoons fresh root ginger, peeled and grated
2 teaspoons ground coriander
1 teaspoon turmeric powder
120ml (4fl oz) apple cider vinegar
60ml (2fl oz) white vinegar
45g (1½oz) soft brown sugar
3–4 mangoes (up to 1.5kg), diced
85g (3oz) raisins, chopped
1 teaspoon finely ground sea salt

Method: In a large saucepan, heat the oil on medium and cook cumin seeds and mustard seeds, stirring until they pop. Add the garlic, onion and ginger. Mix until onions are translucent, then add the ground coriander and turmeric and cook until the spices are fragrant, stirring regularly. In a bowl, mix the vinegars and sugar and then add to the cooking pot. Then add mango, raisins and salt. Stir and simmer uncovered for 1 hour, stirring regularly to prevent the bottom of the chutney from burning. Pour the chutney into hot sterilised jars and seal while hot (see Sterilisation Tips below). Variations of this recipe include adding 1 small red chilli, finely chopped, and you can make the chutney less sweet by adding only 30g (1oz) of brown sugar. For extra Indian spice and a bit of palate intrigue, add ¼ teaspoon of cardamom seeds. (Thanks to Dale for this fantastic modified recipe.)

Sterilisation tips

After cooking chutneys, jams and sauces, immediately store them in hot sterilised jars. Also scoop the mixture into these jars with a sterilised metal spoon or measuring cup. To sterilise jars, their lids and utensils, boil them for 5 to 10 minutes in a very large pot with enough water to cover them. To remove equipment, use tongs (remembering to sterilise the ends only). Seal jars with lids while hot to ensure long shelf life of the product. Product should last for 6 to 12 months if the jars are sterilised correctly.

Sweet Chilli Sauce

SERVES 4, PREPARATION TIME 5 MINUTES (SET ASIDE FOR ½ HOUR BEFORE USING)

This sauce is not your traditional sweet chilli as it is runny like a gourmet Thai dipping sauce. Delish with Vegetable Hand Rolls, spring rolls or Prawn and Sweet Chilli Vegetable Stir-fry. Gluten free if using tamari sauce.

1 small red chilli, finely sliced
1 tablespoon honey, melted
2 tablespoons lime juice
1 tablespoon apple cider vinegar
½ teaspoon tamari sauce (or soy sauce)

Method: Mix all ingredients and set aside for at least ½ hour before serving. Keeps for one week if refrigerated.

Tomato Sauce

MAKES APPROXIMATELY 2 JARS (600G), PREPARATION TIME 10 MINUTES, COOKING TIME 35 MINUTES.

This sauce is bursting with traditional tomato sauce flavour. Gluten free if the mustard used is free of wheat gluten. To make a darker red sauce, add 1 red pepper in the initial cooking phase. Not suitable for people with eczema.

1kg (2lb 4oz) ripe roma tomatoes, roughly chopped
1 large red onion, diced
2 tablespoons soft brown sugar
1 teaspoon fine sea salt
½–1 teaspoon Dijon mustard (to taste)
½ teaspoon paprika (to taste)
100ml (3½fl oz) apple cider vinegar
1 cinnamon stick
1 teaspoon whole allspice
1 teaspoon celery seeds
1 teaspoon black peppercorns
muslin bag or cloth (thin white cotton material is also suitable)

Method: In a large saucepan, combine the tomatoes and onion, and cook on medium heat for 15 minutes or until very soft, stirring occasionally. Remove and briefly purée in batches in a blender (if the mixture is too thick to purée, add the vinegar during this step). Then push through a coarse mesh sieve to remove seeds and skin. Return to a smaller pot and add the sugar, salt, mustard, paprika and vinegar. In a muslin bag, place the cinnamon stick, allspice, celery seeds and peppercorns, and secure the bag tightly. Add the bag to the sauce and bring to the boil. Reduce to a simmer, stirring often and cook for at least 20 minutes, until the mixture reduces and thickens (simmer for up to 40 minutes). Test the mixture and add more mustard and paprika if necessary. Remove muslin bag. Pour the tomato sauce into sterilised jars to ensure long shelf life (see Sterilisation Tips on previous page).

Tasty Salad Dressing

DRESSING SERVES 8–10, PREPARATION TIME 5 MINUTES

This healthy salad dressing is the star ingredient of the Tasty Antioxidant Salad but it can be used with any lettuce-based salad. You can even use it to flavour salad in wraps or burgers. The dressing keeps in the refrigerator for weeks. This recipe is only gluten free if the chutney, sweet chilli sauce and mustard are gluten free.

6 tablespoons flaxseed oil
4 tablespoons apple cider vinegar
2 tablespoons Sweet Chutney (p. 325) or mango chutney
2 teaspoons wholegrain mustard
2 teaspoons sweet chilli sauce (free of artificial additives)
½ teaspoon mild curry powder
salt, pepper

Method: Blend all ingredients together at least 30 minutes before serving.

Omega Salad Dressing

SERVES 8, PREPARATION TIME 5 MINUTES

This sweet and therapeutic salad dressing was specifically designed for people with eczema but anyone can enjoy it. Gluten free.

3 tablespoons flaxseed oil
3 tablespoons apple cider vinegar
1 clove garlic, crushed and finely diced
1 tablespoon real maple syrup

Method: Combine all ingredients and serve on your favourite salad (1 tablespoon per person). This dressing will keep for weeks in the fridge.

Snacks

Vegetable Hand Rolls (raw spring rolls)

SERVES 4 (MAKES 20 ROLLS), PREPARATION TIME 25 MINUTES

Raw spring rolls are a healthy snack or light meal. Bean sprouts are rich in enzymes and this meal is vegetarian if using tofu and it's gluten free if using gluten-free sauce. The Sweet Chilli Sauce on p. 326 makes a perfect dipping sauce to serve with this dish.

2 tablespoons vinegar (white or apple cider)
2 handfuls bean sprouts
3 medium carrots, grated
½ bunch spring onions, ends removed and sliced thinly on the diagonal
45g (1½oz) fresh mint or coriander, chopped
1–2 tablespoons sweet chilli sauce (can be store bought if free of artificial additives)
350g tofu (or cooked chicken), thinly sliced
packet of round rice paper (at least 20 pieces, or 250g)

Method: Add the vinegar to a bowl of water and wash the bean sprouts in the water. Drain and dry with a clean tea towel. In a small bowl, combine grated carrot, spring onions, mint and sweet chilli sauce. Wet another tea towel, wring out excess water and place flat on bench. Then soften rice paper (two at a time) in a large bowl of very warm water, soaking each for 10 seconds. Remove and place flat on damp tea towel. Put 2 tablespoons of carrot mixture on the rice paper near the end closest to you; add slices of tofu and bean sprouts on top, then roll up, tucking the ends in about halfway so they look like cylinders. Serve immediately or store in clingfilm in the fridge for up to 6 hours.

Miso Soup

SERVES 4, PREPARATION TIME 5 MINUTES, COOKING TIME 10 MINUTES.

This vegetarian soup is a quick and tasty snack, and goes well as a side dish to the Vegetable Hand Rolls.

¼ sheet kombu (seaweed), cut into small, thin strips (approx. 1 tablespoon)
1 litre (1¾ pints) water
3 or 4 spring onions, finely chopped
100g (3½oz) soft/silken tofu, diced
2 tablespoons miso paste

Method: Boil kombu in the water for 10 minutes or until seaweed becomes soft, then remove from heat. Add spring onions, tofu and stir in the miso paste (miso should not be boiled). Add a dash of tamari sauce if extra saltiness desired.

B-rich Avocado Salsa

SERVES 4, PREPARATION TIME 10 MINUTES

This tangy salsa is alkalising and rich in B vitamins. Perfect as a snack on sourdough bread or served alongside fish. Not suitable if you have eczema.

1 large avocado, diced
½ red onion, finely diced
1 vine-ripened tomato, seeds removed and diced
90g (3oz) flat leaf parsley, finely chopped
juice of 1 lime
ground black pepper
8 slices sourdough bread, toasted

Method: Combine all main ingredients and serve on sourdough toast.

Avocado Beauty Snack

SERVES 2, PREPARATION TIME 5 MINUTES

This healthy snack is rich in vitamins, minerals and protein.

1 large avocado, halved, seed carefully removed
1 small tin chunky-style tuna
juice of ½ lemon
ground black pepper

Method: Top each avocado half with tuna, lemon and pepper.

Avocado Dip with Dipping Sticks

SERVES 4, PREPARATION TIME 5 MINUTES

A quick and healthy snack that is also ideal for serving at casual social functions. For extra spice, add a dash of cayenne pepper and ¼ red onion, finely diced. Gluten free. Not suitable for those with eczema.

2 large ripe avocados, mashed
3–4 tablespoons lemon juice (1 large lemon)
sea salt and pepper
3–4 large carrots
6 stalks celery
2 red peppers

Method: Blend together the avocado, lemon juice, salt and pepper until smooth. Taste the dip and adjust the seasoning if necessary. Peel the carrots, then halve them lengthwise and cut into sticks. Remove the strings from the celery with a potato peeler, then cut into sticks. Cut the peppers into sticks. Put vegetables on a platter and place dip beside them. Garnish with a sprig of parsley if desired.

Oysters with Dipping Sauce

SERVES 4-6, PREPARATION TIME 5 MINUTES

Oysters are extra special with this decorative dipping sauce. Oysters are a rich source of zinc which is vital for healthy, acne-free skin. For presentation, line your platter with crushed ice before serving. Suitable for all skin conditions.

60ml (2fl oz) lemon juice
240ml (8fl oz) apple cider vinegar
2 tablespoons finely sliced shallots
2 cloves garlic, minced
½ teaspoon sea salt
1 tablespoon finely chopped parsley
24 fresh oysters, on the half shell
1 lemon, sliced into wedges

Method: Mix together the lemon juice, vinegar, shallots, garlic and salt and let stand for 30 minutes before serving. Just before serving, mix in the parsley and check taste to see if it needs seasoning or more lemon. Arrange the oysters on a platter and decorate the platter with lemon wedges. Spoon a teaspoon of the mixture on each oyster if desired and place the dipping bowl on the platter beside the oysters.

Anti-ageing Broth

SERVES 8, PREPARATION TIME 10 MINUTES, COOKING TIME 6 HOURS +

A tasty and super-healthy broth, fantastic for bone, liver and skin health. Bones you can use include 1–2 chicken carcasses or fish, beef or lamb bones. Do not use pork bones. Chicken bones make the tastiest broth but beef and lamb bones with lots of joints make a thicker broth. Bones can be with or without meat still on them. Use feet, ribs, neck and knuckles for a broth rich in collagen (gelatin). You can also use shellfish shells and whole fish carcasses but a seafood-based broth will need to be used up within a couple of days or frozen to preserve freshness. Raw bones and meat may be browned first in an oven to enhance the final flavour of the broth. Gluten free.

bones – 1–2 chicken carcasses or equivalent fish, beef or lamb bones
cold water (start with enough to cover the bones and add more as necessary)
1–2 tablespoons apple cider vinegar (or lemon juice)
1 teaspoon dried mixed herbs (Italian herbs make an aromatic broth)
vegetable scraps – use sweet potato and carrot peel, broccoli ends
1 red onion, finely chopped
1 knob fresh ginger, finely chopped
4 cloves garlic, smashed and finely chopped
60g (2oz) fresh parsley
1 strip kombu or seaweed, cut into strips (optional, to increase metabolism and add extra minerals)
75g (2½oz) chopped cabbage
ground black pepper and quality sea salt (optional)

Method: Combine bones, water, vinegar and dried mixed herbs in a large pot then bring to the boil and simmer for anywhere in between 6–48 hours for chicken bones and 12–72 hours for beef. To reduce cooking time, cut the bones into small pieces after they have softened a bit during cooking. Add vegetable scraps and the other ingredients in the last two hours of cooking (or whenever convenient). Remove any scum that rises to the surface. Add more water as required (up to 3 litres (5 pints) of additional water may be necessary): you will need at least 3¼ litres (5¾ pints) of broth remaining. After cooking, the bones should be brittle and crumbly. Remove the larger bones from the broth and then strain the remainder through a sieve or colander to separate the broth from the bones. Press out extra fluid from the scraps then discard the bones and scraps. After the broth has cooled, remove any fat globules that have set on the surface. The cold broth will gel if sufficient gelatin (collagen) is present, which is ideal but not essential. Add salt and pepper if desired. Chicken or red meat broth will last for approximately 5 days when refrigerated, longer if frozen.

Chicken lunches and dinners

Therapeutic Chicken Soup

SERVES 8, PREPARATION TIME 10 MINUTES, COOKING TIME 30–40 MINUTES

This soup is fantastic for the immune system. Chicken contains cysteine, which helps to reduce mucus associated with colds and flu; garlic and vegetables contain flavonoids and the broth is rich in glycine, calcium and collagen. Leftovers can be frozen in serving- sized containers for up to 2 months. Cayenne pepper gives the soup a hint of spice so omit if serving to children. If you have eczema, omit the corn, cauliflower, cayenne and mushrooms, and add more cabbage, carrot and celery.

1 litre (1¾ pints) water
2L (3½ pints) Anti-ageing Broth (p. 331)
1–2 red onions, finely diced
3 sticks celery, finely chopped
2 cobs corn, kernels shaved off cob
140g (5oz) chopped cauliflower
35g (1oz) finely chopped cabbage
1 carrot, diced
6 cloves garlic, smashed and finely chopped
1 small knob ginger, peeled and finely chopped
1 strip kombu (seaweed), cut into 1cm pieces
4 raw chicken drumsticks, skin removed
4 shitake mushrooms, chopped (optional)
pinch of cayenne pepper (optional)
ground black pepper (optional)

Method: In a large pot, add broth and water (or equivalent stock and water), vegetables, garlic, ginger, kombu and skinless chicken and bring to the boil. If using dried mushrooms, soak them for 5 minutes in boiling water, remove and chop into strips. Then add mushrooms and their soaking water to soup mix. Cook for 30 minutes then remove chicken and allow to marginally cool. Cut the chicken meat from the bones, discard gristle and bones (or freeze them for the next broth), and dice chicken. Return meat to the soup and cook for longer if necessary. Optional: Add a pinch (up to ⅛ teaspoon) of cayenne pepper to add extra flavour and spice to soup (not suitable for small children). Serve with grainy bread.

Chicken and Salad Sandwich

SERVES 4, PREPARATION TIME 10 MINUTES

8 slices grainy bread (such as soya and flaxseed)
1 medium avocado
4 teaspoons Sweet Chutney (p. 325) or Creamy Mayonnaise (p. 323)
300g cooked chicken breast
1 large carrot, grated
150g (5½oz) leafy salad greens, sliced (rocket, baby spinach, cos)
½ sliced red onion (optional)

Method: On four slices of bread spread avocado, and on the other four spread chutney or mayonnaise (mayo must not contain raw egg whites or whole egg). On top of the avocado, place chicken, carrot, lettuce and onion. Close the sandwiches using the other slices of bread and serve.

Chicken and Salad Wrap

SERVES 2, PREPARATION TIME 10 MINUTES, COOKING TIME 6 MINUTES

This wrap gets a 'healthy' hand from the addition of omega-3 rich Creamy Mayonnaise, avocado, alkalising greens and tomato. Enjoy.

½ avocado, mashed
2 tablespoons Creamy Mayonnaise (p. 323) or Aioli (p. 324)
2–4 wholemeal wraps
70g (2½oz) mixed lettuce or baby spinach
½ tomato, sliced
2 chicken thigh fillets, fat trimmed off
1 tablespoon extra-virgin olive oil
Cajun seasoning (optional)
ground black pepper (optional)

Method: Mix the avocado with mayonnaise, adding slightly more mayonnaise if making four wraps, and spread onto the wraps. Then at one end, arrange lettuce and tomato. Season chicken with a small amount of Cajun seasoning and pepper if spicy chicken is desired. Heat oil in a frying pan on high heat and cook chicken for approximately 3 minutes each side or until cooked through (see Cajun Chicken Breast recipe, p. 335). Remove from pan and chop into 3cm slices. Place chicken on top of the salad and roll the flat bread into a cylinder shape. Cut each wrap in half before serving.

A&C-rich Apricot Chicken

SERVES 4, PREPARATION TIME 15 MINUTES, COOKING TIME 50 MINUTES

This unique apricot chicken is a delicious and hearty meal that has a slight spice to it. It's rich in vitamins A and C, and is much healthier than most traditional apricot chicken recipes. It's also gluten free if the stock cube does not contain wheat gluten. Pepper helps increase the antioxidant action of turmeric. Not suitable for children with eczema.

1 teaspoon turmeric
1 teaspoon ground ginger
1 teaspoon Cajun seasoning
600g (1lb 5oz) skinless chicken thigh fillets (or breast), fat trimmed, cut into large pieces
1 x 825g tin of apricot halves in natural juice (no added sugar)
1 knob ginger, peeled and finely grated (1 teaspoon)
4 cloves garlic, crushed and diced
1 tablespoon cornflour
1 vegetable stock cube
1 large onion, sliced chunky style
2 medium carrots, sliced
½ medium red pepper, sliced thinly
1 tablespoon extra-virgin olive oil
300g (10oz) basmati rice (or 400g (14oz) brown rice)
180g (6oz) chopped broccoli (or 2 pieces per person)
ground black pepper

Method: Preheat the oven to 250°C/450°F/gas 8. Mix turmeric, ground ginger and Cajun seasoning and coat the chicken pieces with it. In a frying pan, quickly brown chicken pieces, 1 minute each side but do not cook right through. Remove the chicken from heat and place in a large casserole dish. Set aside 8 apricot halves then purée the remainder and their juice along with the fresh ginger, garlic and cornflour. Dissolve stock cube in 60ml (2fl oz) boiling water then mix stock with apricot purée. Add onion, carrots and pepper to the casserole and top with apricot puree. Cover with lid and cook on high for 10 minutes then reduce heat to 200°C/400°F/gas 6 and cook for a further 30 minutes. During this time bring a large pot of water to the boil and cook the rice. Boil basmati for 10 minutes and brown rice for 15–20 minutes in plenty of water, and in the last minute add broccoli pieces (only boil broccoli for 1 minute so it remains slightly crisp), then drain. Remove the casserole from the heat and stir, then place the remaining apricot halves on top. Cook for a further 5–10 minutes. Remove the casserole dish from the heat and carefully take out the apricot halves and set aside. Serve the casserole on a bed of rice and place 2 apricot halves on top of each serving (for presentation), and add broccoli pieces on the side.

Sweet Chicken Stir-fry

SERVES 4, PREPARATION TIME 15 MINUTES, COOKING TIME 20 MINUTES

This tasty stir-fry will be a favourite with the 'sweet tooth' of the household and children will love it too. The recipe was specifically designed for people with eczema or salicylate sensitivity, although they should favour using papaya instead of salicylate-rich mango. It's rich in antioxidants, protein and cancer-protective indoles, and it's gluten free.

2 tablespoons real maple syrup
4 cloves garlic, minced
600g (1lb 5oz) chicken thigh or breast fillets, fat trimmed and cut into chunks
400g (14oz) brown rice
1 tablespoon extra-virgin olive oil
200g cabbage, finely chopped
100g shallots, finely chopped on the diagonal
200g green beans, ends removed and sliced on the diagonal
3 large sticks celery, finely chopped
good quality sea salt
1 medium-sized mango (or 1 small papaya), skin removed and thinly sliced (if using papaya, cut into chunks)

Method: Mix together the maple syrup and garlic and pour over the chicken pieces. Cook the chicken in its marinade in a large frying pan on medium to high heat for 5 minutes or until it is cooked through. Remove the chicken and remaining marinade from the pan and set aside. Clean the pan in preparation for stir-frying the vegetables. In a medium-sized pot, bring some water to the boil then add the rice and simmer for 15-20 minutes. During the last 2 minutes of cooking, heat the olive oil in the pan and quickly stir-fry the vegetables on a high heat, adding a sprinkle of salt. Continuously stir the vegetables for 1 minute then add the chicken and its marinade for the final minute of cooking. Cook the vegetables for no longer than 2 minutes as you want them to be crisp and tasty. Remove from the heat and stir in half the mango slices. Serve on a bed of rice and garnish with the remaining fruit. If using papaya, do not mix it in with the stir-fry; add it after serving.

Cajun Chicken Breast

SERVES 4, PREPARATION TIME 5 MINUTES, COOKING TIME 5 MINUTES

600g (1lb 5oz) chicken breast fillet, fat trimmed, and halved so pieces are thin
2 tablespoons Cajun seasoning (see p. 336 or buy pre-made)
1 tablespoon extra-virgin olive oil

Method: Coat the chicken pieces with the seasoning. Heat the oil in a large frying pan or grill on medium to high heat and cook the chicken for 3–5 minutes each side or until cooked right through. Serve with a side salad such as Garden Salad (p. 349); Sweet Raspberry, Avocado and Watercress Salad (p. 347) or vegetables and rice.

Cajun Seasoning

This spicy and hot seasoning makes chicken delicious.

Method: Mix together 1 teaspoon paprika, ¼ teaspoon cayenne pepper, a sprinkling of black pepper and finely ground sea salt, 1 teaspoon dried oregano, 1 teaspoon dried thyme and 1 teaspoon garlic powder and store in an airtight jar.

Chicken and Three Veg

SERVES 4, PREPARATION TIME 10 MINUTES, COOKING TIME 20 MINUTES

This is a tasty way to serve chicken and it's accompanied by the goodness of specially selected vegetables for maximum nutrition and flavour. Gluten free if using malt-free soya milk and tamari sauce. If you have eczema, omit Cajun seasoning, cook with butter and use green beans and cabbage instead of broccoli and snow peas.

500g (1lb 2oz) sweet potato, peeled and diced
½ teaspoon tamari sauce (or soy sauce)
80ml (3fl oz) soya milk
ground black pepper (optional)
600g chicken thigh fillet, fat trimmed
2 tablespoons Cajun seasoning *or* wholegrain breadcrumbs, mixed herbs and garlic
1 tablespoon extra-virgin olive oil
300g French green beans or mange tout
300g broccoli, chopped

> **Method**: In a small saucepan, bring some water to the boil and cook the sweet potato for 10 minutes or until very soft, then strain and return the sweet potato to the saucepan. Mash until lump-free then stir in the tamari sauce, soya milk and pepper to make a creamy and tasty mash, and keep the mixture in the saucepan.
> Coat the chicken pieces with the seasoning of your choice – either Cajun seasoning or breadcrumbs, herbs and garlic. Heat the oil in a large frying pan or grill on medium to high heat and cook the chicken for 3–4 minutes each side or until cooked right through. In a steamer, steam the beans or mange tout and broccoli for 2–3 minutes (maximum) – do not overcook the vegetables as they must be slightly crisp. Reheat the mash on the stove top if necessary and serve immediately.

Herb and Garlic Chicken Casserole

SERVES 4, PREPARATION TIME 20 MINUTES, COOKING TIME 1 HOUR

A simple and tasty winter casserole. Gluten free if the stock is free of wheat or gluten. Not suitable for people with eczema.

1 tablespoon extra-virgin olive oil

500g (1lb 2oz) chicken thigh fillets or breast, fat removed and chopped

1 onion, chopped

60g (2oz) corn kernels

4 cloves garlic, minced

150g (5½oz) chopped button mushrooms

120g (3½oz) chopped courgettes

270g (9½oz) chopped sweet potato

115g (3½oz) chopped pumpkin

35g (1oz) chopped Swiss chard

2 tablespoons buckwheat flour (or cornflour)

480–700ml (16–25fl oz) vegetable stock

1 teaspoon dried basil leaves

30g (1oz) fresh parsley, chopped

400g (14oz) cooked basmati rice

Method: Preheat the oven to 220°C/425°F/gas 7. Heat the oil in a frying pan and quickly fry the chicken pieces and onion for 1–2 minutes so they're partially cooked and slightly browned. Remove and place in a large casserole dish. Add all the vegetables, corn and garlic to the dish. In a bowl, mix the flour with 120ml (4fl oz) of cooled stock then pour in the rest of the stock, mix and pour over the casserole. The stock should be approximately 3cm from the top of the dish and not quite covering the vegetables. Add more stock or water if necessary. Sprinkle with basil then cover with a lid. Cook on high heat for 20 minutes then reduce the heat to 180°C/350°F/gas 4 and cook for another 40 minutes or until the vegetables are softened and the chicken cooked and tender. Stir a couple of times during cooking. Remove from heat and stir in parsley and serve on a bed of warm rice in large bowls.

Seafood lunches and dinners

Omega Nicoise Salad

SERVES 4, PREPARATION TIME 15 MINUTES, COOKING TIME 15 MINUTES

This delicious salad is best when using quality chunky style tuna (or freshly cooked tuna or salmon). It's gluten free if the mustard is free of wheat products, and rich in omega-3 if using flaxseed oil in the dressing.

4 free-range eggs (kept in shells)

425g tinned chunky-style tuna, drained

600g (1lb 5oz) baby potatoes, scrubbed and quartered

250g (8oz) small/cherry tomatoes, halved

300g (10oz) baby green beans, ends trimmed, halved

90g (3oz) small black olives, stoned
¼ red onion, peeled, sliced into thin rings
Anchovy dressing:
6 anchovy fillets, drained
80ml (3fl oz) flaxseed oil (or extra-virgin olive oil)
1 tablespoon Dijon mustard
60ml (2fl oz) apple cider vinegar

Method: Place the eggs into a small saucepan and cover with water. Then cover with a lid and bring to the boil. Cook the eggs for 6 minutes then remove from the heat and immediately place the eggs in cold water. After a minute or so, remove the shells then cut the eggs in half and set aside. Boil the potatoes for 3 minutes, then blanch the beans in boiling water for 1 minute only. Remove from heat and place the beans in ice cold water (to keep their colour vivid). Potato can be served warm or cold. To make the anchovy dressing blend all ingredients in a small food processor until combined. Then combine all of the salad ingredients in a large bowl, cover with half the anchovy dressing, then mix gently. Then place chunks of tuna on top, and mix if necessary. Serve, then drizzle with the remaining anchovy dressing. Use within 12 hours and refrigerate if not serving immediately.

Tuna and Avocado Wrap

SERVES 4, PREPARATION TIME 10 MINUTES

Make the mayonnaise yourself so it is rich in omega-3 (see Creamy Mayonnaise recipe, p. 323) or buy a suitable mayonnaise that does not contain whole egg or raw egg white. If you have eczema, omit the avocado, tomato and olives, and instead use cos or iceberg lettuce, shallots, grated carrot and celery.

2 x 185g cans chunky style tuna, drained
1 avocado, sliced and diced
40g (1¼oz) red onion, finely diced
3 tablespoons Creamy Mayonnaise
½ tomato, diced
1 tablespoon chopped Kalamata olives
1 tablespoon lemon juice
ground black pepper (optional)
4 large wholemeal wraps (preservative free)
2 handfuls lettuce of choice, shredded

Method: In a bowl combine tuna, avocado, onion, mayonnaise, tomato, olives, lemon juice and pepper, and mix gently, being careful not to squash the avocado. Lay the wraps out flat and arrange the lettuce on them, then spoon a quarter of the mixture onto each. Roll the wraps into cylinders and cut each wrap in half before serving.

Salmon and Salad Sandwich

SERVES 4, PREPARATION TIME 10 MINUTES

Make the mayonnaise yourself so it's rich in biotin and omega-3 (see p. 323). If you have eczema, use iceberg or cos lettuce and omit the avocado.

375g tinned salmon, drained
1 avocado, sliced and diced
60g (2oz) thinly sliced shallots
3 tablespoons Creamy Mayonnaise
1 stick celery, finely sliced
1 tablespoon lemon juice
ground black pepper (optional)
145g (5oz) leafy greens or lettuce of choice, shredded
8 slices wholegrain bread (preservative free)

Method: In a bowl combine salmon, avocado, shallots, mayonnaise, celery, lemon juice and pepper, and mix gently, being careful not to squash the avocado. Lie the bread flat and arrange lettuce on four of the slices, then spoon a quarter of the mixture onto each. Close each sandwich and cut in half before serving.

Marinated Whole Steamed Trout

SERVES 2, PREPARATION TIME 15 MINUTES (30 MINUTES TO SALT FISH), COOKING TIME 20 MINUTES

Steaming the fish whole is the best way to retain most of the omega-3 goodness. You need a large steamer for this recipe. I use a large steel vegetable steamer, it works just as well as the traditional Japanese basket steamers. If you have eczema, omit the sauce and alternatively season with sea salt and a squeeze of fresh lemon.

1–2 whole rainbow trout (approx. 600g (1lb 5oz), pre-gutted)
sea salt
1 knob ginger, peeled and finely sliced
4 shallots, thinly sliced on the diagonal
½ lemon, washed and cut into thin, flat discs
1 clove garlic, minced
1 bunch Chinese greens of choice
8 pieces broccolini or broccoli (2 small florettes per person)
200g (7oz) basmati rice
Sauce:
1 small knob ginger root, peeled and grated
1 clove garlic, minced
3 tablespoons tamari (or soy) sauce
3 tablespoons fresh lemon juice

1 teaspoon honey
1 tablespoon water
½ small red chilli, thinly sliced (optional)

Method: Rinse the fish and dry with absorbent paper towels, then sprinkle generously with sea salt to firm up the skin, leaving salt on for ½ hour. Meanwhile, place all the sauce ingredients in a small saucepan and simmer for 5 minutes then set aside.

When the trout is ready, wipe off the salt and place lemon slices, ginger and garlic inside the fish. In a saucepan large enough to accommodate the steamer, bring a small amount of water to the boil. Place the fish into the steamer and place the steamer into the saucepan, cover with a lid and steam for 10–15 minutes, depending on size of fish. Do not overcook. When cooked, eyes will be white and insides will be lighter in colour.

Boil the rice for 10 minutes, then drain. In a smaller steamer, steam the greens for 2–3 minutes only; they should be slightly undercooked to retain their brilliant colour and crispness. Reheat the sauce if necessary, then place the fish in a large dish and pour over the sauce and garnish with shallots. Serve with rice and greens.

Thai Baked Fish with Sweet Corn

SERVES 2, PREPARATION TIME 15 MINUTES, COOKING TIME 30 MINUTES

This healthy dish is gluten free if using tamari sauce and gluten-free stock. It can also be served with a small amount of brown or basmati rice. If you have eczema, omit the chilli, tamari sauce and pepper.

2 salmon fillets (or fish of choice)
1 tablespoon chopped lemongrass
2 cloves garlic, crushed and chopped
½ small red chilli, finely sliced
juice of 1 lime
2 tablespoons tamari sauce
1 tablespoon sesame seeds
1 packet baby corn (approx. 8 pieces), halved lengthwise
125ml (4fl oz) natural vegetable stock
1 teaspoon extra-virgin olive oil or coconut oil
1 leek, finely sliced (white part only)
1 stick celery, finely chopped
½ red pepper, finely sliced
60g (2oz) bean sprouts, washed in vinegar and water
1 spring onion, finely sliced on the diagonal
140g (5oz) cooked rice, optional (brown or basmati)

Method: Preheat the oven to 190°C/375°C/gas 5. Place the fish in an ovenproof dish and garnish with lemongrass, garlic and chilli. Mix the lime juice and 1 tablespoon of tamari sauce, and pour over the fish then cover the baking dish with foil and cook for 12–20 minutes, depending on fish thickness. (Note that salmon is beginning to overcook if small white clumps appear on the flesh.)

In a frying pan, toast the sesame seeds for 2 minutes, stirring regularly, being careful not to burn them. Remove seeds from the heat and set aside. In a large frying pan, cook the corn in stock for 5 minutes then drain stock if any left after cooking, leaving the corn in the pan. Add the oil and on high heat stir-fry the corn, leek, celery and pepper for 2 minutes only. Turn off the heat and stir in the sesame seeds, bean sprouts and remaining tamari sauce. Garnish the fish with spring onion, place vegetables on top of rice (if using rice) and serve immediately.

Rainbow Trout with Honey Roasted Vegetables

SERVES 2, PREPARATION TIME 10 MINUTES, COOKING TIME 20 MINUTES

This is the perfect way to roast vegetables with minimal oil and maximum flavour. Trout is succulent and rich in omega-3 when steamed. If you have eczema, use potato, sweet potato, carrot and swedes for roasting. Make sure the stock is free from artificial additives. Gluten free if stock does not contain gluten.

1 tablespoon honey, melted
1 tablespoon extra-virgin olive oil
½–1 teaspoon powdered vegetable stock
1 medium parsnip, sliced into long, thin pieces
2 medium courgettes, sliced chunky on the diagonal
1 large carrot, sliced chunky on the diagonal
1 small sweet potato, peeled and sliced chunky
1 onion, halved
2 whole cloves garlic, peeled (keep whole)
ground black pepper
4 tablespoons fresh thyme leaves, chopped, plus extra for garnish
2 rainbow trout fillets (approx. 400g/14oz), skin removed if desired
½ lemon

Method: Preheat the oven to 240°C/450°F/gas 8. In a large bowl, mix honey, olive oil and powdered stock, making sure honey is runny. Add all the vegetables and garlic cloves and coat with the honey mixture, then transfer vegetables and garlic to a baking pan or shallow dish. Season with pepper and thyme, and bake for 20 minutes, checking regularly to avoid burning.

Place the fish in a steamer, garnish with thyme and steam above rapidly boiling water for 4–5 minutes, until cooked. Remove from the heat immediately and serve alongside roasted vegetables. Squeeze lemon juice over fish and vegetables, and garnish with thyme.

Salmon Steaks with Peas and Mash

SERVES 2, PREPARATION TIME 20 MINUTES, COOKING TIME 20 MINUTES

This is a great way to cook fish for a dinner party. Baking the salmon steaks ensures they remain tender and delish, and the presentation is beautiful. Salmon is a great source of omega-3, and this recipe is gluten free. If you have eczema omit the chilli, corn, tamari sauce and olive oil and alternatively use butter for cooking and cabbage instead of corn.

1 very large sweet potato, peeled and diced
½ teaspoon tamari sauce
60ml (2fl oz) or less calcium-fortified soya milk
ground black pepper (optional)
baking paper
aluminium foil
extra-virgin olive oil
2 salmon steaks, with or without skin (approx. 400g/14oz)
1 large clove garlic, crushed and finely chopped
½ small red chilli, finely chopped into rings
80ml (3fl oz) lemon juice
140g (5oz) frozen green peas
2 whole cobs corn
2 sprigs fresh mint leaves (optional)

Method: Preheat the oven to 200°C/400°F/gas 6. In a small saucepan bring some water to the boil, then boil the sweet potato for 10 minutes or until very soft. Strain and return the sweet potato to the saucepan. Mash until lump-free then stir in the tamari sauce, soya milk and pepper to make a creamy mash, and keep the mixture in the saucepan.

Cut 2 x 30cm long sheets of aluminium foil and cut 2 x 28cm long sheets of baking paper, and place one sheet of baking paper on top of each piece of foil and set aside. Heat a dash of olive oil in a frying pan on high heat and quickly fry the fish to brown the outer layer, for 1 minute each side. Remove the fish and place in the middle of each sheet of baking paper and fold up the edges of the foil and baking paper so they 'cup' the salmon (this is so the marinade does not spill out).

In another pan, heat a little more oil and fry the garlic and chilli. To finish the marinade, add lemon juice to the fried garlic, chilli and oil and mix (discarding any burnt bits), then pour over the fish, placing the chilli on top of the fish for decoration. Close the ends of the foil over the fish to make parcels and set aside in a baking tray. In a medium-sized saucepan, bring some water to the boil and cook the corn for 15 minutes. After the corn has been boiling for 10 minutes, add peas and simmer for 3–4 minutes, then drain. Place the fish parcels in the oven for 8–10 minutes. Check to see if the fish is cooked to your liking. If you would like to cook the fish for longer keep the parcels open and cook for another 2 minutes, then check again and cook for longer if necessary. Tip: if fish develops white clumps on the sides then it is well done or overcooked, however this cooking method should preserve its tenderness. Reheat the mash on the stovetop and serve on plates with corn and peas, leaving room for the fish parcels. Decorate peas with a sprig of fresh mint and pepper if desired. You can either serve the fish inside their parcels for guests to open, or take out of parcels and discard excess lemon marinade.

Seafood Hotpot

SERVES 4, PREPARATION TIME 20 MINUTES, COOKING TIME 15 MINUTES

A winter treat. Choose a low-mercury fish such as salmon, trout, flathead or hake (see Chapter 5, p. 82 for a list of fish to avoid). Gluten free if stock and laksa are free of wheat gluten.

1 tablespoon extra-virgin olive oil
2 medium onions, sliced
1 small knob ginger root, peeled and finely chopped
4 cloves garlic, minced
2 tablespoons laksa paste
125ml (4fl oz) coconut milk
750ml (1¼ pints) vegetable stock
500g (1lb 2oz) fish fillets, skin removed and cubed
350g (12½oz) mussel meat
350g (12½oz) green (uncooked) prawns, peeled
35g (1oz) Swiss chard, finely chopped
1 red pepper, thinly sliced
60g (2oz) bean sprouts, washed in vinegar and water
8 tablespoons fresh coriander, roughly chopped
Sourdough bread or 400g cooked basmati rice (optional)

Method: Heat the oil in a large saucepan and sauté the onion, ginger and garlic until the onion is translucent. Add the laksa paste and coconut milk, and mix. Then add stock and bring to the boil. Add fish, mussels, prawns, Swiss chard and pepper, cover and simmer for 8–10 minutes or until the seafood is cooked. Before serving, stir in the bean sprouts and coriander. A side of toasted sourdough bread or basmati rice goes nicely with this meal.

Prawn and Sweet Chilli Vegetable Stir-fry

SERVES 4, PREPARATION TIME 15 MINUTES, COOKING TIME 25 MINUTES

A fresh-tasting stir-fry that can either be made gourmet-style with homemade Sweet Chilli Sauce (p. 326) or conventionally with shop-bought sweet chilli sauce (choose a sauce that is free of artificial additives). Chop the veggies as thin as possible to ensure quick cooking time and if you don't like coriander, use flat-leaf parsley or Thai basil. Gluten free if the sauce is free of wheat gluten. Not suitable if you have eczema.

1 tablespoon honey, melted (or real maple syrup)
1 clove garlic, minced
1 small red chilli, sliced
1 tablespoon fresh lime juice (1 lime)
800g (1lb 12oz) raw king prawns, peeled and cleaned
350g (12oz) brown rice
1 tablespoon extra-virgin olive oil
1 red onion, thinly sliced
2 medium courgettes, thinly sliced on the diagonal
75g (2½oz) white cabbage, finely chopped
1 medium red pepper, thinly sliced
180g (6oz) bean sprouts, washed in water and vinegar
45g (1½oz) fresh coriander, chopped
4 tablespoons Sweet Chilli Sauce (shop bought or see p. 326)

Method: In a cup, mix the honey, garlic, chilli and lime juice then pour over the prawns and set aside. Bring plenty of water to the boil and cook the rice for 20 minutes, then drain. Meanwhile, in a large frying pan cook prawns in their marinade for 2–3 minutes then remove from the heat, placing both the prawns and the juices aside. Clean the pan, add the oil and heat briefly, being careful not to smoke the oil, then on high heat cook the onion and courgettes for 1 minute only, stirring constantly. Then add the cabbage and red pepper and stir-fry for 1 minute, then add the prawns and leftover juices and stir-fry for 1 more minute only, mixing constantly to prevent burning. Use a timer and do not overcook. If using shop-bought sweet chilli sauce, stir in now.

Turn off the heat and stir in the bean sprouts and coriander. Remove from the heat to prevent further cooking as you want the vegetables to be slightly crisp and tasty. Serve the rice into large bowls then top with stir-fry. If using homemade Sweet Chilli Sauce, sprinkle a tablespoon over each dish, add sea salt if desired and serve immediately.

Creamy Tuna and Mushroom Mornay

SERVES 2, PREPARATION TIME 20 MINUTES, COOKING TIME 10 MINUTES

This creamy dinner is rich in B vitamins, fibre and calcium (if using calcium-fortified soya milk). To make it gluten free, use malt-free soya milk, cornflour and rice bran or buckwheat flour, and serve with brown rice. If you have eczema, omit the mushrooms and use finely chopped celery or shallots instead.

1 tablespoon extra-virgin olive oil

1 onion, chopped

75g (2½oz) small button mushrooms, chopped

2 tablespoons plain wholemeal flour (or cornflour)

2 tablespoons wheat bran (or rice bran or buckwheat flour)

480ml (16fl oz) calcium-fortified soya milk

400g tinned chunky-style tuna (in brine/water)

1 tablespoon chopped parsley

2 tablespoons chopped dill

50g (1¾oz) finely chopped celery

200g (7oz) cooked wholemeal pasta or 135g (5oz) cooked brown rice

Method: Heat oil in a frying pan and lightly fry the onion and mushrooms. Add the flour and wheat bran and stir furiously, cooking for 1–2 minutes. Gradually add the soya milk, stirring continuously to make a white mornay sauce.

Drain the tuna and mash with a fork. Mix the tuna, parsley, dill and celery with the mornay sauce and cook on low heat for a few minutes to develop flavour. Do not overcook. Serve with wholemeal pasta or brown rice and garnish with parsley.

Creamy Salmon Mornay

SERVES 2, PREPARATION TIME 20 MINUTES, COOKING TIME 10 MINUTES

A creamy treat that the kids will love. To make it gluten free, use cornflour, rice bran (or buckwheat flour) and serve with brown rice. Suitable for all skin conditions.

1 tablespoon extra-virgin olive oil

1 onion, chopped

60g (2oz) carrot, finely diced

2 tablespoons plain wholemeal flour (or cornflour)

2 tablespoons wheat bran (or rice bran or buckwheat flour)

480ml (16fl oz) calcium-fortified soya milk

400g tinned salmon (in brine/water)

1 tablespoon chopped parsley

2 tablespoons chopped dill

50g (1¾oz) finely chopped celery

200g (7oz) cooked wholemeal pasta or 140g (5oz) cooked brown rice

Method: Heat oil in a frying pan and lightly fry the onion and carrot. Add the flour and wheat bran and stir furiously, cooking for 1–2 minutes. Gradually add the soya milk, stirring continuously to make a white mornay sauce.

Drain the salmon and mash with a fork (including bones). Mix the salmon, parsley, dill and celery with the mornay sauce and cook on low heat for a few minutes to develop flavour. Add pepper and a dash of sea salt if desired. Do not overcook. Serve with wholemeal pasta or brown rice and garnish with parsley. (Thanks Sue Tierney for this modified recipe.)

Vegetable-based lunches and dinners

Not all of these meals are strictly vegetarian or vegan; some contain Anti-ageing Broth made with chicken bones and the Creamy Mayo is made with egg yolk. See the notes in each recipe for 'vegetarian' meal descriptions if you are a strict vegetarian.

Chickpea Beauty Salad

SERVES 4 AS A SIDE DISH OR 2 AS A LIGHT LUNCH, PREPARATION TIME 10 MINUTES, COOKING TIME 4 MINUTES

A tasty vegetarian meal that is gluten free if using chutney without wheat gluten. High in protein, fibre, antioxidants and other flavonoids. Use good quality mango chutney free of artificial additives or make delicious Sweet Chutney (p. 325).

1 tablespoon extra-virgin olive oil
2 courgettes, thinly sliced on the diagonal
1 x 400g tin of chickpeas, drained and rinsed, discoloured ones removed
½ red onion, thinly sliced into rings
60g (2oz) flat-leaf parsley, chopped
60g (2oz) Sweet Chutney or mango chutney
1 tablespoon fresh lemon juice
1 garlic clove, minced
½ teaspoon ground cumin
½ teaspoon ground coriander
pinch of ground cayenne pepper (spicy)

Method: Heat the olive oil in a frying pan over high heat and quickly add courgettes and cook, turning often, for 2 minutes until slightly browned. Transfer to paper towels to drain.

In a large salad bowl, place the courgettes, chickpeas, onion and parsley. In a small bowl, combine chutney, lemon juice, garlic and spices then mix this dressing into the salad just before serving.

Sweet Raspberry, Avocado and Watercress Salad

SERVES 4, PREPARATION TIME 15 MINUTES

This vegetarian salad is bursting with skin-loving antioxidants and watercress is a good vegetable source of calcium. Gluten free and delicious as a side dish.

2 firm, ripe avocados, skin removed and diced
250g punnet raspberries
1 tablespoon apple cider vinegar
2 tablespoons flaxseed oil
½ teaspoon sea salt
ground black pepper
1 teaspoon honey, heated slightly so it's runny
400g (14oz) lightly packed watercress sprigs, trimmed

Method: Place the avocado and raspberries into a bowl. Make the dressing in a separate bowl by whisking together the vinegar, flaxseed oil, salt, pepper and honey, and spoon over the fruit. Toss gently to avoid squashing the avocado and raspberries. Then line a platter with watercress and pile the fruit on top. (Thanks to Fiona Workman for this adapted recipe.)

Tasty Antioxidant Salad

SERVES 4 (DRESSING SERVES 8–10), PREPARATION TIME 20 MINUTES, COOKING TIME 6 MINUTES

This vegetarian salad is rich in antioxidants and flavour as the name suggests. It's perfect as a side dish with meat, tofu or fish. A must for dinner parties and expect your friends to ask for the recipe afterwards. The dressing keeps in the refrigerator for weeks and goes with most lettuce-based salads. This recipe is only gluten free if the chutney, sweet chilli sauce and mustard are free of wheat gluten.

Dressing:
6 tablespoons flaxseed oil
4 tablespoons apple cider vinegar
2 tablespoons Sweet Chutney (p. 325) or mango chutney
2 teaspoons wholegrain mustard
2 teaspoons sweet chilli sauce (shop bought)
½ teaspoon mild yellow curry powder
salt, pepper
Salad:
250g (approx. 4 handfuls) baby spinach leaves (or ½ rocket, ½ spinach)
2 red apples, grated with skin on
½ red onion, thinly sliced
90g (3oz) grated carrot

90g (3oz) chopped raisins (or sultanas)
60g (2oz) chopped shallots
2 tablespoons sesame seeds
2 tablespoons pine nuts

> *Method*: Preheat the oven to 200°C/425°F/gas 7. Blend all salad dressing ingredients together at least 30 minutes before serving and store in a jar.
>
> Place the seeds and pine nuts on a flat baking tray and toast in the oven until slightly browned (approx. 4 minutes, checking regularly as they burn easily). Remove and allow to cool. Mix all the salad ingredients together and add 3–4 tablespoons of the dressing just before serving. (Thanks to Kerry Meates for this gorgeous recipe.)

Roasted Sweet Potato Salad

SERVES 2 AS A LUNCH OR 4 AS A SIDE SALAD, PREPARATION TIME 10 MINUTES, COOKING TIME 30 MINUTES

> This vegetarian salad is hearty and rich in minerals. It can be served on its own or as a side dish and it's also lovely with the addition one firm green pear, sliced on top. Gluten free.

1 large sweet potato, peel if necessary and diced into bite-sized chunks
1 tablespoon extra-virgin olive oil
3 tablespoons fresh lemon juice
1 small clove garlic, minced
½ teaspoon mild curry powder
ground black pepper
pinch sea salt
1 tablespoon flaxseed oil
200g (7oz) rocket or baby spinach (approx. 2 handfuls)

> *Method*: Preheat the oven to 180°C/350°F/gas 4. Place the sweet potato in a bowl and mix with the olive oil, then place on a baking tray and cook for 30 minutes or until pieces are soft and browned (not mushy). Remove from the oven and set aside. In a large bowl combine the lemon juice, garlic, curry powder, pepper, salt and flaxseed oil. Then add the sweet potato and rocket, and gently mix.

Rich Mineral Salad with Papaya, Dill and Baby Spinach

SERVES 2, PREPARATION TIME 10 MINUTES, COOKING TIME 10 MINUTES

> This vegetarian salad is rich in nutrients: each serve supplies approximately 420mg of calcium (50 per cent of RDI), 342mg of magnesium (100 per cent of RDI), 0.78mg of copper, 14.7mg of iron, 108mg of vitamin C (100 per cent of RDI) and 255mcg of folic acid (100 per cent of RDI). Gluten free.

70g (2½oz) pumpkin seeds
140g (5oz) buckwheat
1 tablespoon extra-virgin olive oil
1 small red onion, peeled and finely chopped
4 cloves garlic, minced
½ papaya, peeled and chopped into small chunks
200g (7oz) baby spinach, washed and finely chopped
juice of 2 fresh limes
4 tablespoons fresh dill, finely chopped
pinch natural sea salt

Method: Preheat the oven to 200°C/400°F/gas 6 and toast the pumpkin seeds for 2–4 minutes until slightly browned, then set aside. In a saucepan bring some water to boil then add the buckwheat and simmer for 5 minutes. Drain and set aside to cool. In a small saucepan, heat the oil and lightly sauté onions and garlic, being careful not to brown or burn them. Remove from the heat and set aside. In a mixing bowl combine all ingredients and serve with protein (such as steamed white fish).

Garden Salad

SERVES 2, OR 4 AS A SMALL SIDE SALAD, PREPARATION TIME 5 MINUTES

A simple, stylish vegetarian salad that will not steal the limelight from your main meal. If you have eczema omit the pepper, olive oil and tomato, and replace with celery, grated carrot and more flaxseed oil. Gluten free.

200g (7oz) mixed lettuce leaves
120g (4½oz) red cabbage, finely shredded
1 small red pepper, finely sliced
2 ripe tomatoes, sliced
2 shallots, thinly sliced on the diagonal
1 teaspoon extra-virgin olive oil
1 teaspoon flaxseed oil
1 tablespoon lemon juice
ground black pepper

Method: Tear the lettuce leaves into bite-sized pieces and mix in a large bowl with the cabbage, pepper, tomatoes and shallots. Then in a cup or jar mix the oils, lemon and pepper. Add the dressing to the salad just before serving.

Spicy Green Papaya Salad

SERVES 3, PREPARATION TIME 30 MINUTES

This spicy vegetarian salad is anti-parasitic and rich in digestive enzymes so it's great for improving gut health. Green papaya/papaw is usually sold at Chinese markets/grocers. If you can't handle the heat omit the chilli. Gluten free.

200g (7oz) green beans, ends trimmed, cut into 3cm lengths
1 medium green papaya, peeled, seeded and grated
120g (4oz) bean sprouts, washed in vinegar and water
45g (1½oz) fresh mint leaves
8 tablespoons fresh coriander leaves
60g (2oz) roasted cashews, chopped, plus extra for garnish
½ small red chilli, finely chopped (optional)
250g punnet cherry tomatoes
Dressing:
½ small red chilli, finely chopped
2 cloves garlic, crushed and chopped
3 tablespoons tamari sauce
juice of 2 limes
2 tablespoons apple cider vinegar

Method: To make the dressing mix the chilli, garlic, tamari sauce, lime juice and apple cider vinegar in a medium screw-lid jar or container then set aside.
Boil some water in a small pot and blanch the beans for 1 minute, then drain and transfer to a bowl filled with ice cold water and soak for 1–2 minutes (this helps to preserve the beans' colour). Drain and put beans in a large bowl and add papaya, bean sprouts, mint, coriander, chilli, tomatoes and cashews. Toss lightly. Serve in large bowls and stir in 2–3 tablespoons of dressing just before serving. Garnish with cashews. Salad will last for 2 days if stored without the dressing. Dressing will last for at least a week.

Roasted Corn and Cauliflower Soup

SERVES 8, PREPARATION TIME 10 MINUTES, COOKING TIME 40 MINUTES

A creamy soup that is great for detoxification thanks to the indole-rich cauliflower. Seaweed such as kombu supplies iodine which can boost metabolism. Gluten free if the stock is gluten free and served with gluten-free bread. To make this a true vegetarian meal, omit the broth and replace with vegetarian stock cubes and water (note that this markedly decreases the nutritional content of the meal). Cauliflower is not suitable for those with eczema.

2 cobs fresh (uncooked) corn

2 red onions, finely diced

4 cloves garlic, minced

1 large leek, thinly sliced (white part only)

2 litres (3½ pints) Anti-ageing Broth (or 700ml (1¼ pints) vegetable stock,
   1.3 litres (2¼ pints) water)

1 large (or 2 small) cauliflower, cut into small chunks

4 dried bay leaves

1 strip kombu/seaweed, cut into pieces

⅛ teaspoon cayenne pepper

ground black pepper

parsley, to garnish

Method: Preheat the oven to 200°C/400°F/gas 6. Shave the kernels off the corn cobs, place them on a baking pan and roast for about 5 minutes until slightly browned. Remove from the oven and set aside.

Add the onion, garlic and leek to a large pot and add 1–2 tablespoons of water. Cook on a medium heat for 2–4 minutes until translucent, stirring often. Add broth (or water and stock), corn, cauliflower, bay leaves and kombu. Cover the pot and bring to the boil. Reduce the heat and simmer for 30 minutes, stirring occasionally. Remove from the heat and take out the bay leaves. Add cayenne pepper and stir (omit cayenne if serving to children). Then purée the soup in small batches with a blender or food processor. Serve and garnish with chopped parsley and pepper if desired.

Therapeutic Veggie Soup

SERVES 8, PREPARATION TIME 10 MINUTES, COOKING TIME 30 MINUTES

This soup is fantastic for the immune system. Garlic and vegetables are rich in flavonoids and the broth is rich in glycine, calcium and collagen. Cayenne pepper gives the soup a hint of spice so omit if serving to children. If you have eczema avoid corn, cauliflower and cayenne, and add more cabbage, carrot and celery. If you're vegetarian, avoid the chicken broth and use vegetarian stock. Leftovers can be frozen in serving-sized containers for up to 2 months.

250g (9oz) red lentils (dried, not tinned)

1 strip kombu (seaweed), cut into 1cm pieces

3 litres (5 pints) Anti-ageing Broth (or vegetarian stock)

1–2 red onions, finely diced

3 sticks celery, finely chopped

2 cobs corn, kernels shaved

180g (6oz) chopped cauliflower

35g (1¼oz) finely chopped cabbage

1 carrot, diced

6 cloves garlic, minced

½ teaspoon finely grated fresh ginger root
1 pinch cayenne pepper (optional)
ground black pepper and sea salt (optional)

Method: Rinse the lentils and discard any that are discoloured. Boil the lentils in plenty of water with half the kombu for 30 minutes. Strain the lentils, rinse and set aside.

Put the broth in a large pot and bring to the boil. Then add all the vegetables, garlic, ginger and the remaining kombu and simmer for 20 minutes. Add the lentils and simmer for an additional 10 minutes if necessary. Add a pinch of cayenne pepper, stir and add salt and pepper if desired. Serve with grainy bread.

Multi-vitamin Dahl (Detox Dahl)

SERVES 2, PREPARATION TIME 10 MINUTES, COOKING TIME 30–40 MINUTES

This vegetarian meal contains turmeric which is rich in flavonoids and the addition of black pepper enhances the flavonoid's cancer-protective abilities. Soak lentils overnight if you have trouble digesting pulses. Kombu also promotes proper digestion of beans and pulses and it may boost metabolism due to its iodine content. Gluten free.

1 tablespoon ghee (clarified butter)
1 red onion, finely chopped
2 teaspoons turmeric
2 teaspoons ground coriander
2 cloves garlic, minced
½ teaspoon dried chilli flakes (optional)
500g red lentils
900ml (30fl oz) water
½ sheet kombu (seaweed), cut into thin strips
2 celery stalks, finely chopped
200g (7 oz) basmati or brown rice
ground black pepper
fresh coriander or parsley, to garnish

Method: Heat the ghee in a large saucepan on medium heat, add the onion and sauté until translucent, about 4 minutes. Add the turmeric, coriander and garlic (and chilli flakes if you want a hot and spicy dahl) and sauté for a further 2 minutes. Rinse the lentils and discard any that are discoloured. Add the water, lentils, kombu and celery to the saucepan and bring to the boil. Reduce the heat and simmer for 25 minutes, until lentils and kombu are soft and the dahl is smooth in consistency, adding extra water if necessary (although do not make the dahl runny).

Boil basmati rice for 10 minutes or brown rice for 15–20 minutes. Serve dahl on a small bed of rice and garnish with coriander and pepper.

Salad Sandwich with Creamy Mayo

SERVES 4, PREPARATION TIME 10 MINUTES

This is not quite vegan as it contains egg yolk so omit the mayonnaise if you are vegan (but you are missing out!). If you have eczema, skip the avocado and favour cos lettuce.

8 slices tinned beetroot, drained (or 1 large beetroot, peeled and grated)
8 slices grainy bread (such as soya and flaxseed)
1 medium avocado, mashed
4 teaspoons Creamy Mayonnaise (p. 323) or Sweet Chutney (p. 325)
1 large carrot, grated
145g (5oz) rocket, baby spinach or cos lettuce
1–2 shallots, sliced thinly on the diagonal
ground black pepper (optional)

Method: Place the beetroot on absorbent paper towels to remove excess moisture. Spread avocado on 4 slices of bread and mayonnaise on the other 4. On top of the avocado place carrot, leafy greens, beetroot and shallots. Season with pepper if desired. Close the sandwich and cut in half before serving.

Falafel Wrap

SERVES 4, PREPARATION TIME 5 MINUTES (IF FALAFEL BALLS AND AIOLI ARE PRE-MADE)

This wrap is a healthy lunchtime meal full of antioxidants. It's easiest to buy your falafel pre-made but if this isn't possible then follow the delicious recipe on page 354. If you have eczema omit the tomato and make your own tomato-free Tabbouli (modify the Tabbouli recipe on p. 354).

1 medium green/Lebanese cucumber
8 cos lettuce leaves, shredded
100g (3½oz) tabbouli or 1 large ripe tomato and ½ onion, diced)
12–16 falafel balls
400g packet wholemeal Lebanese bread or wraps (1–2 wraps per person)
4 tablespoons Aioli (p. 324, contains egg yolk) or Sweet Chutney (p. 325)

Method: Using a vegetable peeler, thinly slice the cucumber into long strips. Place the lettuce, cucumber, tabbouli and falafel onto Lebanese bread and drizzle with aioli or chutney. Roll bread and filling into a cylinder and serve.

Falafel

MAKES 12, PREPARATION TIME 15 MINUTES (PRE-SOAKING OVERNIGHT; SET ASIDE 1 HOUR), COOKING TIME 30–40 MINUTES

Homemade falafel is by far the tastiest and worth the effort. You can use tinned chickpeas if you can't find broad beans. Gluten free and vegetarian.

500g (1lb 2oz) large dried broad beans
30g (1oz) flat-leaf parsley
6 shallots
sea salt
4 cloves garlic, minced
¼ teaspoon cayenne or chilli pepper (or less if you don't like hot spices)
2 teaspoons ground cumin
2 teaspoons ground coriander
1 teaspoon baking powder
2 tablespoons extra-virgin olive oil

Method: Soak the beans in water overnight then remove their skins. Rinse the beans, drain well and dry on a clean tea towel. Finely chop the parsley and shallots – to ensure they are fine enough, chop in a food processor, then set aside. Blend the beans in a food processor until smooth, the longer the better. Add salt, garlic, cayenne pepper, cumin, coriander and baking powder and process until the paste is soft and sticks together. Mix in the parsley and shallots and set aside mixture for 1 hour.

Make small 3cm balls with the mixture. Then heat the oil and using a spatula gently place the balls in the oil and slightly flatten the falafel as you fry them. Cook until golden brown, turning once and drain on absorbent paper towels.

Tabbouli

SERVES 4, PREPARATION TIME 30 MINUTES

This is a vegetarian cracked wheat salad with parsley, onion and tomatoes. It is highly alkalising and rich in antioxidants. To make it gluten free exclude the burghul. If you have eczema, leave out the tomato.

2 tablespoons burghul (cracked wheat)
3 firm ripe tomatoes (approx. 250g/9oz), diced
1 bunch flat-leaf parsley (approx. 250g/9oz), finely chopped
2 shallots, finely chopped
2–3 teaspoons lemon juice
2 teaspoons extra-virgin olive oil

Method: Soak the cracked wheat in hot water for 10 minutes, then drain and blot with absorbent paper. Mix the cracked wheat with the tomato and leave for 20 minutes to absorb the juices. Then mix in the parsley, shallots, lemon juice and oil. Serve in wraps, burgers and sandwiches or as a side salad.

Tropical Vegetarian Stir-fry

SERVES 2, PREPARATION TIME 15 MINUTES, COOKING TIME 10 MINUTES

This colourful stir-fry is a tropical taste sensation. Undercook the veggies so they are crisp. If you're not vegetarian, this stir-fry is also fantastic with 500g of chopped chicken thigh fillets (marinated in tamari sauce and garlic). Gluten free if using tamari sauce. Tempeh is more nutritious than tofu. Not suitable if you have eczema.

3 slices pineapple, core removed, cut into chunks
300g (10½oz) marinated tempeh (or tofu), diced
tamari sauce (or soy sauce)
200g (7oz) basmati rice
1 tablespoon extra-virgin olive oil
½ onion, thinly sliced
1 small knob ginger root, grated
3 cloves garlic, minced
250g (9oz) mange tout, strings removed and chopped
80g (2½oz) cooked corn kernels
red pepper, thinly sliced
35g (1oz) Swiss chard or spinach, thinly sliced
90g (3oz) carrot, peeled and finely sliced
60g (2oz) chopped shallots
30g (1oz) roasted cashews (unsalted)

Method: Place the pineapple chunks on absorbent paper towels and blot to remove excess moisture. Marinate the tempeh in tamari sauce if not pre-marinated, then heat in a small frying pan and set aside. In a saucepan, bring plenty of water to the boil and simmer the rice for 8 minutes. Check rice regularly: if the water boils dry then turn off the heat, stir the rice and cover with a lid.

In a large frying pan or wok, heat the oil and quickly fry the onion and ginger for 1 minute only (set timer). Then on high heat add the garlic, mange tout, corn, pepper, Swiss chard and carrot, and quickly fry for 1 minute only. Vegetables must remain crisp. Then add the tempeh, pineapple, shallots and cashews, and fry for a further 1 minute only, stirring constantly to avoid burning. Serve on a small bed of rice and top with the desired amount of tamari sauce. Leftovers can be used in a salad or chicken wrap the next day.

Rich Mediterranean Pasta

SERVES 4, PREPARATION TIME 15 MINUTES, COOKING TIME 35 MINUTES

A fresh and decorative Mediterranean pasta that will satisfy. Vegetarian and rich in low GI carbohydrates. Not suitable if you have eczema.

2 tablespoons apple cider vinegar
2 tablespoons extra-virgin olive oil
6 Roma tomatoes, halved
sea salt
1 large red onion, cut into chunks
6 cloves garlic, peeled and left whole
2 medium courgettes, thinly sliced on the diagonal
1 red pepper, sliced
1–2 teaspoons dried basil
ground black pepper
500g (1lb 2oz) coloured vegetable pasta (large spirals)
2 tablespoons fresh parsley, finely chopped
90g (3oz) Kalamata olives
80ml (3fl oz) fresh lemon juice

Method: Preheat the oven to 220°C/425°F/gas 7. Place the vinegar and 1 tablespoon of oil in a bowl and mix before adding the tomatoes and a sprinkle of salt. Toss to coat, then place the tomatoes on a large flat baking dish or tray and roast for 10 minutes. Place the onion, whole garlic cloves, courgettes and pepper in a bowl, then drizzle with 1 tablespoon of olive oil and sprinkle with basil and pepper. Mix, then add the vegetables to the same dish as the tomato (cooking to one side, so as not to combine juices). Cook for a further 20–25 minutes until the vegetables are soft and turning slightly golden, mixing occasionally to promote even cooking. Once cooked, remove from the oven.

Cook the pasta in a large saucepan of boiling salted water (add salt to pasta now instead of salting the meal later). Boil the pasta for the time recommended by the manufacturer or until al dente. Drain the pasta and place on top of cooked vegetables and mix, coating the pasta with the remaining oils. Stir in parsley, olives, lemon juice and pepper, and mix. Serve hot.

Creamy Chickpea Curry

SERVES 2, PREPARATION TIME 10 MINUTES, COOKING TIME 15 MINUTES

This tasty vegetarian curry is rich in cancer-protective flavonoids, enhanced by the addition of black pepper. Kombu is added to promote proper digestion of the chickpeas. This recipe is not suitable for people with eczema or rosacea. Omit the chilli if you don't like spicy foods. Add some Sweet Chutney on serving for extra sweetness.

1 tablespoon coconut oil (or ghee or olive oil)
1 large red onion, chopped
2 cloves garlic, minced
1 tablespoon ginger root, grated or finely chopped
1 large carrot, diced
1 teaspoon turmeric
1 teaspoon garam masala
½–1 small red chilli, chopped
400g (14oz) brown rice (uncooked)
400g (14oz) chickpeas (freshly cooked or tinned)
120ml (4fl oz) coconut milk
1 strip kombu, cut into 1cm lengths
1 x 400g tin chopped tomatoes
120ml (4fl oz) vegetable stock (or 1 vegetable stock cube in 120ml hot water)
1 teaspoon honey
8 tablespoons fresh coriander, chopped (extra for garnish)
ground black pepper

Method: Heat the oil in a large saucepan and the sauté onion for 1 minute. Add the garlic, ginger, turmeric, garam masala, carrot and chilli and cook for 1–2 minutes. In another saucepan bring plenty of water to the boil and cook the rice for 15–20 minutes.

To the spices add the chickpeas, coconut milk, kombu, tomatoes (with juice), stock and honey. Simmer on low heat for 10-15 minutes, stirring occasionally. Mix in the coriander and serve on a bed of rice. Add pepper, garnish with extra coriander and a tablespoon of Sweet Chutney on the side, if desired.

Colourful Non-fried Rice

SERVES 4, PREPARATION TIME 15 MINUTES, COOKING TIME 15 MINUTES

Fried rice is just as tasty when you skip the oil and frying part. This recipe can be made with the addition of marinated tofu or egg; however egg will have to be fried (but this can be done without oil). This recipe is gluten free if using tamari sauce. Basmati rice makes it a low GI dish (other white rice is high GI and not suitable).

400g (14oz) basmati rice
1 litre (1¾ pints) water
4 eggs, lightly beaten or 250g (9oz) firm tofu, diced
140g (5oz) frozen peas
1 large carrot, diced
160g (5½oz) corn kernels
3 stalks spring onions, chopped (green and white parts)

1 small green pepper, diced
tamari sauce (or soy sauce)
2 tablespoons fresh parsley, finely chopped
2 tablespoons shop-bought sweet chilli sauce (optional)
ground black pepper (optional)

Method: If using tofu, marinate it for at least 10 minutes in tamari sauce. Boil the rice in the water, simmering on low for 8–10 minutes or until rice boils dry. Check the rice regularly while cooking: once water is absorbed, switch off heat, stir and cover with a lid for the remaining cooking time. The rice needs to end up cooked but partially dry so it's not sticky. If after 10 minutes of cooking there is water left with the rice then drain and set aside on a tray to air dry.

Cook the eggs in batches in a small non-stick frying pan – you want the egg to look like a flat pancake or crêpe. Flip the egg and briefly cook the second side, being careful not to burn. Remove and cut 3cm strips and set aside. In a small pot, boil the peas for 2 minutes then add carrots and blanch for 1 minute, then drain and add the vegetables to the rice. Marinated tofu can be briefly heated in the microwave or fried without oil for 2–4 minutes. Add cooked egg, corn, spring onions, pepper, parsley and tamari sauce (taste test to determine how much tamari is necessary). Mix in sweet chilli sauce and ground black pepper if desired.

Annie's Decadent Veggie Bake

SERVES 12 (FREEZE LEFTOVERS), PREPARATION TIME 30–40 MINUTES (IT'S QUICK AND EASY ONCE YOU KNOW THE RECIPE), COOKING TIME 1 HOUR

This tasty recipe is rich in fibre, protein and flavonoid-rich herbs, and each layer is flavoured with a different combination of spices. You can freeze leftovers for up to 3 months so it's very handy for busy people. Use two medium or large, deep baking trays. The corn, carrot, broccoli and cauliflower can be fresh or frozen (360g (13oz) frozen mixed vegetables for convenience). If you don't eat egg use an egg substitute. This recipe is not suitable for people with eczema. Lovely with Sweet Chutney spread on top before serving.

1 large aubergine, thinly sliced
4 large courgettes, thinly sliced
extra-virgin olive oil
6 cloves garlic, minced
2 large onions, sliced into chunks
2 x 400g tins red kidney beans, drained and rinsed
400g tinned lentils, drained and rinsed
400g tinned chickpeas, drained and rinsed (discoloured peas removed)
2 x 400g tins chopped tomatoes
1 x 500g jar tomato-based sauce or pasta sauce
6 large free-range eggs, lightly beaten

160g (5½oz) corn kernels
120g (4oz) chopped carrots
90g (3oz) finely chopped broccoli
90g (3oz) finely chopped cauliflower
spices such as fresh parsley, dried oregano or basil
3 large sweet potatoes
Chinese five spice (finely ground aniseed, cinnamon, cloves, fennel and black pepper)
1 x large box lasagne sheets (at least 375g/13oz)
800g potatoes, scrubbed and thinly sliced (keep skin on)
60ml (2fl oz) soya milk
mild curry powder

Method: Preheat the oven at moderate heat (180°C/350°F/gas 4), or on high heat if oven-baking the aubergine and courgettes. Aubergine mix: Coat the aubergine and courgettes with 2 tablespoons of olive oil and a sprinkling of salt, and grill, barbecue or bake on high heat until cooked (may take 20 minutes). Meanwhile, in a large wok or frying pan cook the garlic and the onion for 2–3 minutes until the onion is translucent, remove from the heat and mix with the aubergine and courgettes in a large bowl.

Tomato mix: In a very large wok or frying pan add beans, lentils, chickpeas, chopped tomato and tomato-based sauce, and simmer for 10 minutes. Then add the beaten eggs and stir. Add the remaining frozen or fresh veggies (corn, carrots, broccoli and cauliflower) into the tomato mix and cook for a further 5 minutes. You can also add parsley and oregano or basil if desired.

Now prepare your first layer: place your two deep baking dishes on the bench and spray with olive oil. Then peel and thinly slice the sweet potatoes and line the bottom of both trays with them. Now pour half of the tomato mix into both baking dishes and spread evenly, saving half the tomato mix for another layer. Place a single layer of lasagne sheets on top. The next layer is the aubergine mix: Spread evenly onto baking trays and sprinkle with Chinese five spice. Then place a layer of lasagne sheets on top. Now build the third layer: Place the last of the tomato mix on top, spread evenly, then top with a layer of thinly sliced potato. Baste with a small amount of soya milk to prevent the potato from drying out, sprinkle with curry powder and bake in the oven for 40–50 minutes. Test with a knife or skewer to make sure all layers are cooked. Serve with Sweet Chutney on top if desired, and a side of Garden Salad. To store leftovers, let cool overnight so the veggie bake sets and then cut into meal-sized pieces and freeze. (Thanks Annie Bloom for this modified recipe.)

Tasty Vegetable Casserole

SERVES 4, PREPARATION TIME 10 MINUTES, COOKING TIME 50 MINUTES

A soupy vegetarian casserole suitable for everyone including those with eczema and gluten intolerance (check to see if stock you use is gluten free).

1 onion, chopped
50g (1¾oz) chopped celery
75g (2½oz) chopped cabbage
270g (9¼oz) chopped sweet potato
120g (4oz) chopped carrot
250g (9oz) tinned haricot beans, drained and rinsed
250g (9oz) tinned kidney beans, drained and rinsed
2 tablespoons buckwheat flour (or cornflour)
480–700ml (16–35fl oz) vegetable stock
4 cloves garlic, minced
1 teaspoon dried mixed herbs (such as basil and oregano)
30g (1oz) fresh parsley, finely chopped
400g (14oz) cooked basmati rice

Method: Preheat the oven to 220°C/425°F/gas 7. Place all the vegetables and beans in a large casserole dish. In a bowl, mix the flour with 120ml (4fl oz) of cold stock until lump-free, then add 350ml (12fl oz) of stock and the garlic, mix then pour over the casserole. Stock should be approximately 3cm from top and not quite covering vegetables. Add more stock if necessary. Sprinkle with mixed herbs then cover with a lid. Cook on high heat for 10 minutes then reduce the oven temperature to 180°C/350°F/gas 4 and cook for another 40 minutes or until the vegetables are softened. Stir a couple of times during cooking. Remove from the oven and stir in the parsley. Serve in large bowls on a bed of warm rice.

Red meat lunches and dinners

Steak Sandwich

SERVES 2, PREPARATION TIME 10 MINUTES, COOKING TIME 5 MINUTES

This steak sandwich gets its healthy status by containing omega-3 rich Aioli (p. 324) and wholegrain bread. To increase meal size, serve sandwiches with a side salad such as Garden Salad (p. 349).

1 tablespoon extra-virgin olive oil
1 small onion, sliced into rings
2 x minute steaks (thin slices of sirloin or fillet steak) (approx. 200g)
sea salt and ground black pepper (optional)

4 slices wholegrain bread, toasted
70g (2½oz) rocket or lettuce of choice, chopped
1 medium carrot, grated
1 vine-ripened tomato, sliced
2 tablespoons Aioli or Tomato Sauce (p. 326)

> **Method**: Heat the oil in a large frying pan and cook the onion on medium heat
> for 2 minutes, until slightly translucent, then remove from heat. Increase the
> heat to high and when pan is hot quickly cook the steaks, adding salt and pepper
> if desired. Depending on the thickness of the steaks, cooking time will be approx-
> imately 1 minute or less for each side. Spread the toast with aioli. Place lettuce
> on two slices then add carrot, tomato, steak and onion, and close the sandwich.
> Cut in half before serving.

Healthy Hamburger

SERVES 4, PREPARATION TIME 25 MINUTES, COOKING TIME 10 MINUTES

Hamburgers are much healthier if made at home as you can choose quality mince
and use wholegrain buns. These burgers are also delish with the addition of a slice of
fresh pineapple and rocket can be used instead of cos lettuce. Use a coffee or seed
grinder to make the breadcrumbs. Use a stock cube that is free of artificial additives.

500g (1lb 2oz) extra lean minced beef
½ medium onion, finely diced
1 large carrot, grated
2 slices wholegrain bread, lightly toasted and made into breadcrumbs
3 cloves garlic, minced
1 vegetable stock cube, crumbled
1 teaspoon dried mixed herbs
15g (½oz) parsley, finely chopped
1 egg, lightly beaten
1 tablespoon extra-virgin olive oil
½ medium onion, cut into rings
4 large wholemeal buns (preservative free)
2 tablespoons Sweet Chutney (p. 325) or Tomato Sauce (p. 326)
4 cos lettuce leaves, halved
1 fresh tomato, sliced (optional)
1 fresh beetroot, grated (or 8 slices tinned beetroot)

> **Method**: Combine the beef, diced onion, 30g (1oz) of carrot, breadcrumbs, garlic,
> stock, dried herbs, parsley and egg (and add a tablespoon of water if necessary) and
> mix. Form four large meat patties and cook on medium heat for 4–5 minutes each
> side, using a grill, frying pan or barbecue pre-greased with olive oil. At the same
> time, sauté the onion rings for 2–3 minutes, until translucent.

Split the buns in half and, if desired, toast the insides under the grill for 1–2 minutes until slightly browned, then remove and spread buns with chutney or sauce. Put two layers of lettuce on each bun plus the meat patty, onion rings, remaining carrot, tomato and beetroot. Close the buns and serve immediately.

Beef Barley Soup

SERVES 4, PREPARATION TIME 10 MINUTES, COOKING TIME 60 MINUTES

This soup is for meat lovers and it's ideal for a cold winter's night. Barley contains gluten.

1 tablespoon extra-virgin olive oil
250g (9oz) stewing beef, fat trimmed, cut into chunks
1 medium onion, diced
2 carrots, thinly sliced
2 sticks celery, finely chopped
3 garlic cloves, crushed and finely diced
1.5 litres (30fl oz) Anti-ageing Broth (or vegetable stock)
100g (3½oz) barley, rinsed
2 teaspoons fresh thyme, chopped

Method: Add half the oil to a large saucepan and cook the meat on high heat until browned, for 3–5 minutes. Then transfer to paper towels to drain. Reduce to medium heat, add the remaining oil and cook the onion until translucent. Then add carrots, celery and garlic and cook for a further 3 minutes, stirring as necessary. Add 240ml (8fl oz) of broth and mix with pan juices then add the remaining broth and bring to the boil. Add the barley, meat and thyme and simmer for 40–50 minutes until meat is tender and barley cooked. Serve with grainy toast if desired.

Lean Meat and Three Veg

SERVES 4, PREPARATION TIME 20 MINUTES, COOKING TIME 25 MINUTES

This tasty lamb dish is balanced with specially selected vegetables. Gluten free if using tamari sauce and malt-free soya milk. If you have eczema exclude the tamari sauce, broccoli and Swiss chard, and use sea salt and chopped cabbage.

2 medium sweet potatoes (approx. 500g/1lb 2oz), peeled and diced
500g (1lb 2oz) lean lamb cuts of choice (lean cutlets, chops)
1 teaspoon dried rosemary
300g (10½oz) yellow beans or green beans
300g (10½oz) broccoli or Swiss chard, chopped
80ml (3fl oz) soya milk
½ teaspoon tamari sauce (or soy sauce)
ground black pepper

Method: Preheat the oven to 250°C/500°F/highest gas mark. In a saucepan, boil the sweet potato for 10 minutes or until very soft, then strain and return the sweet potato to the saucepan. Mash the sweet potato until lump-free then stir in tamari sauce, soya milk and pepper to make a creamy and tasty mash, and keep the mixture in the saucepan. Place the meat in a shallow baking dish and sprinkle with rosemary then cook in the oven for 8–10 minutes on each side, checking to see when desired amount of cooking has been achieved. In a steamer, cook the beans and broccoli or Swiss chard for 2–3 minutes (maximum). Set the timer so you don't overcook the vegetables; they must be slightly crisp. Reheat the mash on stove top if necessary and serve immediately.

Lamb Stir-fry

SERVES 2, PREPARATION TIME 15 MINUTES, COOKING TIME 25 MINUTES

This crispy and tasty stir-fry is gluten free and has a slight nutty taste from the toasted sesame seeds. Keep the vegetables thinly sliced for best effect and you can also serve each meal with 70g (2oz) of cooked brown rice if you want more energy carbs.

1 tablespoon sesame seeds
4 lean lamb chops, fat trimmed
1 teaspoon dried mint flakes
1 tablespoon extra-virgin olive oil
150g (5½oz) mushrooms, thinly sliced
200g (7oz) cabbage, finely chopped
3 stalks shallots, sliced on the diagonal
1 small red pepper, thinly sliced
1 large carrot, halved and thinly sliced into strips
¼ teaspoon dried chilli flakes
150g (5½oz) bean sprouts, rinsed in vinegar and water

Method: Preheat the oven to 250°C/500°F/highest gas mark. In a frying pan, toast the sesame seeds on high for 2 minutes until slightly browned then remove from heat. Place the chops in an ovenproof dish, sprinkle with mint flakes and bake in the oven for 8–10 minutes each side. After cooking, place the meat on paper towels to drain.

Heat the oil in a hot frying pan and quickly fry the mushrooms, cabbage, shallots, pepper, carrot and chilli flakes for no more than 2 minutes (vegetables must be slightly crisp). Then stir in the bean sprouts and sesame seeds and serve beside lamb or slice lamb and place on top of stir-fried vegetables.

Slow Roasted Lamb with Steamed Greens

SERVES 4, PREPARATION TIME 15 MINUTES, COOKING TIME 40 MINUTES

2 medium sweet potatoes (approx. 500g), peeled and sliced
extra-virgin olive oil
1 tablespoon fresh rosemary, chopped
sea salt
1 tablespoon honey, melted
2 tablespoons wholegrain mustard
cracked black pepper
2 tablespoons chopped parsley, plus extra for garnish
8 large lean lamb cutlets, fat trimmed
4 large leaves Swiss chard, chopped
8 pieces chopped broccoli (approx. 250g)
1 bunch asparagus, ends trimmed

Method: Preheat the oven to 220°C/425°F/gas 7. Sprinkle the sweet potato with 1 tablespoon of olive oil, rosemary and sea salt, and mix. Then arrange on a baking tray and cook in the oven for 20 minutes.

In a bowl, make the honey marinade by combining honey, mustard, pepper and parsley and set aside. Preheat a large frying pan on high heat and sear the lamb cutlets for 1 minute only, until meat is sealed. Remove the cutlets from the pan and spread the honey marinade on them. Place the cutlets on a separate baking tray and reduce the oven temperature to 150°C/300°F/gas 2. Roast the lamb and sweet potato for 20 minutes or until cooked to your liking. Meanwhile, to ensure asparagus ends are tender, use a potato peeler to peel the outer layer of ends to expose lighter, more tender flesh (approximately 3cm from the end). Using a saucepan that has a steamer attached, bring some water to the boil and 3 minutes before lamb has finished cooking, steam the greens for 2–3 minutes on high heat. Remove the greens to preserve crispness and colour. Place the sweet potato and greens on serving plates and top with lamb cutlets. Garnish with parsley.

Lamb's Fry in Rich Tomato

SERVES 4, PREPARATION TIME 15 MINUTES (SOAKING TIME 1 HOUR), COOKING TIME 30 MINUTES

Lamb's fry is a rich source of protein, iron, zinc, B vitamins and vitamin A. Ideal for people with anaemia. Only use organic lamb's fry as the non-organic variety may contain pesticides. If you can't find lamb's fry at your butcher, use another lean cut of lamb. Not suitable for eczema and may not be suitable if you're pregnant due to the high vitamin A content.

500–600g (1lb 2oz–1lb 5oz) lamb's fry, preferably skinned
50g (1¾oz) wholemeal plain flour
finely ground sea salt and pepper
80ml (3fl oz) extra-virgin olive oil
1 medium onion, chopped
2 cloves garlic, minced
3 spring onions, chopped on the diagonal
250ml (8fl oz) vegetable stock
415g tinned chopped tomatoes
1 sachet (2 tablespoons) tomato paste
1 tablespoon wholegrain mustard
30g (1oz) fresh parsley, finely chopped
6 large Swiss chard leaves, chopped
8 pieces chopped broccoli (approx. 250g)
4 yellow squash, halved

Method: If the lamb's fry has the skin on, soak for 1 hour in enough water to cover it (this will make it easier to remove the skin). Drain, pat dry and remove skin. Slice thinly, then coat the slices with flour and season with salt and pepper. Then heat some of the oil in a large frying pan or electric pan on medium to high heat and cook the lamb's fry for 1–2 minutes each side. Do not overcook: the outside should be slightly crispy and the inside mostly cooked. Cook in two batches if necessary and add extra oil as needed. Remove and place on paper towels. Do not wash the pan.

To the same pan add the onion and garlic, and cook for 1 minute. Then add shallots, stock, tomatoes and tomato paste, stirring in any brown bits from the bottom of the pan. Cook until the mixture reduces to a thick sauce. Stir in mustard and parsley and season with salt and pepper if necessary. Then add the cooked lamb's fry and allow to sit for 2 minutes. Using a saucepan that has a steamer attached, bring some water to the boil and 3 minutes before the lamb's fry is ready steam the Swiss chard, broccoli and squash for 2–3 minutes on high heat. Remove immediately to avoid overcooking, garnish with parsley or spring onions and serve. (Thanks to Joy for this lovely recipe.)

Desserts and sweet treats

Stewed Pears with Vanilla Soya Custard

SERVES 4, PREPARATION TIME 5 MINUTES, COOKING TIME 15 MINUTES

This dessert is delicious, sophisticated and easy to make. Use juice that is sugar and preservative free. Suitable for people with eczema (preferably use pear juice). Gluten free if the soya milk is malt free. The soya custard contains B vitamins and calcium. (If you have blood sugar problems, sprinkle this dessert with cinnamon as maple syrup is high GI.)

500ml (18fl oz) apple or pear juice
500ml (18fl oz) water
6 pears, peeled, cored and halved
Custard:
5 free-range egg yolks
3 tablespoons real maple syrup
500ml (18fl oz) calcium-fortified soya milk
1 vanilla bean, cut lengthways and opened
3 cardamom pods, pressed
sprinkle of carob powder

Method: Place the apple juice and water in a large saucepan and bring to the boil. Add the pears and simmer for 10 minutes, until the pears are soft. Remove the pears and place three halves in each dessert bowl and set aside.

In a small bowl, lightly beat the egg yolks then add the maple syrup, mix and set aside. Then in a small saucepan add the soya milk, vanilla bean and cardamom pods, bring to the boil and simmer for 5 minutes, stirring continuously. While mixing, add the egg yolks and stir until the custard thickens (this should take less than 1 minute). Remove from the heat before curdling occurs. Remove pods and bean, and pour custard over the pears. For presentation, sprinkle a tiny amount of carob powder over each dessert before serving. You can use the leftover egg whites in an omelette (modify the Tasty Omelette recipe on p. 316).

Poached Apple Surprise

SERVES 2, PREPARATION TIME 2 MINUTES, COOKING TIME 15 MINUTES

The surprise is it's simple and tasty. Use juice that is sugar and preservative free. Gluten free. If you have blood sugar problems sprinkle this dessert with cinnamon.

500ml (18fl oz) apple juice
500ml (18fl oz) water
2 green apples, peeled and cored

1 teaspoon real maple syrup
sprinkle of ground flaxseeds

> **Method**: Place the apple juice and water in a saucepan and bring to the boil. Add the apples and simmer for 15 minutes, until soft. Remove the apples and place in dessert bowls. Decorate with maple syrup and flaxseeds, or Vanilla Soya Custard (see Stewed Pears with Vanilla Soya Custard, opposite). Serve warm.

Tangy Papaya Cups

SERVES 2, PREPARATION TIME 2 MINUTES

> This healthy and light dessert (or snack) tastes fantastic and contains alkalising lime, banana and flaxseeds. Gluten free. If you have eczema, reluctantly omit the lime juice.

1 large ripe papaya, halved and seeds removed
1 ripe banana, sliced
juice of 1 lime
2 teaspoons ground flaxseeds

> **Method**: Fill the papaya halves with chopped banana and sprinkle with lime juice and ground flaxseeds.

Mango Ice

SERVES 4, PREPARATION TIME 5 MINUTES, FREEZING TIME AT LEAST 2 HOURS

> Mangoes are rich in vitamins and make a great frozen dessert.

2 large ripe mangoes, peeled and sliced
4 teaspoons ground flaxseeds

> **Method**: Divide the mango slices into four small containers and freeze. Before serving, sprinkle with flaxseeds. Frozen mango can also be used in smoothies.

Sweet Banana and Carob Spread

SERVES 2, PREPARATION TIME 5 MINUTES

> A fab children's snack or dessert. Spread on French Toast (p. 312), Banana Cake (p. 368) or drizzle over fruit. You can also double or triple the recipe and freeze it in popsicle containers, or freeze for half an hour to make a light 'pudding'. Very suitable for people with eczema. For Banana Cake filling, use 6 bananas, 3 tablespoons maple syrup, 1 tablespoon carob powder and vanilla essence.

2 large ripe bananas, mashed
1–2 teaspoons carob powder (less is best)
2 teaspoons real maple syrup
dash of real vanilla essence

Method: Combine all ingredients and using a beater, mix on high until smooth and creamy. (Thanks to Lynda Spencely for this modified recipe.)

Rhubarb Crumble

SERVES 6, PREPARATION TIME 10 MINUTES, COOKING TIME 30 MINUTES

This dessert is just gorgeous and it has half the sugar of regular crumbles. If you have eczema, modify this recipe and use sliced or tinned pear instead of rhubarb. Cinnamon assists with keeping blood sugar levels steady.

1 large bunch rhubarb, chopped
60ml (2fl oz) lemon juice
1 tablespoon soft brown sugar
1 tablespoon water
½ teaspoon cinnamon
Topping:
70g (2½oz) plain wholemeal flour
1 tablespoon wheat bran or wheat germ
pinch of salt
¼ teaspoon baking soda/bicarbonate of soda
100g (3½oz) rolled oats
1 tablespoon soft brown sugar
1 tablespoon whole flaxseeds
60ml (2fl oz) extra-virgin olive oil

Method: Preheat the oven to 180°C/350°F/gas 4. Arrange the diced rhubarb in a 20cm square baking dish and sprinkle with lemon juice, sugar, water and cinnamon. To make the topping, combine in a bowl the flour, wheat bran, salt and baking soda. Then add oats, sugar, whole flaxseeds and oil, and mix until crumbly. Add another tablespoon of oil if necessary (if the mixture looks too dry). Spread evenly over the rhubarb and top with a sprinkling of cinnamon if desired. Bake for 30 minutes or until the rhubarb is stewing and soft, and topping is lightly golden. Serve warm.

Banana Cake

SERVES 8 OR MAKES APPROX. 12 SMALL MUFFINS, PREPARATION TIME 10 MINUTES, COOKING TIME 10–20 MINUTES

With less sugar and more wholemeal, this cake is bordering on being healthy. Think of this cake as a party treat or suitable birthday cake for children with eczema. To counteract some of the acid effect produced by ingesting sugar, flour and saturated fat, have a glass of Green Water afterwards.

90g (3oz) soft brown sugar
125g (4½oz) unsalted butter, left to soften

2 free-range eggs, lightly beaten
3 medium very ripe bananas, mashed
290g (10oz) wholemeal self-raising flour
pinch of salt
½ teaspoon bicarbonate of soda
3 tablespoons calcium-fortified soya milk
Sweet Banana and Carob Spread (p. 367, triple quantity)
sprinkling of icing sugar (if it's a birthday cake)

Method: Preheat the oven to 180°C/350°F/gas 4. Beat the brown sugar and butter together to a cream. Add the eggs and beat well, then add the mashed banana and beat. In a separate bowl combine the flour, soda and salt, and mix. Fold in the dry ingredients with the banana mix and add soya milk to form a soft dough. Divide the mixture into two greased and floured 18cm sandwich tins or loaf dishes (the mixture will not cook properly in one large tin). Alternatively, bake as small muffins. Cake baking time is 20–25 minutes; muffins will be cooked in less than 10 minutes. Test with a skewer. Cool on a wire rack. If desired, turn one layer of the cake upside down and top with Sweet Banana and Carob Spread, then place the other layer on top (right side up). Sprinkle with a small amount of icing sugar for presentation. If not eating immediately, cake slices are extra lovely when heated for 10 seconds in the microwave. Store refrigerated in a sealed container.

Carrot Cake

SERVES 8, PREPARATION TIME 10 MINUTES, COOKING TIME 30 MINUTES

This cake is dairy free and full of carrot goodness. However, to counteract some of the acid effect produced by ingesting sugar and flour, have a glass of Green Water afterwards.

145g (5oz) plain wholemeal flour
90g (3oz) soft brown sugar
1 teaspoon bicarbonate of soda
1 teaspoon baking powder
pinch of salt
1 teaspoon cinnamon
120ml (4fl oz) extra-virgin olive oil
2 free-range eggs, lightly beaten
1 teaspoon real vanilla essence
240g (9oz) grated carrot
100g (3½oz) grated green apple
2 tablespoons water (if necessary)

Method: Preheat the oven to 150°C/300°F/gas 2. In a mixing bowl combine the flour, sugar, soda, baking powder, salt and cinnamon. Stir in the oil, eggs and vanilla and beat well until smooth. Add the carrot and apple, and water if mixture is not quite wet enough. Mix well then pour into a greased 23cm x 13 cm loaf dish. Cook on the lower shelf in the oven for 30 minutes, checking to see when cooked from 20 minutes onwards. Test with a skewer. Allow to cool slightly before removing the cake from the dish. Store refrigerated in a sealed container.

Appendix 3

Recipes for natural cleaning products

Vinegar cleaning spray

Vinegar is anti-bacterial and cuts through grease, making it a great all-purpose cleaning spray (although do not use on marble surfaces). You'll need:

1 x empty spray bottle
equal parts water and white vinegar

Baking Soda

Baking soda is the original all-purpose scrub. Sprinkle some onto a damp cloth and use it as a scrub on bathroom and kitchen surfaces. Perfect for cleaning the bath.

Acknowledgments

Many people have helped me to finetune this book and I am very grateful for their time, wisdom and assistance. Firstly, I'd love to say a huge thank you to my writer's agent Selwa Anthony and also Exisle Publishing for believing in me and my book – I could not have completed this project without your support. I'd like to thank my editors Anouska Jones and Karen Gee for doing a great job editing *The Healthy Skin Diet*. I also had some early editing assistance from Sue Tierney, Joy Fischer, Alice Hocking, Katie Ashton and Louise Roberts – thanks guys; I really appreciate your invaluable advice! Sophie Gabriel, author of *Breathe for Life*, put a lot of time and effort into finetuning Chapter 19, 'Beauty breathing', and I am forever grateful that she freely shared her extensive knowledge on breathing training with me. It has made a huge difference to my own health and stamina. Thanks to my biochemistry teacher Helen Stevenson for her information on prostaglandins, which I've included in Chapter 4. I also received valuable skin-care information from cosmetic physician Dr Van Huynh-Park, Snezna Kerekovic, Bahar Etminan and Ray Thatcher. There are hundreds of awesome scientific studies on skin care and skin health and I really appreciate the scientific researchers who have allowed their findings to be published on the net. I'd also like to thank author Tara Moss for forwarding my book 'aspirations' on to her writer's agent Selwa. And I'd love to thank Jon, Ayva, Jack and the rest of my family for your patience and infinite support.

For Mum and Dad,
thanks for everything.

Notes

Chapter 2

1. British Association of Dermatology website, 'Social importance of skin', retrieved 17 March 2006: http://www.bad.org.uk/public/skin/social/
2. ibid.
3. Pennisi, E. 2005, 'Why do humans have so few genes?', *Science Magazine*, vol. 309, no. 5731, retrieved 18 March 2006: http://www.sciencemag.org/cgi/content/full/309/5731/80
4. U.S. Department of Energy, Office of Science, Human Genome Project Information website, 'How many genes are in the human genome?', retrieved 18 March 2006: http://www.ornl.gov/sci/techresources/Human_Genome/faq/genenumber.shtml
5. Cordain, L. et. Al. 2002, 'Acne vulgaris, a disease of western civilisation', *Archives of Dermatology*, vol. 138, no. 12, pp 1584-1590.
6. Cordain. L. 2005, 'Implications for the role of diet in acne', *Seminars in Cutaneous Medicine and Surgery*, vol. 24, no. 2, reprinted in *Rosacea News* 'Could rosacea be caused by diet?'
7. Cordain, L., et al., 2005, 'Origins and Evolution of the Western Diet: health implications for the 21st century', *American Journal of Clinical Nutrition*, vol. 81, pp 341–54.
8. 'Acne vulgaris, a disease of western civilisation', *Archives of Dermatology*, op. cit.
9. 'Implications for the role of diet in acne', *Seminars in Cutaneous Medicine and Surgery*, op. cit.
10. Sardi, B. 2004, 'Yuzurihara, the village of long life, reveals its secrets', Knowledge of Health Inc., retrieved 10 April 2006: http://www.knowledgeofhealth.com/pdfs/yuzurihara.pdf
11. 'Implications for the role of diet in acne', *Seminars in Cutaneous Medicine and Surgery*, op. cit.
12. 'Acne vulgaris, a disease of western civilisation', *Archives of Dermatology*, op. cit.

Chapter 3

1. Guerrero, A., 2005, *In Balance for Life*, chapters 1, 3 and 5, Square One Publishing, New York.
2. Robbins, A. 2001, 'Pure energy live', *Get the Edge*, The Anthony Robbins Companies, California.
3. ibid.
4. *In Balance for Life*, op. cit.
5. ibid.
6. ibid.
7. ibid.
8. *Get the Edge*, op. cit.
9. *In Balance for Life*, op. cit.
10. ibid.
11. ibid.
12. Higgins, E.M. and du Vivier, A.W.P. 1994, 'Cutaneous disease and alcohol misuse', *British Medical Bulletin*, vol. 50, no. 1, pp 85-98.
13. Vander Straten, M., et al., 2001, 'Tobacco use and skin disease,' *Southern Medical Journal*, retrieved 20 April 2006: http://www.medscape.com/viewarticle/410808_print
14. ibid.
15. Sarin, C.L., Austin, J.C. and Nickel, W.O. 1974, *Journal of the American Medical Association*, vol 229, in Vander Straten M. et. al, 2001, 'Tobacco use and skin disease', *Southern Medical Journal*.
16. Saavedra, J.M., Harris, G.D. and Finberg, L. 1991, 'Capillary refilling (skin turgor) in the assessment of dehydration', *Archives of Pediatrics & Adolescent Medicine*, vol. 145, no. 3 pp 296–298.
17. Chek, P., 2004, *How to Eat, Move and Be Healthy!*, C.H.E.K Institute, San Diego.
18. World Health Organization website, 'The big guns of resistance', *Infectious disease report*, retrieved 21 January 2007: http://www.who.int/infectious-disease-report/2000/ch4.htm
19. World Health Organization website, 2007, 'Frequently asked questions about worms', *Soil transmitted helminths*, retrieved 21 January 2007: http://www.who.int/worm-control/statistics/faqs/en/index1.html
20. ibid.

21. Cassavant, M.C., et. al. 2006, 'Investigation of antibiotic and antioxidant properties of leaf extracts from Juglans nigra, Quercus alba, and Quercus rubra,' OLCC-McClain. Retrieved 21 January 2007: http://acs.confex.com/acs/mwrm06/techprogram/P38759.HTM

22. Clark, A.M., et. al. 2006, 'Antimicrobial activity of juglone,' *Phytotherapy Research*, vol. 4, no. 1, pp 11-14.

23. Briozzo, J., et. al., 1989, 'Antimicrobial activity of clove oil dispersed in a concentration of sugar solution,' *The Journal of Applied Bacteriology*, vol.66, no. 1, pp 69-75.

24. Winkler, C., et. al. 2005, 'Extracts of pumpkin (cucurbita pepo L.) seed suppress stimulated peripheral blood mononuclear cells in vitro,' *American Journal of Immunology*, vol. 1, no. 1, pp 6-11, retrieved 22 January 2007 http://www.scipub.us/fulltext/aji/aji116-11.pdf

25. Jayaprakasam, B. et. al. 2003, 'Anticancer and antiinflammatory activities of cucurbitacins from cucurbita andreana,' *Cancer Letters*, vol. 189, no. 1, pp 11-16.

26. Caili, F., et. al. 2006, 'A review on pharmacological activities and utilization technologies of pumpkin,' *Plant Foods for Human Nutrition*, vol. 61, no. 2, pp 70-7.

27. Shelef, L.A. 1984, 'Antimicrobial effects of spices,' *Journal of Food Safety*, vol. 6, no. 1, pp 29-44.

28. Snyder, P. 1997, 'Antimicrobial effects of spices and herbs,' Hospitality Institute of Technology and Management, St Paul, Minnesota

29. Dorman, H.J.D. and Deans, S.G., 2000, 'Antimicrobial agents from plants: antibacterial activity of plant volatile oils,' *Journal of Applied Microbiology*, vol. 88, pp 308-16.

30. De, M., et. al. 1999, 'Antimicrobial screening of some Indian spices,' *Phytotherapy Research*, vol. 13, no. 7, pp 616-18.

31. Pitchford, P., 1993, *Healing with Whole Foods*, (revised edn), chapter 7, North Atlantic Books, Berkeley, California.

32. Murray, M. and Pizzorno J. 1998, *Encyclopaedia of Natural Medicine*, (2nd edn), Little, Brown & Company, London.

33. *In Balance for Life*, op. cit.

34. World Health Organization website, *Soil transmitted helminths*.

35. Hawrelak, J. 2003, 'Probiotics: choosing the right one for your needs,' *Journal of the Australian Traditional-Medicine Society*, vol. 9, no. 2, pp. 67-75.

36. ibid.

37. ibid.

38. ibid.

39. *In Balance for Life*, op. cit.

40. ibid.

41. *Seminars in Cutaneous Medicine and Surgery*, op. cit., pp 84-91.

42. 'Acne vulgaris, a disease of western civilisation,' *Archives of Dermatology*, op. cit., pp 1584-90.

43. Boelsma, E. 2003, 'Human skin condition and its association with nutrient concentrations in serum and diet,' *American Journal of Clinical Nutrition*, vol. 77, no. 22 pp 348-55.

44. Baumann, L. 2005, 'How to prevent photoaging?' *Journal of Investigative Dermatology*, vol. 125, no. 4, pp xii-xiii.

45. Purba, M., et.al. 2001, 'Skin wrinkling: can food make a difference?' *Journal of the American College of Nutrition*, vol. 20, no. 1, pp 71-80.

46. Podda, M. and Grundmann-Kollmann, M. 2001, 'Low molecular weight antioxidants and their role in skin ageing,' *Clinical & Experimental Dermatology*, vol. 26, no. 7. pp 578–582

Chapter 4

1. Erasmus, U. 1993, *Fats that Heal, Fats that Kill*, chapter 8, Alive Books, Burnaby, BC, Canada.

2. ibid.

3. Horrocks, L.A. and Yeo, Y.K. 1999, 'Health benefits of Docosahexaenoic (DHA)' *Pharmacological Research*, vol. 40, no. 3, pp 211–225

4. *Fats that Heal, Fats that Kill*, op. cit.

5. Manku, M.S. et. al., 1982, 'Reduced levels of prostaglandin precursors in the blood of atopic patients: defective delta-6-desaturase function as a biochemical basis of atopy,' *Prostaglandins Leukotrienes & Medicine*, vol. 9, no. 6, pp 615–628

6. Samuelsson, B. 1983, 'Leukotrienes: mediators of immediate hypersensitivity reactions and inflammation,' *Science*, vol. 220, no 4597, pp 568-75.

7. Ruzicka, T. 1989, 'Leukotrienes in atopic eczema', *Acta Dermato-Venereologica Supplementum*, vol. 144, p48-9, retrieved 10 November 2006: www.ncbi.nlm.gov/pubmed/

8. Fogh, K., et. al. 1989, 'Eicosanoids in skin of patients with atopic dermatitis: prostaglandin E2 and leukotrienes B4 are present in biologically active concentrations', *Journal of Allergy and Clinical Immunology*, vol. 83, no. 2 pt. 1, pp 450-5.

9. Dixon R.A.F., et. al. 1990, 'Requirement of 5-lipoxygenase-activating protein for leukotriene synthesis', *Nature*, vol 343, pp 282-4.

10. Qiu, H. et. al. 2006, 'Expression of 5-lipoxygenase and leukotrienes A4 hydrolase in human atherosclerotic lesions correlates with symptoms of plaque instability', *PNAS*, vol. 103, no 21, pp 8161-6.

11. Fauler, J. and Frolich, J.C. 1989, 'Cardiovascular effects of leukotrienes', *Cardiovascular Drugs and Therapy*, vol. 3, no. 4, pp 499-505.

12. Christman, B.W., et. al. 1992, 'An imbalance between the excretion of thromboxane and prostacyclin metabolites in pulmonary hypertension', *New England Journal of Medicine*, vol. 327, no. 2, pp 70-5.

13. Walsh, S.W. 1984, 'Pre-eclampsia: an imbalance in placental prostacyclin and thromboxane production', *American Journal of Obstetrics and Gynecology*, vol. 152, no. 3, pp 335-40.

14. 'Leukotrienes: mediators of immediate hypersensitivity reactions and inflammation,' *Science*, op. cit.

15. Srivastava, K.C. 1984, 'Aqueous extracts of onion, garlic and ginger inhibit platelet aggregation and alter arachidonic acid metabolism', *Biomedica Biochimica Acta*, vol. 43, no. 8-9, pp S335-46.

16. Hong, J., et. al. 2004, 'Modulation of arachidonic acid metabolism by curcumin and related beat-diketone derivatives', *Carcinogenesis*, vol. 25, no. 9, pp 1671-9.

17. Nijveldt, R.J., et. al. 2001, 'Flavonoids: a review of probable mechanisms of action and potential applications', *American Journal of Clinical Nutrition,*' vol. 74, pp 418-25.

18. Eskew, M.L. et. al. 1989, 'Effects of inade-quate vitamin E and/or selenium nutrition on the release of arachidonic acid metabolites in rat alveolar macrophages', *Prostaglandins*, vol. 38, no. 1, pp 79-89.

19. Ferrandiz, M.L. and Alcaraz, M.J. 1991, 'Anti-inflammatory activity and inhibition of arachidonic acid metabolism by flavonoids', *Inflammation Research*, vol. 32, no. 3-4, pp 283-8.

20. Leitzmann, M.F., et. al. 2004, 'Dietary intake of n-3 and n-6 fatty acids and the risk of prostate cancer', *American Journal of Clinical Nutrition*, vol. 80, pp 204-16.

21. Hansen Petrik, M.B., et. al. 2000, 'Antagonism of arachidonic acid is linked to the antitumorigenic effect of dietary eicosapentaenoic acid in apc min/+ mice', *Journal of Nutrition*, vol. 130, pp 1153-8.

22. Bangyan, L., et. al. 1994, 'Antithetic relationship of dietary arachidonic acid and eicosapentaenoic acid on eicosanoid production in vivo', *Journal of Lipid Research*, vol. 35, pp 1869-77.

23. List compiled from product packaging and Kirschmann, G.J. and Kirschmann, J.D. 1996, *Nutrition Almanac*, (4th edn), McGraw Hill Book Co, Singapore.

24. Barham, J.B., et. al. 2000, 'Addition of eicosapentaenoic acid to y-linolenic acid-supplemented diets prevents serum arachidonic acid accumulation in humans,' *Journal of Nutrition*, vol. 130, pp 1925-31.

25. 'Antithetic relationship of dietary arachidonic acid and eicosapentaenoic acid on eicosanoid production in vivo', *Journal of Lipid Research*, op. cit.

26. 'Dietary intake of n-3 and n-6 fatty acids and the risk of prostate cancer', *American Journal of Clinical Nutrition*, op. cit.

27. 'Antagonism of arachidonic acid is linked to the antitumorigenic effect of dietary eicosapentaenoic acid in apc min/+ mice,' *Journal of Nutrition*, op. cit.

28. *Fats that Heal, Fats that Kill*, op. cit.

29. Higdon, J. 2005, 'Essential Fatty Acids', Linus Pauling Institute, Oregon State University, retrieved 13 November 2006: http://lpi.oregonstate.edu/infocenter/othernuts/omega3fa

30. Fats that Heal, Fats that Kill, op. cit.

31. 'Essential fatty acids', Linus Pauling Institute, Oregon State University. retrieved 13

November 2006: http://lpi.oregonstate.edu/infocenter/other-nuts/omega3fa

32. Fortin, P.R., et. al. 1995, 'Validation of a meta-analysis: the effects of fish oil in rheumatoid arthritis', *Journal of Clinical Epidemiology*, vol. 48, no. 11, pp 1379-90.

33. Daviglus, M.L., et. al. 1997, 'Fish consumption and the 30-year risk of fatal myocardial infarction', *New England Journal of Medicine*, vol 336, no. 15, pp 1046-53.

34. SanGiovanni, J.P. and Chew, E.Y. 2005, 'The role of omega-3 long-chain polyunsaturated fatty acids in health and disease of the retina', *Progress in Retinal & Eye Research*, vol. 24, no. 1, pp 87-138.

35. *Fats that Heal, Fats that Kill*, op. cit.

36. Fito, M., et. al. 2000, 'Protective effect of olive oil and its phenolic compounds against low density lipoprotein oxidation', *Lipids*, vol. 35, no. 6, pp 633-8.

37. Deiana, M., et. al. 1999, 'Inhibition of peroxynitrite dependent DNA base modification and tyrosine nitration by the extra virgin olive oil-derived antioxidant hydroxytyosol', *Free Radical Biology & Medicine*, vol. 26, no. 5-6, pp 762-9.

38. Murakoshi, M., et. al. 1992, 'Inhibition by squalene of the tumor-promoting activity of 12-0-tetradecanolyphorbol-13-acetate in mouse skin carcinogenesis', *International Journal of Cancer*, vol. 52, no. 6, pp 950-2.

39. Persson, E., et. al. 2003, 'Influence of antioxidants in virgin olive oil on the formation of heterocyclic amines in fried beefburgers', *Food & Chemical Toxicology*, vol. 41, no. 11, pp 1587-97.

40. ibid.

Chapter 5

1. Pashko, L.L. and Schwartz, A.G. 1992, 'Reversal of food restriction-induced inhibition of mouse skin tumour promotion by adrenalectomy', *Carcinogenesis*, vol. 13, no. 10, pp 1925-8.

2. Birt, D.F., et. al. 1999, 'Glucocorticoid mediation of dietary energy restriction inhibition of mouse skin carcinogenesis', *Journal of Nutrition*, vol. 129, supplement pp 517S-574S.

3. Kritchevsky, D. 1999, 'Caloric restriction and experimental carcinogenesis', *Toxicological Sciences*, vol. 52, pp 13-16.

4. Kritchevsky, D. 1995, 'The effect of over-and undernutrition on cancer', *European Journal of Cancer Prevention*, vol. 4, no. 6 pp 445-51.

5. Reiter, R.J. 1995, 'The pineal gland and melatonin in relation to aging: a summary of the theories and of the data', *Experimental Gerontology*, vol. 30, no. 3-4, pp 199-212.

6. Reiter, R.J., et. al. 1995, 'A review of the evidence supporting melatonin's role as an antioxidant', *Journal of Pineal Research*, vol. 18, no. 1, pp 1-11.

7. Armstrong, S.M. and Redman, J.R. 1991, 'Melatonin: a chronobiotic with anti-aging properties?' *Medical Hypotheses*, vol. 34, no. 4, pp 300-309.

8. Pierpaoli, W. and Maestroni G.J. 1987, 'Melatonin: a principle neuroimmunoregulatory and anti-stress hormone: its anti-aging effects', *Immunology Letters*, vol. 16, no. 3-4, pp 355-61.

9. 'The pineal gland and melatonin in relation to aging: a summary of the theories and of the data,' *Experimental Gerontology*, op. cit.

10. 'Melatonin: a chronobiotic with anti-aging properties?' *Medical Hypotheses*, op. cit.

11. Reiter, R.J. 1995, 'Oxygen radical detoxification process during aging: the functional importance of melatonin,' *Aging*, vol. 7, no. 5, pp 340-51.

12. Roth, G.S., et. al. 2001, 'Dietary caloric restriction prevents the age-related decline in plasma melatonin levels of rhesus monkeys', *Journal of Endocrinology & Metabolism*, vol. 86, no. 7, pp 3292-5.

13. ibid.

14. 'Glucocorticoid mediation of dietary energy restriction inhibition of mouse skin carcinogenesis', *Journal of Nutrition*, op. cit.

15. 'The effect of over-and undernutrition on cancer', *European Journal of Cancer Prevention*, op. cit.

16. 'Oxygen radical detoxification process during aging: the functional importance of melatonin', *Aging*, op. cit.

17. 'Dietary caloric restriction prevents the age-related decline in plasma melatonin levels of rhesus monkeys', *Journal of Endocrinology & Metabolism*, op. cit.

18. Mattison, J.A., et. al. 2003, 'Calorie restrictions in rhesus monkeys', *Experimental Gerontology*, vol. 38, no 1-2, pp 35-46.

19. Stokkan K.A., et. al. 1991, 'Food restriction retards aging of the pineal gland', *Brain Research*, vol. 545, no. 1-2, pp 66-72.

20. Lumb, K and Tan , K. 2007, 'Melanoma – anyone can be affected', *Sunday* programme, retrieved 12 March 2007: www.ninemsm.com.au

21. Brand-Miller, J., Foster-Powell, K. and Colagiuri, S. 2002, *The New Glucose Revolution*, Hodder Headline Australia, Sydney.

22. ibid.

23. ibid.

24. 'Implications for the role of diet in acne', *Seminars in Cutaneous Medicine and Surgery*, op. cit.

25. Smith, R., et. al. 2004, 'The effects of short-term altered macronutrient status on acne vulgaris and biochemical markers of insulin sensitivity', *Asia Pacific Journal of Clinical Nutrition*, vol. 13, (supplement), ppS67

26. 'Acne vulgaris, a disease of western civilisation', *Archives of Dermatology*, op. cit.

27. *The New Glucose Revolution*, op. cit.

28. ibid.

29. ibid.

30. *Nutrition Almanac*, op. cit.

31. *The New Glucose Revolution*, op. cit.

32. Coeliac Society of Australia website, 'Information about coeliac disease', retrieved 20 November 2006: http://www.coeliac.org.au/index.htm

33. ibid.

34. Diegelmann, R. F. 2001, 'Collagen Metabolism,' *Wounds,* vol. 13, no. 5, pp 177-82.

35. Siebecker, A. 'Traditional bone broth in modern health and disease', *Townsend Letter,* Feb/Mar 2005 issue.

36. Gong, H. 2004, 'Ocular surface in zn-deficient rats', *Ophthalmic Research*, vol. 36, no. 3, pp 129-38.

37. 'Traditional bone broth in modern health and disease', *Townsend Letter*, op. cit.

38. Kang, Y, et. al. 1999, 'Hyaluronan suppresses fibronectin fragment-mediated damage to human cartilage explant cultures by enhancing proteoglycan synthesis', *Journal of Orthopaedic Research*, vol. 17 no. 6. pp 858-69.

39. Murad, H. 2005, *The Cellulite Solution*, introduction, Piatkus, London.

40. 'Hyaluronan suppresses fibronectin fragment-mediated damage to human cartilage explant cultures by enhancing proteoglycan synthesis', *Journal of Orthopaedic Research*, op. cit.

41. *The Cellulite Solution*, op. cit.

42. McCarthy, M.F. 1996, 'Glucosamine for wound healing', *Medical Hypotheses*, vol. 47, no. 4, pp 273-5.

43. *The Cellulite Solution*, op. cit.

44. Ghersetich, I., et. al., 1994, 'Hyaluronic acid in cutaceous intrinsic aging', *International Journal of Dermatology*, vol. 33, no. 2, pp 119–22

45. McDevitt, C.A., et. al. 1989, 'Cigarette smoke degrades hyaluronic acid', *Lung*, vol. 167, no. 4, pp 237-45.

46. 'Glucosamine for wound healing', *Medical Hypotheses*, op. cit.

47. Thompson, R.W., et. al. 1975, 'Alterations of porcine skin acid mucopolysaccharides in zinc deficiency', *Journal of Nutrition*, vol. 105, no 2, pp 154-60.

48. Moscatelli, D. and Rubin, H. 1977, 'Hormonal control of hyaluronic acid production in fibroblasts and its relation to nucleic acid and protein synthesis', *Journal of Cellular Physiology* vol. 91, no 1, pp79-88.

49. Sardi, B., 2004, 'Yuzurihara, the village of long life, reveals its secrets', Knowledge of Health Inc., retrieved 10 April 2006: http://www.knowledgeofhealth.com/pdfs/yuzurihara.pdf

50. ibid.

51. ibid.

52. 'Traditional bone broth in modern health and disease,' *Townsend Letter*, op. cit.

53. ibid.

Chapter 6

1. Reiter, R.J. 1995, 'Oxygen radical detoxification process during aging: the functional importance of melatonin', *Aging*, vol. 7, no. 5, pp 340-51.

2. Roth, G.S., et. al. 2001, 'Dietary caloric restriction prevents the age-related decline in

plasma melatonin levels of rhesus monkeys', *Journal of Endocrinology & Metabolism.*

3. Bonds, C.L. and Lucia, M.A. 2006, 'Sleep disorders', University of California, LA, retrieved 2 March 2007: http://emedicine.com/med/TOPIC609.HTM

4. Jaivin, L. 2006, 'Let's sleep on it,' *Sunday Telegraph*, 13 August.

5. 'Sleep disorders', University of California, op. cit.

6. 'Let's sleep on it', *Sunday Telegraph*.

7. ibid.

8. ibid.

9. ibid.

Chapter 7

1. BBC News, 2006, 'Exercise cuts skin cancer risk', 12/5/2006. http://news.bbc.co.uk/2/hi/health/4764535.stm

2. Masumura, S., et. al. 1992, 'The effects of season and exercise on the levels of plasma poly-unsaturated fatty acids and lipoprotein cholesterol in young rats', *Biochimica et Biophysica Acta*, 1125 pp 292-6.

3. Tortora, G.J. & Grabowski. S.R. 2000, *Principles of Anatomy and Physiology*, (9th edn), chapter 22, John Wiley & Sons, New York.

Chapter 8

1. Patils, S., et. al. 1995, 'Quantification of sodium lauryl sulfate penetration into the skin and underlying tissue after topical application – pharmacological and toxicological implications', *Journal of Pharmaceutical Sciences*, vol. 84, no. 10, pp 1240-4.

2. Gloor, M. et. al. 2004, 'On the course of the irritant reaction after irritation with sodium lauryl sulphate', *Skin Research & Technology*, vol. 10, no. 3, pp 144-8.

3. Cowley, N.C. and Farr, P.M. 1992, 'A dose-response study of irritant reactions to sodium lauryl sulphate in patients with seborrhoeic dermatitis and atopic eczema', *Acta Dermato-Venereologica*, vol. 72, no. 6, pp 432-5.

4. Leveque, J.L., et. al. 1993, 'How does sodium lauryl sulfate alter the skin barrier function in man? A multiparametric approach', *Skin Pharmacology*, vol. 6, no. 2, pp 111-15.

5. 'A dose-response study of irritant reactions to sodium lauryl sulphate in patients with seborrhoeic dermatitis and atopic eczema', *Acta Dermato-Venereologica.*

6. National Institute of Health website, 2007, Household Products Database, 'DMDM hydantoin', retrieved 4 March 2007: http://hpd.nlm.nih.gov/cgi-bin/household/brands?tbl=chem&id=711

7. Carstens, J. 2006, 'The ugly side of beauty products', *Nature & Health*, October/November issue, pp 24-7.

8. De Groot, A.C. and Frosch, P.J. 1997, 'Adverse reactions to fragrance', *Contact Dermatitis*, vol. 36, no. 2, p 57.

9. Pugazhendhi, D., et. al. 2005, 'Oestrogenic activity of p-hydroxybenzoic acid (common metabolite of parabens esters) and methyl-paraben in human breast cancer cell lines', *Journal of Applied Toxicology*, vol. 25, no. 4, pp 301-309.

10. Darbre. P.D. et. al. 2004, 'Concentrations of parabens in human breast tumours', *Journal of Applied Toxicology*, vol. 24, no. 1. pp5–13

11. Harvey, P.W. and Everett, D.J. 2004, 'Significance of the detection of esters of p-hydroxybenzoic acid (parabens) in human breast tumours', *Journal of Applied Toxicology*, vol. 24, no. 1. pp 1–4

12. 'Adverse reactions to fragrance', *Contact Dermatitis*, op. cit.

13. Kitigawa S, Li H, Sato S. 1997, 'Skin permeation of parabens in excised guinea pig dorsal skin, its modification by penetration enhancers and their relationship with n-octanol/ water partition coefficients', *Chemical & Pharmaceutical Bulletin (Tokyo)*, vol. 45, pp 1354-7.

14. 'Significance of the detection of esters of p-hydroxybenzoic acid (parabens) in human breast tumours', *Journal of Applied Toxicology*, op. cit.

15. 'Adverse reactions to fragrance', *Contact Dermatitis*, op. cit.

16. De Groot, A.C. et. al. 1987, 'Contact allergy to cocamide DEA and lauramide DEA in shampoos', *Contact Dermatitis*, vol. 16, no. 2, p 117.

17. Lanigan, R.S. and Andersen, F.A. 1999, 'Final report on the safety assessment of cocamide MEA', *International Journal of Toxicology*, vol. 18, no. 2, pp 9-16.

18. ibid.
19. Ortho Evra, 'The birth control patch', retrieved 13 March 2007: www.orthoevra.com/html/pevr/about.jsp;jsessionid=K5K3FRTLR2BFICQPCCGTC0YKB2IIQNSC?
20. Begoun, P. 2002, *The Beauty Bible*, (2nd edn), chapter 2, Beginning Press, Seattle.
21. Tung, R.C., et. al. 2000, '_-hydroxy acid-based cosmetic procedures: guidelines for patient management', *American Journal of Clinical Dermatology*, vol. 1, no. 2, pp81-8.
22. Fartasch, M., et. al. 1997, 'Mode of action of glycolic acid on human stratum corneum: ultrastructural and functional evaluation of the epidermal barrier', *Archives of Dermatological Research*, vol. 289, no. 7, pp404-409.
23. Athar, M. and Nasir S.M. 2005, 'Taxonomic perspective of plant species yielding vegetable oils used in cosmetics and skin care products', *African Journal of Biotechnology*, vol. 4, no. 1, pp 36-44, retrieved 14 November 2006: http://www.academicjournals.org/AJB/PDF/Pdf2005/Jan/Athar%20and%20Nasir.pdf
24. Dweck, A.C. 2000, 'Functional botanicals – their chemistry and effects', International Cosmetic Expo, Miami, Florida.
25. ibid.
26. Thomsen M. 2001, *Phytotherapy Desk Reference*, (2nd edn), Institut For Phytoterapi, Australia.
27. 'Taxonomic perspective of plant species yielding vegetable oils used in cosmetics and skin care products', *African Journal of Biotechnology*, op. cit.
28. *Phytotherapy Desk Reference*.
29. Wille, J., et. al. 2003, 'Palmitoleic acid isomer in human skin sebum is effective against gram-positive bacteria', *Skin Pharmacology and Physiology*, vol. 16, no. 3, pp 176–87
30. 'Taxonomic perspective of plant species yielding vegetable oils used in cosmetics and skin care products', *African Journal of Biotechnology*, op. cit.
31. Wang, Z.Y., et. al. 1991, 'Protection against ultraviolet B radiation induced photocarcinogenesis in hairless mice by green tea polyphenols', *Carcinogenesis*, vol. 12, no. 8, pp 1527-30.
32. Santosh, K., et. al. 2000, 'Green tea and skin', *Archives of Dermatology*, vol. 136, no. 8, pp 989-94.
33. 'Taxonomic perspective of plant species yielding vegetable oils used in cosmetics and skin care products', *African Journal of Biotechnology*, op. cit.
34. Moreno, J.A., et. al. 2003, 'Effect of phenolic compounds of virgin olive oil on LDL oxidation resistance', *Medicina Clinica*, vol. 120, no. 4, pp 128-31.
35. Budiyanto, A., et. al. 2000, 'Protective effect of topically applied olive oil against photocarcinogenesis following UVB exposure of mice', *Carcinogenesis*, vol. 21, no. 11, pp 2085-90.
36. ibid.
37. Pareja, B. and Kehl, H. 1990, 'Contribution to the identification of the active principles of Rosa aff rubiginosa', *Anales de la Real Academia de Farmacia*, Institute de Espana, vol. 56, no. 2, pp 283-94.
38. 'Taxonomic perspective of plant species yielding vegetable oils used in cosmetics and skin care products', *African Journal of Biotechnology*, op. cit.
39. 'Palmitoleic acid isomer in human skin sebum is effective against gram-positive bacteria', *Skin Pharmacology and Physiology*, op. cit.
40. 'The ugly side of beauty products', *Nature & Health*, op. cit.
41. Griffiths, C.E.M. 2001, 'The role of retinoids in the prevention and repair of aged and photoaged skin', *'Clinical and Experimental Dermatology*, vol. 26, no. 7. pp 613–18
42. 'The ugly side of beauty products', *Nature & Health*, op. cit.

Chapter 9

1. Rexbye, H., et. al. 2006, 'Influence of environmental factors on facial ageing', *Oxford Journals*, vol. 35, no. 2, pp 110-15.
2. Akiba, S., et. al. 1999, 'Influence of chronic UV exposure and lifestyle on facial skin photo-aging – results from a pilot study', *Journal of Epidemiology*, vol. 9, no. 6. S136–42
3. The Cancer Council Australia website, 2004, 'All about skin cancer', retrieved 21 September 2006:

http://www.cancer.org.au/content.cfm?randid=960742

4. ibid.

5. BBC News, 2006, 'Exercise cuts skin cancer risk'.

6. The Cancer Council Australia website, 2004, 'All about skin cancer'.

7. BBC News, 2006, 'Exercise cuts skin cancer risk'.

8. The Cancer Council Australia website, 2004, 'All about skin cancer'.

9. BBC News, 2006, 'Exercise cuts skin cancer risk'.

10. Haywood, R., et. al. 2003, 'Sunscreens inadequately protect against ultraviolet-A-induced free radicals in skin: implications for skin aging and melanoma?' *Journal of Investigative Dermatology*, vol. 121, no. 4, pp 862-8.

11. National Cancer Institute (US) website, 2005, 'What you need to know about skin cancer', retrieved 21 September 2006: http://www.cancer.gov/cancertopics/wyntk/skin/page13

12. The Cancer Council Australia, 2004, 'All about skin cancer'.

13. National Cancer Institute (US) website, 2005, 'What you need to know about skin cancer'.

14. ibid.

Chapter 10

1. Robbins, A, 2001, *Get the Edge: A 7 day programme to transform your life*, Robbins Research International, San Diego, CA

Chapter 11

1. Kern, D. 2006, 'What is acne? What are pimples?', retrieved 23 August 2006: www.acne.org

2. National Institute of Arthritis and Musculoskeletal and Skin Disorders (NIAMS) website, 'Questions and answers about acne', retrieved 24 August 2006: http://www.niams.nih.gov/hi/topics/acne/acne.htm

3. Cotterill, J.A. and Cunliffe, W.J. 1997, 'Suicide in dermatological patients', *British Journal of Dermatology*, vol. 137, no. 2, p 246.

4. Purvis, D., et. al. 2006, 'Acne, anxiety, depression and suicide in teenagers: a cross-sec-

tional survey of New Zealand secondary school students,' *Journal of Paediatrics and Child Health*, vol. 42, no. 12.

5. Kilkenny, et. al. 1998, 'The prevalence of common skin conditions in Australian school children: 3. acne vulgaris', *British Journal of Dermatology*, vol. 139, no. 5, p 840.

6. Plunkett, A et. al. 1999, 'The frequency of non-malignant skin conditions in adults in central Victoria, Australia', *International Journal of Dermatology*, vol. 38, no. 12, p 901.

7. Enshaieh, S., et. al. 2007, 'The efficacy of 5% topical tea tree oil gel in mild to moderate acne vulgaris: a randomized double-blind placebo-controlled study', *Indian Journal of Dermatology, Venereology and Leprology*, vol. 73, no 1, pp 22-5.

8. 'Acne, anxiety, depression and suicide in teenagers: a cross-sectional survey of New Zealand secondary school students', *Journal of Paediatrics and Child Health*, op. cit.

9. Wooltorton, E. 2003, 'Accutane (isotretinoin) and psychiatric adverse effects', *Canadian Medical Association Journal*, vol 168, no. 1, p 66.

10. 'The efficacy of 5% topical tea tree oil gel in mild to moderate acne vulgaris: a randomized double-blind placebo-controlled study', *Indian Journal of Dermatology, Venereology and Leprology*, op. cit.

11. ibid.

12. Tortora, G.J. and Grabowski. S.R. 2000, *Principles of Anatomy and Physiology*, (9th edn), chapters 2, 5 and 22, John Wiley & Sons, New York.

13. ibid.

14. ARL Pathology, 2006, Practitioner Manual, Melbourne.

15. *Principles of Anatomy and Physiology*, op. cit.

16. ibid.

17. ibid.

18. ibid.

19. Michaelsson, G., Juhlin, L. and Vahlquist, A. 1977, 'Effects of oral zinc and vitamin A in acne', *Archives of Dermatology*, vol. 113, no. 1, pp 31-6.

20. ibid.

21. Weimar, V.M., et. al. 1978, 'Zinc sulfate in acne vulgaris', *Archives of Dermatology*, vol. 114, no, 12. Retrieved 24 August 2006:

http://archderm.ama-assn.org/cgi/content/abstract/144/12/1776

22. Adebamowo, C.A., et. al. 2005, 'High school dietary dairy intake and teenage acne', *Journal of the American Academy of Dermatology*, vol. 52, no. 2, pp 360-2.

23. Östman, E. M., et. al. 2001, 'Inconsistency between glycemic and insulinemic responses to regular and fermented milk products', *American Journal of Clinical Nutrition*, vol. 74, no. 1, pp 96-100.

24. Hoyt, G, Hickey, M. S. and Cordain L. 2005, 'Dissociation of the glycaemic and insulinaemic responses to whole and skimmed milk', *British Journal of Nutrition*, vol. 93, pp 175-7.

25. 'Effects of oral zinc and vitamin A in acne', *Archives of Dermatology*, op. cit.

Chapter 12

1. Rosenbaum, M. et. al. 1998, 'An exploratory investigation of the morphology and biochemistry of cellulite', *Plastic and Reconstructive Surgery*, vol. 101, no. 7, pp 1934-9.

2. Dr.Hauschka Skin Care, 'Viewing cellulite holistically' (Booklet).

3. Murad, H. 2005, *The Cellulite Solution*, Introduction, Piatkus, London.

4. PRD Health, 'Phosphatidylcholine', retrieved 5 October 2006: www.pdrhealth.com/drug_info/nmdrugprofiles/ nutsupdrugs/pho_0288.shtml

5. Kirschmann, G.J. and Kirschmann, J.D. 1996, *Nutrition Almanac*, (4th edn), section VIII, McGraw Hill Book Co, Singapore.

6. ibid.

7. *The Cellulite Solution*, op. cit.

8. ibid.

9. Kang, Y, et. al. 1999, 'Hyaluronan suppresses fibronectin fragment-mediated damage to human cartilage explant cultures by enhancing proteoglycan synthesis', *Journal of Orthopaedic Research*, vol. 17 no. 6. pp 858-69.

10. Thompson, R.W., et. al. 1975, 'Alterations of porcine skin acid mucopolysaccharides in zinc deficiency', *Journal of Nutrition*, vol. 105, no 2, pp 154-60.

11. Moscatelli, D. and Rubin, H. 1977, 'Hormonal control of hyaluronic acid production in fibroblasts and its relation to nucleic acid and protein synthesis', *Journal of Cellular Physiology*, vol. 91, no 1, pp 79-88.

Chapter 13

1. The Merck Manual, section 10, chapter 111, retrieved 23 March 2006: http://www.merck.com/mrkshared/mmanual/section10/chapter111/111d.jsp

2. ibid.

3. Cowley, N.C. and Farr, P.M. 1992, 'A dose-response study of irritant reactions to sodium lauryl sulphate in patients with seborrhoeic dermatitis and atopic eczema', *Acta Dermato-Venereologica*, vol. 72, no. 6, pp 432-5.

4. Gloor, M. et. al. 2004, 'On the course of the irritant reaction after irritation with sodium lauryl sulphate', *Skin Research & Technology*, vol. 10, no. 3, pp 144-8.

5. American Family Physician, 2003, 'Tea tree oil shampoo in treatment of dandruff', retrieved 6 September 2006: http://www.aafp.org/afp/20030501/tips/2.html

6. Pitchford, P. 1993, *Healing with Whole Foods*, chapter 50, North Atlantic Books, Berkeley, California.

7. Recipe adapted from Breedlove, G. 1998, *The Herbal Home Spa*, Storey Books, North Adams, US

8. Adapted from www.earthclinic.com

9. *Healing with Whole Foods*, op. cit.

Chapter 15

1. Eczema Association of Australasia website, retrieved 23 March, 2006: http://www.eczema.org.au/ info/facts.html

2. David, T.J. 2000, 'Adverse reactions and intolerances to foods', *British Medical Bulletin*, vol. 56, no. 1, pp 34-50.

3. Wrong Diagnosis website, 'Prevalence of eczema', retrieved 12 January 2006: http://www.wrongdiagnosis.com/e/eczema/stats-country.htm

4. Eczema Association of Australasia website.

5. National Eczema Society statistic.

6. ibid.

7. 'Adverse reactions and intolerances to foods', *British Medical Bulletin*, op. cit.

8. Dengate, S. 2001, *The Failsafe Cookbook: Reducing food chemicals for calm happy families*, chapter 1, Random House, Sydney.

9. Buttriss, J., (ed) 2002, 'Adverse reactions to food', *British Nutrition Foundation*, Blackwell Science, London.

10. Manku, M.S., et. al. 1982, 'Reduced levels of prostaglandin precursors in the blood of atopic patients: defective delta-6-desaturase function as biochemical basis for atopy', *Prostaglandins, Leukotrienes and Medicine*, vol. 9, no. 6, pp 615-28.

11. 'Reduced levels of prostaglandin precursors in the blood of atopic patients: defective delta-6-desaturase function as biochemical basis for atopy', *Prostaglandins, Leukotrienes and Medicine*, op. cit.

12. Banni, S., et. al. 1996, 'Characterization of conjugated diene fatty acids in milk, dairy products, and lamb tissues', *The Journal of Nutritional Biochemistry*, vol. 17, no. 3, pp 150-55.

13. Sausenthaler, S. et. al. 2006, 'Margarine and butter consumption, eczema and allergic sensitization in children', *Pediatric Allergy and Immunology*, vol. 17, no. 2, pp 85-93.

14. Eczema Association of Australia website.

15. 'Adverse reactions and intolerances to foods', *British Medical Bulletin*, op. cit.

16. Swain, A.R., Soutter, V.L. and Loblay, R.H. 2002, *Friendly Food*, Royal Prince Alfred Hospital Allergy Unit, Murdoch Books, Sydney.

17. Eczema Association of Australasia website.

18. British Association of Dermatologists website, Nottingham Eczema Team, 2000, 'Salt water baths and eczema', retrieved [AQ: date needed]: www.bad.org.uk

19. *The Failsafe Cookbook*, op. cit.

20. There are two detoxification phases that occur in the liver: Phase I detoxification is an enzyme reaction where salicylates and other chemicals are made into water soluble substances. This phase can make a substance *more* toxic. Then phase II detoxification should occur as your liver converts these toxic substances into harmless water soluble substances so they can safely be removed from the body. If your phase II reactions are poor then you can get all sorts of health problems including eczema.

21. *The Failsafe Cookbook*, op. cit.

22. ibid.

23. Cork, M., 2006, 'Emollients Information Sheet', National Eczema Society (UK). retrieved 27 November 2006: http://www.eczema.org/emolienttherapy.pdf

24. Proksch, E., et. al. 2006, 'Skin barrier function, epidermal proliferation and differentiation in eczema', *Journal of Dermatological Science*, vol. 43, no. 3, pp 159-69.

25. Siddappa, K. 2003, 'Dry skin conditions, eczema and emollients in their management', *Indian Journal of Dermatology, Venereology and Leprology*, vol. 69, no. 2, pp 69-75.

26. Cork, M., et. al. 'New understanding of the predisposition to atopic eczema and sensitive skin', retrieved 27 November 2006: www.allergyuk.org

27. De Paepe, K., et. al. 2002, 'Repair of acetone- and sodium lauryl sulphate-damaged human skin barrier function using topically applied emulsions containing barrier lipids', *Journal of the European Academy of Dermatology and Venereology*, vol. 16, no. 6 pp 587-94.

28. Cowley, N.C. and Farr, P.M. 1992, 'A dose-response study of irritant reactions to sodium lauryl sulphate in patients with seborrhoeic dermatitis and atopic eczema', *Acta Dermato-Venereologica*, vol. 72, no. 6, pp 432-5.

29. Gloor, M. et. al., 2004, 'On the course of the irritant reaction after irritation with sodium lauryl sulphate,' *Skin Research & Technology*, vol. 10, no. 3, pp 144-8.

30. 'Repair of acetone- and sodium lauryl sulphate-damaged human skin barrier function using topically applied emulsions containing barrier lipids', *Journal of the European Academy of Dermatology and Venereology*, op. cit.

31. Jones, M. 1998, *Your Child: Eczema*, chapter 5, Element Books. Shaftsbury, Dorset, Great Britain

32. 'Repair of acetone- and sodium lauryl sulphate-damaged human skin barrier function using topically applied emulsions containing barrier lipids', *Journal of the European Academy of Dermatology and Venereology*, op. cit.

33. Williams, H.C., et. al. 1995, 'Skin moisturisers in atopic eczema', retrieved 27 November 2006, British Association of Dermatologists website retrieved 27 November 2006:

http://www.bad.org.uk/public/leaflets/other_atopic_-_skin.asp

34. 'Repair of acetone- and sodium lauryl sulphate-damaged human skin barrier function using topically applied emulsions containing barrier lipids', *Journal of the European Academy of Dermatology and Venereology*, op. cit.

35. Levin, C. and Maibach, H. 2002, 'Exploration of alternative and natural drugs in dermatology', *Archives of Dermatology*, vol. 138, pp 207-11.

36. Gehring, W., et. al. 1999, 'Effect of topically applied evening primrose oil on epidermal barrier function in atopic dermatitis as a function of vehicle', *Arzneimittel-forschung*, vol. 49, no. 7, pp 635-42.

37. Muhlebach, S., et. al. 1996, 'Successful therapy of salicylate poisoning using glycine and activated charcoal', *Schweisische Medizinische Wochenschrift*, vol. 126, no 49. Abstract, retrieved 28 November 2006: www.ncbi.nlm.nih.gov/sites/entrez?db=pubmed&uid=8999500&cmd=showdetailview&indexed=google

38. Patel, D.K., et. al. 1990, 'Depletion of plasma glycine and effect of glycine by mouth on salicylate metabolism during aspirin overdose', *Human & Experimental Toxicology*, vol. 9, no. 6, pp 389-95.

39. ARL Pathology, 2006, Practitioner Manual, Melbourne, VIC, Australia.

40. Orthoplex, 2007, dosages for glycine.

41. Hawrelak, J. 2003, 'Probiotics: choosing the right one for your needs', *Journal of the Australian Traditional-Medicine Society*, vol. 9, no. 2, pp 67-75.

42. ibid.

43. Baugh, C.M., Malone, J.H. and Butterworth, C.E. 1968, 'Human Biotin Deficiency', *American Journal of Clinical Nutrition*, vol. 21, pp 173-82.

44. ibid.

45. ibid.

46. ibid.

47. Manku, M.S., et. al. 1984, 'Essential fatty acids in the plasma phospholipids of patients with atopic eczema', *British Journal of Dermatology*, vol. 110, no. 6, pp 64-8.

48. Horrobin, D.F. 1989, 'Essential fatty acids in clinical dermatology', *Journal of the American Academy of Dermatology*, vol. 20, no. 6, pp 1045-53.

49. Horrobin, D.F. 2000, 'Essential fatty acid metabolism and its modification in atopic eczema', *American Journal of Clinical Nutrition*, vol. 71, pp 367S-72S.

50. Berbis, P., et. al. 1990, 'Essential fatty acids and the skin', *Allergie et Immunologie*, vol 22, no. 6, pp 225-31, retrieved 27 November 2006 from PubMed database. http://www.ncbi.nlm.nih.gov/sites/entrez

51. Erasmus, U. 1993, *Fats that Heal, Fats that Kill*, chapter 57, Alive Books, Burnaby, BC, Canada

52. Masumura, S., et. al. 1992, 'The effects of season and exercise on the levels of plasma poly-unsaturated fatty acids and lipoprotein cholesterol in young rats', *Biochimica et Biophysica Acta*, 1125 pp 292-6.

Chapter 16

1. Levin, C. and Maibach, H. 2002, 'Exploration of alternative and natural drugs in dermatology', *Archives of Dermatology*, vol. 138, pp 207-11.

2. Gehring, W., et. al. 1999, 'Effect of topically applied evening primrose oil on epidermal barrier function in atopic dermatitis as a function of vehicle'. *Arzneimittel-forschung*, vol. 49, no. 7, pp 635-42.

3. Orthoplex, 2007, dosages for glycine.

4. Young, P., 'Salicylate' summary for UKPID, IPCS INTOX Databank retrieved 13 September 2006: http://www.intox.org/databank/documents/pharm/salicy/ukpid14.htm

5. 'Probiotics: choosing the right one for your needs', *Journal of the Australian Traditional-Medicine Society*, op. cit.

6. ibid.

7. Uauy, R., et. al. 2000, 'Essential fatty acids in visual and brain development', *Lipids*, vol 36, no. 9, pp 885-95.

8. Sausenthaler, S. et. al., 2006, 'Margarine and butter consumption, eczema & allergic sensitization in children', *Pediatric Allergy and Immunology*, vol. 17, no. 2, pp 85–93

9. Sanitarium Education Service leaflet, 'Ready for Solids'.

10. Treffers, S. 1999, *Food Additives*, Hartrade, Queensland.

Chapter 17

1. Mansburg, G. 2004, 'Eczema and psoriasis', *Journal of Complementary Medicine*, vol. 3, no. 3, pp 26-32.
2. Psoriasis Association (UK) website, 'What is Psoriasis?', retrieved 23 March 2006: www.psoriasis-association.org.uk/ultra.html
3. National Psoriasis Foundation website, 2006, 'About psoriasis, statistics', retrieved 23 March 2006: www.psoriasis.org/about/stats/
4. Psoriasis Association statistic.
5. Australian Institute of Health and Welfare (AIHW), 2004, 'Heart, stroke and vascular disease – Australian facts'.
6. National Psoriasis Foundation website.
7. ibid.
8. ibid.
9. Medem: Medical Library, 2005, 'News from the American Medical Association: smoking associated with the severity of psoriasis', retrieved 28 March 2006: http://www.medem.com/medlb/article_detaillb.cfm
10. Cohen, D., 'Complete Psoriasis Relief', retrieved 16 August 2006: http://newyork-bodyscan.com/psoriasis.html
11. Boreham, D.R, Gasmann, H.C. and Mitchel, R.E. 1995, 'Water bath hyperthermia is a simple therapy for psoriasis and also stimulates skin tanning in response to sunlight', *International Journal of Hyperthermia*, vol. 11, no. 6, pp 745-54.
12. ibid.
13. Staberg, B., et. al. 1987, 'Abnormal vitamin D metabolism in patients with psoriasis', *Acta Dermato-Venereologica*, vol. 67, no. 1, abstract, retrieved 22 August 2006 from PubMed database: http://www.ncbi.nlm.nih.gov/sites/entrez
14. 'Complete Psoriasis Relief', op. cit.
15. ibid.
16. ibid.
17. Wille, J., et. al. 2003, 'Palmitoleic acid isomer in human skin sebum is effective against gram-positive bacteria', *Skin Pharmacology and Physiology*, vol. 16, no. 3, abstract.
18. Athar, M. and Nasir S.M. 2005, 'Taxonomic perspective of plant species yielding vegetable oils used in cosmetics and skin care products', *African Journal of Biotechnology*, vol. 4, no. 1, pp 36-44.
19. Murray, M. and Pizzorno, J. 1998, *Encyclopedia of Natural Medicine*, (2nd edn), 'Psoriasis', Little, Brown & Company, London
20. ibid.
21. ibid.
22. ibid.
23. ibid.
24. ibid.
25. Zlatkov, N.B., et. al. 1984, 'Free fatty acids in the blood serum of psoriatics', *Acta Dermato-Venereologica*, vol. 64, no. 1. pp22–5
26. Erasmus, U. 1993, *Fats that Heal, Fats that Kill*, section 6-7, Alive Books., Burnaby, BC, Canada
27. Seville, R.H. 1997, 'Psoriasis and stress', *British Journal of Dermatology*, vol. 97, no. 3, pp 297-302.

Chapter 18

1. Australasian College of Dermatologists website, 'What is Rosacea?', retrieved 23 March 2006: http://www.dermcoll.asn.au/rosacea.pdf
2. National Institute of Arthritis and Musculoskeletal and Skin Disease website, 'Questions and answers about rosacea', retrieved 23 March 2006: http://www.niams.nih.gov/hi/topics/rosacea/rosacea.htm#ros_a
3. Nase, G. 2005, 'Beating rosacea, vascular, ocular and acne forms', retrieved 16 August 2006: http://www.drnase.com/research_rosacea_articles.htm
4. Wilkin, J., et al. 2002, 'Standard classification of rosacea: report of the National Rosacea Society expert committee on the classification and staging of rosacea', *Journal of the American Academy of Dermatology*, vol. 46, no. 4, pp 584-7.
5. Nase, G. 2005, 'Facial rosacea: vascular basis of the disorder', retrieved 18 August 2006: http://www.drnase.com/vascular_basis.htm
6. ibid.
7. ibid.
8. ibid.
9. Rosacea Support Group website, 2006, 'Histamine containing or triggering foods', retrieved 18 August 2006: http://rosacea-sup-

port.org/australian

10. Swain, A.R., Soutter, V.L. and Loblay, R.H. 2002, *Friendly Food*, Royal Prince Alfred Hospital Allergy Unit, Murdoch Books, Sydney.

11. Tidwell, J. 'Allergies, histamine in food,' retrieved 18 August 2006: http://allergies.about.com/cs/histamine/a/aa071000a.htm

12. *Friendly Food*, op. cit.

13. Robbins, A. 2001, *Get the Edge*, The Anthony Robbins Companies, California.

14. Rosacea Support Group website, 2006, 'Exercise influence', retrieved 18 August 2006: http://www.rosacea-research.org/wiki/index.php/Exercise_Influence

15. Nase, G. 2005, 'Facial rosacea: vascular basis of the disorder', op. cit.

16. Rosacea Support Group website.

17. Masumura, S., et. al. 1992, 'The effects of season and exercise on the levels of plasma poly-unsaturated fatty acids and lipoprotein cholesterol in young rats', *Biochimica et Biophysica Acta*, 1125 pp 292-6.

Chapter 19

1. Tortora, G.J. & Grabowski, S. 2000, *Principles of Anatomy and Physiology*, (9th edn), chapters 17 and 22, John Wiley & Sons, New York.

2. ibid.

3. Pitchford, P. 1993, *Healing with Whole Foods*, chapter 27, North Atlantic Books, Berkeley, California.

4. Gabriel, S. 2000, *Breathe for Life*, Hardie Grant Books, South Yarra.

5. *Principles of Anatomy and Physiology*, op. cit.

6. Chek, P, 2004, *How to Eat, Move, and Be Healthy!* chapter 6, C.H.E.K Institute, San Diego.

7. *Breathe for Life*, op. cit.

8. ibid.

9. ibid.

10. ibid.

Chapter 20

1. Crossroads Institute, 'Brainwaves and EEG: The language of the brain', retrieved 20 June 2006: www.crossroadsinstitute.org/eeg.html

2. ibid.

3. Robbins, A. 2001, *Get The Edge*, Robbins Research International.

Appendix 1

1. Dengate, S. 2001, *The Failsafe Cookbook: reducing food chemicals for calm happy families*, chapter 1, Random House, Sydney.

2. Swain, A.R., Soutter, V.L. and Loblay, R.H. 2002 *Friendly Food*, Royal Prince Alfred Hospital Allergy Unit, Murdoch Books, Sydney.

Index